Historical Aspects of Critical Illness and Critical Care Medicine

Guest Editors

ANAND KUMAR, MD
JOSEPH E. PARRILLO, MD

CRITICAL CARE CLINICS

www.criticalcare.theclinics.com

Consulting Editors
RICHARD W. CARLSON, MD, PhD
MICHAEL A. GEHEB, MD

January 2009 • Volume 25 • Number 1

SAUNDERS an imprint of ELSEVIER, Inc.

W.B. SAUNDERS COMPANY
A Division of Elsevier Inc.

Elsevier Inc. • 1600 John F. Kennedy Blvd., • Suite 1800 • Philadelphia, Pennsylvania 19103-2899

http://www.theclinics.com

CRITICAL CARE CLINICS Volume 25, Number 1
January 2009 ISSN 0749-0704, ISBN-13: 978-1-4377-0463-1, ISBN-10: 1-4377-0463-8

Editor: Patrick Manley

© **2009 Elsevier** ■ **All rights reserved.**

This journal and the individual contributions contained in it are protected under copyright by Elsevier, and the following terms and conditions apply to their use:

Photocopying
Single photocopies of single articles may be made for personal use as allowed by national copyright laws. Permission of the Publisher and payment of a fee is required for all other photocopying, including multiple or systematic copying, copying for advertising or promotional purposes, resale, and all forms of document delivery. Special rates are available for educational institutions that wish to make photocopies for non-profit educational classroom use.

For information on how to seek permission visit www.elsevier.com/permissions or call: (+44) 1865 843830 (UK)/(+1) 215 239 3804 (USA).

Derivative Works
Subscribers may reproduce tables of contents or prepare lists of articles including abstracts for internal circulation within their institutions. Permission of the Publisher is required for resale or distribution outside the institution. Permission of the Publisher is required for all other derivative works, including compilations and translations (please consult www.elsevier.com/permissions).

Electronic Storage or Usage
Permission of the Publisher is required to store or use electronically any material contained in this journal, including any article or part of an article (please consult www.elsevier.com/permissions). Except as outlined above, no part of this publication may be reproduced, stored in a retrieval system or transmitted in any form or by any means, electronic, mechanical, photocopying, recording or otherwise, without prior written permission of the Publisher.

Notice
No responsibility is assumed by the Publisher for any injury and/or damage to persons or property as a matter of products liability, negligence or otherwise, or from any use or operation of any methods, products, instructions or ideas contained in the material herein. Because of rapid advances in the medical sciences, in particular, independent verification of diagnoses and drug dosages should be made.

Although all advertising material is expected to conform to ethical (medical) standards, inclusion in this publication does not constitute a guarantee or endorsement of the quality or value of such product or of the claims made of it by its manufacturer.

Critical Care Clinics (ISSN: 0749-0704) is published quarterly by Elsevier Inc., 360 Park Avenue South, New York, NY 10010-1710. Months of issue are January, April, July, and October. Business and Editorial Offices: 1600 John F. Kennedy Blvd., Suite 1800, Philadelphia, PA 19103-2899. Customer Service Office: 6277 Sea Harbor Drive, Orlando, FL 32887-4800. Periodicals postage paid at New York, NY and additional mailing offices. Subscription prices are $222.00 per year for US individuals, $366.00 per year for US institution, $111.00 per year for US students and residents, $274.00 per year for Canadian individuals, $454.00 per year for Canadian institutions, $320.00 per year for international individuals, $454.00 per year for international institutions and $161.00 per year for Canadian and foreign students/residents. To receive student/resident rate, orders must be accompanied by name of affiliated institution, date of term, and the *signature* of program/residency coordinator on institution letterhead. Orders will be billed at individual rate until proof of status is received. Foreign air speed delivery is included in all *Clinics* subscription prices. All prices are subject to change without notice. POSTMASTER: Send address changes to *Critical Care Clinics*, Elsevier Periodicals Customer Service, 11830 Westline Industrial Drive, St. Louis, MO 63146. **Customer Service: 1-800-654-2452 (US). From outside of the US, call 1-314-453-7041. Fax: 1-314-453-5170. E-mail: journalscustomerservice-usa@elsevier.com (for print support), journalsonlinesupport-usa@elsevier.com (for online support).**

Reprints. For copies of 100 or more of articles in this publication, please contact the Commercial Reprints Department, Elsevier Inc., 360 Park Avenue South, New York, NY 10010-1710. Tel.: 212-633-3812; Fax: 212-462-1935; E-mail: reprints@elsevier.com.

Critical Care Clinics is also published in Spanish by Editorial Inter-Medica, Junin 917, 1er A, 1113, Buenos Aires, Argentina.

Critical Care Clinics is covered in *MEDLINE/PubMed (Index Medicus)*, *EMBASE/Excerpta Medica, Current Concepts/ Clinical Medicine, ISI/BIOMED*, and *Chemical Abstracts*.

Printed and bound by CPI Group (UK) Ltd, Croydon, CR0 4YY
Transferred to Digital Print 2011

Contributors

CONSULTING EDITORS

RICHARD W. CARLSON, MD, PhD
Chairman, Department of Internal Medicine, Marcopia Medical Center; and Professor, Department of Medicine, Mayo Graduate School of Medicine, Phoenix, Arizona

MICHAEL A. GEHEB, MD
Professor, Department of Medicine, and Vice President, Clinical Programs, Oregon Health & Sciences University, Portland, Oregon

GUEST EDITORS

ANAND KUMAR, MD
Associate Professor, Section of Critical Care Medicine, Section of Infectious Diseases, Associate Professor of Medicine, Medical Microbiology and Pharmacology/Therapeutics, University of Manitoba, Manitoba, Winnipeg, Canada; and Associate Professor of Medicine, Section of Critical Care Medicine, Section of Infectious Diseases, Robert Wood Johnson Medical School, University of Medicine and Dentistry of New Jersey, Camden, New Jersey

JOSEPH E. PARRILLO, MD
Professor of Medicine, Robert Wood Johnson Medical School, University of Medicine and Dentistry of New Jersey; Chief, Department of Medicine, Edward D. Viner, MD Chair, Department of Medicine; and Director, Cooper Heart Institute Cooper University Hospital Camden, New Jersey

AUTHORS

CARRIE E. ALLISON, MD
Trauma/Critical Care Fellow, Department of Surgery, Oregon Health & Science University, Portland, Oregon

ROBERT E. ARIANO, PharmD
Associate Professor, Department of Pharmacology & Therapeutics, University of Manitoba, Winnipeg, Manitoba, Canada

DEAN D. BELL, MD, FRCPC
Associate Professor, Department of Anesthesia, University of Manitoba, Winnipeg, Manitoba, Canada

THOMAS P. BLECK, MD, FCCM
Professor of Neurological Sciences, Neurosurgery, Medicine, and Anesthesiology, Associate Chief Medical Officer (Critical Care), Rush Medical College, Chicago, Illinois

SAQIB I. DARA, MD, FCCP
Consultant in Critical Care Medicine, Al Rahba Hospital - Johns Hopkins International, Abu Dhabi, United Arab Emirates

R.P. DELLINGER, MD
Director, Division of Critical Care Medicine; and Professor, Department of Medicine,
Cooper University Hospital, Camden, New Jersey

J. CHRISTOPHER FARMER, MD, FCCM
Professor of Medicine and Consultant in Critical Care Medicine, Associate Dean, Mayo
School of Graduate Medical Education, Mayo Clinic College of Medicine; Associate Chair,
Department of Medicine, Mayo Clinic College of Medicine; and Associate Director,
Program in Translational Immunovirology and Biodefense, Mayo Clinic College of
Medicine, Rochester, Minnesota

DUANE FUNK, MD, FRCP(C)
Assistant Professor of Anesthesiology and Critical Care, University of Manitoba, Manitoba, Winnipeg, Canada

FREDRIC GINSBERG, MD
Assistant Professor of Medicine, Robert Wood Johnson Medical School at Camden,
University of Medicine and Dentistry of New Jersey; and Director Heart Failure Program,
Director, Nuclear Cardiology, Cooper University Hospital, Camden, New Jersey

AKE GRENVIK, MD, PhD, FCCM
Distinguished Service Professor of Critical Care Medicine, Department of Critical Care
Medicine, University of Pittsburgh, Pittsburgh, Pennsylvania

ANAND KUMAR, MD
Associate Professor, Section of Critical Care Medicine, Section of Infectious Diseases,
Associate Professor of Medicine, Medical Microbiology and Pharmacology/Therapeutics,
University of Manitoba, Manitoba, Winnipeg, Canada; and Associate Professor
of Medicine, Section of Critical Care Medicine, Section of Infectious Diseases, Robert
Wood Johnson Medical School, University of Medicine and Dentistry of New Jersey,
Camden, New Jersey

R. BRUCE LIGHT, MD
Professor of Medicine and Medical Microbiology, University of Manitoba, Winnipeg,
Manitoba

PETER K. LINDEN, MD
Professor of Critical Care Medicine, Director of Abdominal Organ Transplant Intensive
Care unit, University of Pittsburgh Medical Center, Department of Critical Care Medicine,
Pittsburgh, Pennsylvania

JOHN M. LUCE, MD
Professor, Department of Medicine, University of California, San Francisco; and Chief
Medical Officer and Member, Division of Pulmonary and Critical Care Medicine, San
Francisco General Hospital, San Francisco, California

RIZWAN A. MANJI, MD
Cardiac Sciences Program, University of Manitoba, Winnipeg, Manitoba, Canada

JOSEPH E. PARRILLO, MD
Professor of Medicine, Robert Wood Johnson Medical School, University of Medicine and
Dentistry of New Jersey; Chief, Department of Medicine, Edward D. Viner, MD Chair,
Department of Medicine; and Director, Cooper Heart Institute Cooper University Hospital
Camden, New Jersey

BOJAN PAUNOVIC, MD, FRCPC
Assistant Professor, Department of Medicine, University of Manitoba, Winnipeg, Manitoba, Canada

MICHAEL R. PINSKY, MD CM, Dr hc, FCCP, FCCM
Vice Chair, Academic Affairs, Department of Critical Care Medicine, Professor of Critical Care Medicine, Bioengineering, Cardiovascular Diseases and Anesthesiology, University of Pittsburgh, Pittsburgh, Pennsylvania

NITIN PURI, MD
Critical Care Fellow, Division of Critical Care Medicine, Department of Medicine, Cooper University Hospital, Camden, New Jersey

VINOD PURI, MD
Director, Division of Critical Care Medicine (Rtd), Department of Surgery, Providence Hospital, Southfield, Michigan

GIUSEPPE RISTAGNO, MD
Weil Institute of Critical Care Medicine, Rancho Mirage, California

WANCHUN TANG, MD
Weil Institute of Critical Care Medicine, Rancho Mirage; Keck School of Medicine of the University of Southern California, Los Angeles, California

DONALD D. TRUNKEY, MD, FACS
Professor, Department of Surgery, Oregon Health & Science University, Portland, Oregon

MAX HARRY WEIL, MD, PhD
Weil Institute of Critical Care Medicine, Rancho Mirage; Keck School of Medicine of the University of Southern California, Los Angeles, California; and Northwestern University Medical School, Chicago, Illinois

DOUGLAS B. WHITE, MD, MAS
Assistant Professor, Department of Medicine, University of California, San Francisco; and Member, Division of Pulmonary and Critical Care Medicine and Program in Medical Ethics, University of California, San Francisco, California

KENNETH E. WOOD, DO
Professor, Department of Medicine; Professor, Department of Anesthesiology; Senior Director of Medical Affairs; and Director, Critical Care Medicine and Respiratory Care, Section of Pulmonary and Critical Care Medicine, University of Wisconsin Hospital and Clinics, Madison, Wisconsin

RYAN ZARYCHANSKI, MD, FRCPC
Assistant Professor, Department of Medicine, University of Manitoba, Winnipeg, Manitoba, Canada

Contents

Cardiac arrest represents a dramatic event that can occur suddenly and often without premonitory signs, characterized by sudden loss of consciousness and breathing after cardiac output ceases and both coronary and cerebral blood flows stop. Restarting of the blood flow by cardiopulmonary resuscitation potentially re-establishes some cardiac output and organ blood flows. This article summarizes the major events that encompass the history of cardiopulmonary resuscitation, beginning with ancient history and evolving into the current American Heart Association's commitment to save hearts.

The appropriate starting point for a history of neurocritical care is a matter of debate, and the organization of facts and conjectures about it must be somewhat arbitrary. Intensive care for neurosurgical patients dates back to the work of Walter Dandy at the Johns Hopkins Hospital in the 1930s; many consider his creation of a special unit for their postoperative care to be the first real ICU. The genesis of neurocritical care begins in prehistory, however. This article gives a predominantly North American history, with some brief forays into the rest of the world community of neurointensivists.

Solid organ transplantation is one of the most remarkable and dramatic therapeutic advances in medicine during the past 60 years. This field has progressed initially from what can accurately be termed a "clinical experiment" to routine and reliable practice, which has proven to be clinically effective, life-saving and cost-effective. This remarkable evolution stems from a serial confluence of: cultural acceptance; legal and political evolution to facilitate organ donation, procurement and allocation; technical and cognitive advances in organ preservation, surgery, immunology, immunosuppression; and management of infectious diseases. Some of the major milestones of this multidisciplinary clinical science are reviewed in this article.

Critical care medicine is a young specialty and since its inception has been heavily reliant upon technology. Invasive monitoring has its humble beginnings in the continuous monitoring of heart rate and rhythm. From the development of right heart catheterization to the adaption of the echocardiogram for use in shock, intensivists have used technology to monitor hemodynamics. The care of the critically ill has been buoyed by investigators who sought to offer renal replacement therapy to unstable patients and worked to improve the monitoring of oxygen saturation. The evolution of mechanical ventilation for the critically ill embodies innumerable technological advances. More recently, critical care has insisted upon rigorous testing and cost-benefit analysis of technological advances.

Significant progress in critical care medicine has been the result of tireless
observation, dedicated research, and well-timed serendipity. This article
provides a historical perspective for four meaningful therapies in critical
care medicine: blood transfusion, fluid resuscitation, vasopressor/inotro-
pic support, and antibiotics. For each therapy, key discoveries and events
that have shaped medical history and helped define current practice are
discussed. Prominent medical and social pressures that have catalyzed
research and innovation in each domain are also addressed, as well as
current and future challenges.

Because they provide potential benefit at great personal and public cost,
the intensive care unit (ICU) and the interventions rendered therein have
become symbols of both the promise and the limitations of medical technology. At the same time, the ICU has served as an arena in which many of
the ethical and legal dilemmas created by that technology have been defined and debated. This article outlines major events in the history of ethics
and law in the ICU, covering the evolution of ICUs, ethical principles, informed consent and the law, medical decision-making, cardiopulmonary
resuscitation, withholding and withdrawing life-sustaining therapy, legal
cases involving life support, advance directives, prognostication, and futility and the allocation of medical resources. Advancement of the ethical
principle of respect for patient autonomy in ICUs increasingly is in conflict
with physicians' concern about their own prerogatives and with the just
distribution of medical resources.

This article discusses the history of the ICU and critical care medicine
(CCM). It also discusses the certification of critical care nurses and allied
health professionals, as well as CCM societies and congresses, education
and board certification, evidence-based CCM, research and publications,
and future challenges to the field.

THE CLINICS ARE NOW AVAILABLE ONLINE!

Access your subscription at:
www.theclinics.com

Dedication

To Aparna and Gale.

Crit Care Clin 25 (2009) xii
doi:10.1016/j.ccc.2009.02.001
0749-0704/09/$ – see front matter © 2009 Elsevier Inc. All rights reserved.

Preface

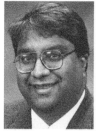 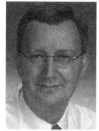

Anand Kumar, MD   Joseph E. Parrillo, MD
Guest Editors

"If I have seen farther than others, it is because I have stood on the shoulders of giants."

Sir Isaac Newton
Letter to Robert Hooke (15 February 1676)

Critical care medicine is a young subspecialty. Many of the early titans of the discipline have lived and worked well within the memory of senior members of the profession. Contrary to popular professional perception, however, the origins of critical care do not begin with the polio epidemics that necessitated the development of positive pressure ventilation in the 1950s or with the introduction of the balloon-tipped, flow-guided, thermodilution cardiac output-capable pulmonary artery catheter in the 1970s. Rather, the genesis of critical care medicine is built on a base of other disciplines stretching back through generations of physicians, many of whose names are now only familiar to scholars of the history of medicine. Well know healers, physicians, and scientists, such as Galen, Harvey, Crile, and Cournand, and lesser known lights, such as Guthrie, Goltz, Henderson, Bradley, van Meenerem, Dotter, Carrel, Waldenburg, and Murray each in their own way set the foundations for the birth and development of critical care medicine.

This discipline, at the cutting edge of technology in medicine, has advanced tremendously in recent decades. Given the speed with which the field is developing it is very easy to focus only on the road ahead, ignoring the path already travelled. It is difficult to know where critical care medicine is going as a subspecialty, however, without understanding how it came to be at its present point.

Central to understanding critical care medicine's professional past is an examination of the challenges and contributions of its predecessors as they forged the path now followed. We are aware of no such similar effort as it relates to critical care medicine and hope that illumination of the footsteps of our professional forebears provides direction for future progress in the field.

Crit Care Clin 25 (2009) xiii–xiv
doi:10.1016/j.ccc.2009.01.001
0749-0704/09/$ – see front matter © 2009 Published by Elsevier Inc.

"Nescire autem quid ante quam natus sis acciderit, id est semper esse puerum."
"He who knows only his own generation remains always a child."
Marcus Tullius Cicero
Roman philosopher, statesman, and orator (106 BC–43 BC)

Anand Kumar, MD
Section of Critical Care Medicine
Health Sciences Centre, JJ 399
700 William Ave
Winnipeg, Manitoba, Canada
R3E-0Z3

Joseph E. Parrillo, MD
Department of Medicine
Robert Wood Johnson Medical School
University of Medicine and Dentistry of New Jersey
Cooper Heart Institute
Cooper University Hospital, D384
One Cooper Plaza
Camden, NJ 08103, USA

E-mail addresses:
akumar61@yahoo.com (A. Kumar)
Parrillo-Joseph@CooperHealth.edu (J.E. Parrillo)

The History and Evolution of Circulatory Shock

Rizwan A. Manji, MD[a], Kenneth E. Wood, DO[b], Anand Kumar, MD[c,d],*

KEYWORDS

• History • Shock • Hypovolemic • Cardiogenic • Distributive

Claudius Galen, the famous second-century Greek physician, taught that there were two kinds of blood. "Nutritive blood" was formed in the liver from ingested food. This blood was carried by the veins to all parts of the body to be consumed as fuel. "Vital blood" was produced by the heart, traveled through the arteries, and carried "vital spirits." Recirculation of blood via a cardiac pumping mechanism was not part of his conceptual framework. This view of the cardiovascular system was accepted as doctrine for millennia. William Harvey (1578–1657),[1] the court physician to King Charles I and King James I, in his 1628 treatise, "Exercitatio Anatomica de Motu Cordis et Sanguinis in Animalibus,"[2] questioned Galen's concepts and set the path to the modern understanding of cardiovascular physiology and hemodynamics. He described how the heart functions as a pump to maintain the recirculation of blood in the arteries and veins. Harvey stated, "The blood in the animal body moves around in a circle continuously, and that the action or function of the heart is to accomplish this by pumping. This is the only reason for the motion and beat of the heart." Understanding the basics of circulation was the first step in understanding shock.

The history of shock starts with traumatic injury and much of the history of shock relates to the history of traumatic shock. A "posttraumatic syndrome" was recognized by the early Greeks, including Hippocrates and Galen. It was not until the 1740s, however, that that the term, *shock*, came into clinical use. In the late 1700s, Woolcomb, Hunter, and Latta, among others, provided clinical descriptions of shock and death caused by shock. The question of why a wounded soldier who had modest visible blood

a Cardiac Sciences Program, University of Manitoba, Winnipeg, Manitoba, Canada
b Section of Pulmonary and Critical Care Medicine, University of Wisconsin Hospital and Clinics, Madison, WI, USA
c Sections of Critical Care Medicine and Infectious Diseases, University of Manitoba, Winnipeg, Manitoba, Canada
d Section of Critical Care Medicine, Cooper Hospital/University Medical Center, Robert Wood Johnson Medical School, University of Medicine and Dentistry, New Jersey, Camden, NJ, USA
* Corresponding author. Section of Critical Care Medicine and Infectious Diseases, University of Manitoba, Winnipeg, Manitoba, Canada.
E-mail address: akumar61@yahoo.com (A. Kumar).

Crit Care Clin 25 (2009) 1–29
doi:10.1016/j.ccc.2008.12.013
0749-0704/08/$ – see front matter © 2009 Elsevier Inc. All rights reserved.

losses would succumb was not always clear.[3] The idea that soldiers could die from a mysterious, indefinable condition, later termed "shock", a process not synonymous with hemorrhage, was a novel concept.

A French surgeon, Henri Francois LeDran (1685–1770), in "A Treatise of Reflections Drawn from Experience with Gunshot Wounds" (1731), coined the word, *choc*, to indicate a severe impact or jolt that often led to death. Review of the original article, however, reveals that his use of the term was in reference to the original injury itself (as in a jolt or blow [ie, the initial physical injury]), not to a posttraumatic syndrome. The British physician Clarke's mistranslation of LeDran's term introduced the term, "shock", to the English language to indicate the sudden deterioration of a patient's condition with major trauma and wounds. The term was initially used to denote any state characterized by physical collapse.

The English surgeon, George James Guthrie,[4] was the first to use the word to specifically denote physiologic instability in 1815. Edwin A. Morris,[5] however, who began to popularize the term, using it in his 1867 Civil War text, "A Practical Treatise on Shock After Operations and Injuries." He defined it as "a peculiar effect on the animal system, produced by violent injuries of any cause, or from violent mental emotions." Before Morris popularized the term, "shock", a variety of colorful terminology often was used to describe the phenomenon, including "sudden vital depression," "great nervous depression," and "final sinking of vitality."

TECHNOLOGY

There have been several technologic advancements that have assisted physicians and scientists in understanding and treating shock. Among them, two monitoring methods stand out: the ability to measure blood pressure with the sphygmomanometer and the ability to measure cardiac output (CO) and filling pressures using a balloon-tipped, flow-directed pulmonary artery catheter. To a great extent, these devices have been the used as basis of the development of the defining characteristics of shock.

Sphygmomanometer

The first known records of blood pressure measurements were obtained by Stephen Hales[6] (1677–1761), a member of the British clergy who had no formal training in medicine and who measured the blood pressure of a horse in 1706 at Cambridge. In 1733, he published the book, *Haemastaticks*, in which he described his technique of inserting a brass tube into the femoral artery of a horse and connecting it to vertical glass tube. Arterial blood rose to a level of over 8 feet in the glass tube. After putting the tube into a vein, the blood rose only inches. This led to the discovery that blood circulated because of a pressure gradient between the arteries and veins. Hales[7] used the same technique to perform the first right and left heart catheterizations in a mammal. In 1828, J.L.M. Poiseuille, the French physiologist and mathematician, reduced Hales' bulky apparatus by having blood push against a reservoir of a substance heavier than blood (ie, mercury). Normal blood pressure would support a column of mercury no more than 200 mm high.[7,8] In 1847, Carl Ludwig modified the Poiseuille instrument by attaching a pen to a float on top of the mercury column that traced fluctuations of pressure on a revolving drum.[7,8] This was called a kymograph and became popular for keeping a permanent record of the pressure fluctuations. Karl Vierordt[9,10] designed a sphygmograph that drew pulse tracings without penetrating an artery but did not directly measure blood pressure, a predecessor to the modern sphygmomanometer. His device measured blood pressure noninvasively by using the principle that blood pressure was equivalent to the amount of force required to obliterate the pulse. The instrument required that physicians pile up weights over an artery until the pulse tracing ceased, impractical for clinical use. Fortunately, S.S. von Basch[11] subsequently developed the first relatively accurate clinical sphygmomanometer in 1881 and in 1896, Scipione Riva-Rocci[12] introduced the now familiar instrument that collapses vessels by means of an inflatable cuff which became generally adopted in 1903 after some additional modifications (**Fig. 1**).

In the early days of shock research, it was not clear which parameter (pulse rate, pulse strength, level of consciousness, skin temperature, and so forth) was the most relevant for the diagnosis and monitoring of shock. Lockhart Mummery and George Washington Crile[8,13] (a famous surgeon-scientist in the 1800s and one of the founders of the Cleveland Clinic in 1920), proposed that low blood pressure was the central and defining feature of shock. Crile, one of the first experimental physiologists to systematically study shock, produced the seminal treatise, "An Experimental Research into Surgical Shock," in 1899.[14] In this volume, he discussed his 138 animal experiments causing shock by means that had been observed in humans: laceration or incision, crush injury, manipulation of organs during operations, scalding, electrical injury, and gunshot wounds. He measured arterial and venous blood pressures, respiration, and heart rate. He also tested many remedies then used to combat shock, including cocaine and atropine.[8,14] Respected physicians and physiologists of that

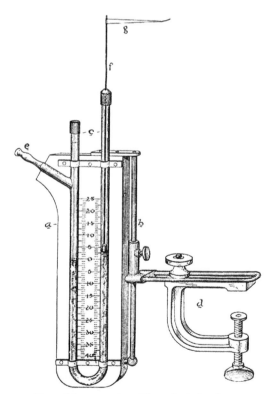

Mercurial manometer with graduated scale.

Fig. 1. Mercury sphygmomanometer (circa 1905).

era, including Harvey Cushing (the father of modern neurosurgery), Lockhart Mummery, Henry W. Cook, John B. Briggs, and Theodore C. Janeway, assisted Crile in winning acceptance of the importance of blood pressure monitoring in critical illness.[8,13,15]

Although invasive arterial blood pressure monitoring in the critically ill has become the standard of practice in recent decades, the importance of the development of noninvasive blood pressure assessment for defining shock at the turn of the century has never been surpassed.

Cardiac Output Assessment and the Pulmonary Artery Catheter

Although Hales is credited with the first right and left heart catheterizations in 1711, the Frenchmen, Bernard, a physician (in 1844), and Chauveau and Marey, a veterinarian and physician, respectively (in 1861), produced the first tracings of the right and left ventricles (both groups of studies in horses) (**Fig. 2**).[7,16–18] Human catheterization was to follow. In the early twentieth century, medical dogma suggested that the introduction of a catheter into a human heart would uniformly result in immediate death. Despite this, Bleichroder and colleagues[19] performed right heart catheterization on themselves in 1905 while trying to find ways to deliver medical therapy closer to target organs. No contemporaneous tracings or radiographs were taken, however, and the work faded into obscurity. In the summer of 1929, a 25-year-old surgical resident, Werner Forssmann (1904–1979), working in a hospital in Berlin, Germany, introduced a ureteral catheter into his left basilic vein and threaded it up 30 cm (against the explicit instructions of his surgical chairman). Obtaining a radiograph, he saw that the catheter had reached his shoulder.[7,20,21] He then advanced the catheter to 60 cm and found that it was in the right ventricular cavity. The radiograph taken was the first documented evidence of right heart catheterization in a human (**Fig. 3**). The historical significance of this event has been well documented. A notable but little noticed element in this episode, however, is the fact that, to perform the procedures required (including venous cutdown), Forssmann had to restrain and tie down the surgical nurse, Gerda

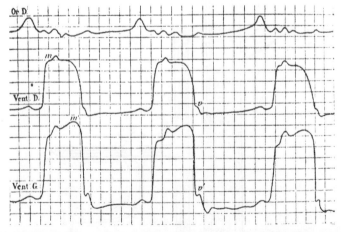

Fig. 2. Tracings of one of the earliest cardiac catheterizations (horse) by Chauveau and Marey (1863). Right atrium (*top*), right ventricle (*middle*); and, left ventricle (*bottom*). (*From* Chauveau JBA, Marey EJ. Appareils et experiences cardiographiques: demonstration nouvelle du mecanisme des mouvements deu coeur par l'emploi des instruments enregistreurs a indications continues. Mem Acad Med 1863;26:268–319.)

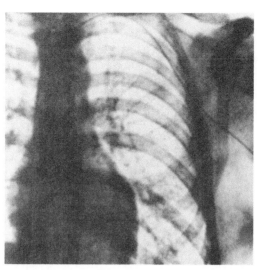

Fig. 3. Original radiograph of Forssmann's placement of a catheter into his right atrium. (*From* Forssmann W. The catheterization of the right side of the heart. Klin Wochenschr 1929;8[2085]:2087. With kind permission from Springer Science+Business Media.)

Ditzen, charged with supervision of the operating room during the procedure.[7,21] In the 1940s, Andre Cournand (**Fig. 4**) (1895–1988) and Dickinson Richards (1895–1973)[22–25] obtained right heart and pulmonary artery pressures of normal individuals and of patients who had heart failure. The studies done of right heart catheterization earned Cournand and Forssmann the Nobel Prize in Medicine and Physiology in 1956.[7,26]

Although the techniques for vascular catheterization were developing, there also were significant success in measuring human CO. A scientific basis for noninvasively measuring CO based on blood and lung oxygen concentrations dates back to Fick[27] in 1870. Indirect measurements of CO were made by Grisham and Masters[28] using pulse wave analysis in 1941 and by Starr and Wood[29] using ballistocardiographic methods in 1943. It was the work of Hamilton in 1929, however, who adapted Stewart's[30,31] indicator dye technique for human application that opened the door to the first clinically relevant studies of CO. Cournand and colleagues[24] used the technique to assess CO in traumatic shock during World War II whereas the first attempts to measure CO in myocardial infarction (using indocyanine green dye dilution) was described in 1951 by Gilbert and colleagues[32] and Freis and colleagues.[33] The first use of this technique for assessment of the hemodynamics of septic shock also is credited to Gilbert and colleague[34] during the 1950s.

The work by these early investigators and scientists eventually culminated in the development of the flow-directed, balloon-tipped, thermodilution CO-capable pulmonary artery catheter. Even though this catheter's creation is attributed to H.J.C. Swan (1922–2005) and William Ganz (1919–present), several earlier investigators provided the immediate groundwork for this development. Charles Dotter, who later gained acclaim as the inventor of angioplasty, described the first balloon-tipped pulmonary artery catheter in 1951 whereas Lategola described a soft (but not balloon-tipped) flow-directed pulmonary artery catheter in 1953.[7,35–37] Both catheters were able to obtain pulmonary artery occlusion pressures in animals but did not have thermomodilution capability. R.D. Bradley[38] was the first to describe the use of a miniature flow-directed pulmonary artery catheter in critically ill patients in 1964. The first thermodilution-derived CO catheter

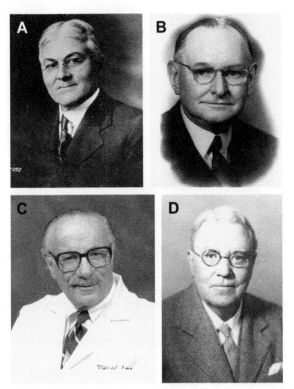

Fig. 4. Major figures in shock research during the nineteenth and twentieth centuries: (*A*) George Washington Crile (1864–1943), (*B*) Carl Wiggers (1883–1962), (*C*) Max Harry Weil (1927–present) (*Courtesy of* The American Physiological Society, Bethesda, MD; with permission.), and (*D*) Walter B. Cannon (1871–1945).

was described by Fegler[39] in anesthetized animals in 1954 but not until 14 years later did Bradley, in collaboration with M.A. Branthwaite,[40] describe the assessment of CO by thermal dilution in humans using a thermistor mounted on the tip of his earlier catheter device. Absent a balloon tip, this device did not "float" in the circulation and thus could not readily traverse the pulmonic valve into the pulmonary artery or provide a pulmonary artery occlusion pressure to estimate left ventricular end-diastolic pressure.

The eponymously named modern, balloon-tipped, flow-directed catheter now in ICUs throughout the world, was developed by Swan and Ganz. As the story goes, Swan's conception of the flow-directed pulmonary artery catheter occurred "in a brief moment of enlightenment during an outing with his children in Santa Monica."[41] Swan is reported to have noted that among many sedentary boats, a boat with a spinnaker sail catching the wind was flying by the others. Swan apparently hypothesized that a balloon attached to the end of a highly flexible catheter might, like a sail, facilitate the safe passage of the catheter into the pulmonary artery. Lategola and Rahn[37] also used the sail analogy ("As the catheter is slowly advanced into the jugular vein, the partially inflated balloon, *acting like a sail*, is swept into the right heart by the blood flow.") [*emphasis added*] in their published work almost 2 decades earlier. Ganz[42–44] initially conducted the experiments with the balloon-tipped, thermodilution-capable catheter in dogs and found that the catheter floated through the right heart into the pulmonary artery and wedged itself in a small pulmonary arterial branch. The use of this device was documented in 1970 in *The New England Journal of Medicine*.[42] The Swan-Ganz catheter has since had a central role in shock research and in clinical ICU practice.

DEFINITIONS

Definitions of shock have paralleled the prevalent concepts regarding pathophysiology, which in turn often correlated with advancements in technology used to assess the condition. In the 1700s and 1800s, there was no understanding of pathophysiology. Definitions of shock essentially were descriptive in nature. Travers (1826) provided what might be the first etiologic definition of shock as "species of functional concussion...The influence of the brain over the organ of circulation is deranged or suspended." In 1867 Furneaux Jordan,[45] a British surgeon, described a patient who had shock: "...as pale, as motionless, as indifferent to the outward world as if the injury had already terminated in death. The pallor of the skin has the sickly white hue which only bloodless human skin is capable of presenting. The ruddiness of the lips is gone...The surface of the body is everywhere cold to the touch...Small drops of moisture lie on the skin, especially on the forehead....It is commonly said that the action of the heart is accelerated; it is certainly enfeebled, the pulse being irregular and intermittent....Most inspirations are shallow and of varying degrees of rapidity." In 1895, John Collins Warren[46] described shock as a "momentary pause in the act of death" characterized by an "imperceptible" or "weak, thread-like" pulse and a "cold, clammy sweat." In 1876, Samuel Gross described shock as a "manifestation of the rude unhinging of the machinery of life."[47]

In the early 1900s, after the introduction of the sphygmomanometer, hypotension was used to define shock. The belief held by notable physicians of the time (in particular the influential Crile) (see **Fig. 4**), that shock was the result of a disorder of the nervous system, led to definitions focused on "nervous collapse." Surgeons[48] defined shock as a bodily reaction to the wound: "severe...injuries...are followed by a train of phenomena known as shock, or a general perturbation of the nervous system." In the 1930s and 1940s, as it became clearer that blood volume was a central issue in traumatic shock, the definitions incorporated these beliefs. Alfred Blalock (see **Fig. 4**)[49] wrote, "shock is a peripheral circulatory failure resulting from a discrepancy in the size of the vascular bed and the volume of the intravascular fluid." Carl Wiggers (see **Fig. 4**),[50] in the 1950s, suggested that "shock is a syndrome that results from a depression of many functions, but in which reduction of the effective circulating blood volume is of basic importance, and in which impairment of the circulation steadily progresses until it eventuates in a state of irreversible circulatory failure." With this definition, Wiggers introduced the critical concept that shock could become irreversible, the underpinning of the golden hour concept that underlies so much shock research and therapy today. With the understanding that other disease processes (besides trauma) could cause shock, Simeone,[51] in the 1960s, defined shock as "a clinical condition characterized by signs and symptoms, which arise when the cardiac output is insufficient to fill the arterial tree with blood, under sufficient pressure to provide organs and tissues with adequate blood flow." Given further advancements, Kumar and Parrillo[52] have defined shock as the "state in which profound and widespread reduction of *effective* tissue perfusion leads first to reversible, and then if prolonged, to irreversible cellular injury." There can be no doubt future definitions of shock will continue to evolve as new insights develop.

CLASSIFICATION

Like the definitions, the classification systems for shock have evolved over time. In the early eighteenth century, shock was intrinsically related to trauma. There were initially no distinctions made between hemorrhagic shock and traumatic shock. The idea of a shock syndrome without trauma did not exist. By the mid- to late 1800s, physicians noted that some wounded soldiers who did not have shock at the outset of injury developed a secondary shock, or "wound" shock.[3,53] In retrospect, many of these cases likely were related to posttraumatic hypovolemia resulting from tissue edema or infection, but at the time the cause was entirely unclear. Sepsis as a distinct cause of shock initially was proposed by Laennec (1831)[54] and subsequently supported by Boise (1897).[55] In 1934, Fishberg and colleagues[56] introduced the concept of primary cardiogenic shock resulting from myocardial infarction.

In the early 1900s, as the scientific community came to realize that there were other forms of shock not primarily related to trauma, a broader classification system emerged. Blalock suggested a four-group classification system: (1) oligemic (ie, hypovolemic)-type (primary decline in blood volume), (2) neurogenic (primary loss of vascular tone), (3) vasogenic (primary arteriolar and capillary dilatation), and (4) cardiogenic.[57–59] With continued research into the causes of shock, a more elaborate classification system arose. In 1967, Weil[60] (see **Fig. 4**) proposed seven categories of shock: hypovolemic, cardiogenic, bacteremic (ie, septic), hypersensitivity (ie, anaphylactic), neurogenic, obstructive, and endocrine. Weil[61] later proposed a reclassification of shock grouping the seven previous categories into a simpler scheme with only four categories: hypovolemic, cardiogenic, distributive, and obstructive. Hinshaw and Cox[62] delineated the hemodynamic profiles of these forms of shock in 1972. They described (1) hypovolemic shock, resulting from a decreased circulating blood volume in relation to the total vascular capacity and characterized by a reduction of diastolic filling pressures and volumes; (2) cardiogenic shock, related to cardiac pump failure resulting from loss of myocardial contractility or functional myocardium or structural or mechanical failure of the cardiac anatomy and characterized by elevations of diastolic filling pressures and volumes; (3) extracardiac obstructive shock, involving obstruction to flow in the cardiovascular circuit and characterized by impairment of diastolic filling or excessive afterload; and (4) distributive shock, caused by loss of vasomotor control resulting in arteriolar and venular dilation and (after resuscitation with fluids) characterized by increased CO with decreased systemic vascular resistance (SVR). This four-category classification system, suggested by Weil and Shubin and whose hemodynamic profiles were described by Hinshaw and Cox, is the basis of the broad classification system used today.

HISTORY OF SHOCK RESEARCH

This review discusses some of the highlights in the development of the understanding of hypovolemic shock, particularly as a consequence of trauma; cardiogenic shock resulting from acute myocardial infarction (AMI); and distributive (ie, septic) shock. The study of shock for many years was the study of victims of injury (as a result of war, accident, or surgery). This review, therefore, has a larger section on the development of ideas related to traumatic/hypovolemic shock than other areas.

Hypovolemic/Traumatic Shock

Nervous system dysfunction
The predominant pathophysiologic theory regarding the genesis of shock from approximately the mid-1800s to World War I was that of nervous system dysfunction.

As nerves were the only anatomic structures believed ubiquitous throughout the body,[8] clinicians and investigators concluded that only a disorder of the nervous system could account for the variety of clinical signs and symptoms encountered with shock. Crile was the most prominent advocate of this theory. Bernard, Brown-Sequard, Goltz, Mitchell, Fischer, and G.H. Groeningen were among the other well-known clinicians and physiologists advancing this position. Their view is reflected in the emphasis on psychologic influences in many of the early shock definitions. James C. Mumford,[63] for example, observed in 1891 that shock could follow "violent mental emotion" in addition to a variety of physical ailments. In 1817, John Hunter (a British surgeon)[64] proposed that entire body "sympathized" with wounded part whereas Astley Cooper,[65] a British surgeon, in 1928 said there was "irritation," leading to "the remote effects of injury." In 1827, Guthrie[66] stated that after any wound, there was a general "constitutional alarm" that harmed organs distant from the site of injury. Frank E. Bunts[8] in 1891 stated, "While some difference of opinion exists as to what proportion of the nervous system is primarily affected, yet most are agreed, I believe, that shock is the result of a sudden violent impression upon some part of the nervous system, acting not alone, as some would have us believe, upon the heart but upon the entire blood vascular system."

There were several reasons why nervous system dysfunction won early uncritical acceptance as the cause of the clinical manifestations of shock. First, several nervous system findings, such as altered state of consciousness, anxiety, and muscular weakness, are manifested by patients who have shock. Second, many surgeons believed, as noted by Bunts, that individual psychologic differences influenced severity of shock with worse outcomes in those who had excessive fear toward operation than those who approached operation more calmly.[8] Similarly, William Gibson[67] in 1824 suggested that psychologic condition may have been the reason that similar wounds in different people produced widely varying reactions. These observations and the knowledge that people could faint on hearing bad news or on witnessing an unpleasant event provided further support to the notion that shock was a nervous system disorder. Third, given the understanding of human physiology at the time, other mechanisms by which an injury in one part of body could affect distant sites or how so many different injuries could produce the single clinical picture of shock were not readily apparent.[8] As a consequence, the concept of nervous system failure as the cause of shock became widely accepted despite the paucity of direct evidence.

By the mid–nineteenth century, a body of knowledge began to emerge indicating that the heart and vasculature were under nervous control.[8,68] This insight set the stage for the scientific theories that followed proposing a physiologic basis for the proposition that physical injury could lead to nervous dysfunction-induced shock.

In 1861, Friedrich Leopold Goltz[69,70] made a connection between nerves and the heart. Goltz performed an experiment in which he repeatedly tapped the abdomen of a frog. This caused "overstimulation" of the vagus nerve resulting in cardiac asystole with pooling blood in the splanchnic veins. The underlying idea was that exhaustion of the stimulatory nerves resulted in shock in these experimental animals. Based on the work of Goltz, Hermann Fischer,[71] in 1870, argued that wound injury produced a reflex paralysis of the vasomotor nerves, especially to the splanchnic vessels leading to pooling of blood in the abdominal vessels. These theories quickly were adopted by clinicians of the era. In 1864, Mitchell and colleagues[72] made the connection between vasomotor nerves and injuries causing shock in the text, "Gunshot Wounds and Other Injury of Nerves:" "Recalling the fact that irritation of the vasomotor nerves is capable of producing contraction of the blood vessels, [some have] inferred that when an external nerve is violently or permanently excited, it may be able to produce contraction of the capillary vessels of the nerve centers and thus give rise to paraly-sis....We suppose, first, the existence of an exterior nerve lesion, secondly a conse-quent irritation of the vasomotor nerves in a limited part of the spine; contraction of its capillaries, anemia, nutritive changes, and [shock]." At the turn of the century, Samuel Meltzer put a different spin on the nature of nervous dysfunction in shock. The clinically minded Meltzer, observed that many organs, including the heart, are regulated by two sets of nerves, one which excites and one which inhibits, and argued that the general depression seen in shock might be the result not of the exhaustion of excitatory nerves but rather of the predominance of inhibitory nerve activity. Providing an experimental example, Meltzer[73,74] noted that the normally rhythmic contractions of intestinal peristalsis ceased immediately when he cut the skin of an animal. As no time elapsed in which excitatory nerves could become exhausted, Meltzer concluded that inhibitor nerves produced the inactivity. He suggested a similar explanation for all the depressed bodily functions in shock.

Given the competing theories of the time, it is no surprise that the clinical terms frequently used to describe this "nervous dysfunction" of shock included "over-stim-ulation," "paralysis," "under-stimulation," and "depression."[8,75] The use of these contradictory terms was reflective of the fact that no clear consensus existed on whether or not nervous system activity required support or suppression. Based on the varying views of the nature of nervous dysfunction as the source of shock, drugs used to combat shock included stimulants and depressants, depending on which type of injury to the nerves was suspected. Strychnine, a stimulant producing convulsions and widely used as a tonic, was William Halstead's[8] therapeutic mainstay. Some surgeons suggested goading the nervous system with electric current. For those who believed the nervous system was overstimulated from wound injury, a patient's nerves could be rested with alcohol, opium, or sleep.[8,76]

Crile was one of the earliest investigators to systematically study shock. He origi-nally was a major proponent of the theory of vasomotor exhaustion initially proposed by Goltz[69,70] and modified by Groeningen[8] to suggest "exhaustion" occurred in the brainstem. Many of Crile's early experiments in the late 1800s involved incising the flesh of an unanesthetized animal (presumably cutting cutaneous nerves) and assess-ing the blood pressure response. Crile found that immediately after the initial incision, there was a reflex fluctuation of blood pressure believed the normal response of the animal to interruption of a sensory nerve. Later in the experiment, after hours of manip-ulation and with the animal in shock, further incisions failed to elicit any further reflex fluctuation. This was interpreted by Crile as evidence of exhaustion of the vasomotor center after repeated insults to the animal. He believed that once the vasomotor center was exhausted and failed, large vessels would relax, blood pressure would fall precip-itously, and blood would pool in the great veins. This would lead to reduced venous return to the heart, which would cause it to beat erratically leading to clinical shock.[8] In 1899, "An Experimental Research into Surgical Shock" by Crile[14] suggested that local anesthesia might reduce shock by preventing damaging impulses from reaching the brainstem. In 1901, in "An Experimental and Clinical Research into Certain Prob-lems relating to Surgical Operations," Crile recommended cocaine for its ability to block reflex fluctuations in blood pressure.[8] Continuing to believe that nervous impulses were responsible for the lowered blood pressure and shock, he claimed that cocaine hindered "the passing of such afferent impulses, thereby preventing effects upon the respiration, the heart, or the vasomotor mechanism – ie, shock."[8]

During his subsequent studies, Crile tested, alone and in combination, strychnine, alcohol, digitalis, saline solutions, adrenalin, nitrates, and a rubber pressure suit. In test after test, only adrenalin, saline solution, and the pressure suit consistently raised pressure.[8] Notably, Crile's pressure suit was the progenitor of the later flight suits used for fighter pilots and astronauts to combat the impact of high g-force maneuvers and of medical antishock trousers. Based on his own work, Crile[77] recommended that surgeons use limited amounts of saline solution and adrenaline to raise blood pressure for management of traumatic shock (an approach that has found a place in modern practice).

In view of the later data that Crile published, other investigators began to question whether or not vasomotor exhaustion existed or played a role in the pathogenesis of shock; however, controversy on this issue persisted for decades from the late 1800s to World War I. Several experiments in the early 1900s helped put the question of "nervous failure" of vasomotor responsiveness as a cause of shock to rest. A key experiment overlooked by Crile and other advocates of the theory of vasomotor paralysis was performed by Henry H. Janeway[78] in 1914. Janeway surmised that if the theory of vasomotor exhaustion was correct, then shock should be able to be induced by simply overstimulating major nerves in an animal not in shock. This critical experiment failed to reproduce shock and, along with other key studies, that showed an absence of medullary damage in shock[79] helped convince investigators that the nervous system dysfunction was a manifestation rather than a cause of the syndrome. Despite these results, the final studies on the question of "nervous dysfunction" as a cause of shock did not occur until 1956.[80,81]

Circulating volume loss

The primary competing hypothesis to nervous system dysfunction as the cause of shock was loss of circulating blood volume. Overt hemorrhage generally was conceded to cause shock but the relationship of decreased circulating blood volume to shock absent overt hemorrhage was uncertain. The earliest insights regarding the potential role of fluid deficiency in shock dates back to the attempts by Thomas Latta[82] in 1832 to resuscitate shock due to cholera-induced volume loss with intravenous fluids. This idea generally was ignored until Goltz[70] suggested that death from hemorrhage was the result of loss of intravascular volume rather than red blood cells 32 years later. By the late 1880s to 1890s, the observation had been made that intravenous fluid replacement of lost blood could cure patients who were hypotensive and in shock from overt hemorrhage,[83–85] although this therapy would not become the standard of care for decades.

Despite this, the importance of giving fluid in shock states other than those associated with overt hemorrhage was not appreciated, perhaps because the nervous system dysfunction theory of shock was pervasive at that time. Further, the understanding of cardiac hemodynamics was in its infancy and it was not understood that even if there was venous pooling in abdominal veins, fluid infusion still could increase venous return, forward flow, and blood pressure. In the early 1900s through World War I, the central importance of fluid administration to treat dehydration and hypovolemia began to emerge. Therapy of shock typically might have included normal salt solution (rectally and subcutaneously) and strychnine (1/60 g) along with best rest and passive warming. In some cases, fluid (water) was given orally or rectally.[3,8,86] It was only in most urgent cases that intravenous route was believed necessary.

In the early 1900s, efforts were made to examine circulating blood volume and demonstrate that blood volume was decreased in nonhemorrhagic traumatic shock. Yandell Henderson and coworkers[87] first suggested in 1908 that a decrease in venous return and CO was responsible for the decline in arterial blood pressure in traumatic shock. Unfortunately, they have rarely received credit for this insight because the proposal was embedded in the "acapnia" theory of shock (ie, that low levels of carbon dioxide were responsible for hypotension). Given the study design, these experiments likely represent the first examination of what would become known as obstructive shock. Henderson's model of shock required overventilation of his animals to create positive intrathoracic pressure resulting in decreased venous return. At the time, Henderson believed that it was hypocapnia-mediated venous pooling that caused the shock in the model.

In 1915, Keith and coworkers[88,89] aand Robertson and Bock[90] at John Hopkins developed and used a crude technique to measure blood volume in the field by injecting the dye, vital red, which is retained intravascularly in the plasma compartment. In their series of war-related clinical studies, the concentration of dye in the blood was measured several minutes after initial injection. From the concentration of dye in the sample, they were able to calculate the volume of blood in the body.[88,89] They found that if blood volume was approximately 75% or greater of the expected value, the blood pressure was essentially normal. If the blood volume was decreased to 65% to75% of normal, then the systolic blood pressure was 70 to 80 mm Hg and the patient showed evidence of clinical shock. If the blood volume was 50% to 60% of normal, then many patients were very ill and almost pulseless. In making these observations, they concluded that the decrease in blood volume clearly produced shock and that severity of hypotension correlated with the degree of blood loss. Effective circulating blood volume was a central factor in the pathogenesis of traumatic shock. This work was reinforced by the early animals studies of the famous cardiovascular physiologist, Wiggers,[91] who was able to demonstrate that traumatic "surgical" shock was most akin to severe hemorrhage in the marked decrease in blood and central venous pressure. This series of studies by Keith was a remarkable achievement that presaged Wiggers'[92,93] work on the nature of irreversible shock in his canine hemorrhagic shock model almost 25 years later.

Knowing that decreased effective volume was important, investigators then needed to determine where plasma volume was redistributed in traumatic shock patients who were not obviously bleeding. One hypothesis was that blood pooled in the abdominal veins during shock and essentially became unable to contribute to circulating blood volume (termed, *intravascular hemorrhage*), an extension of the theories of Goltz[70] and later supported by Crile.[94] The idea that a patient in shock "bled" into his own abdominal veins, however, primarily stemmed from Fischer's[71] animal experiments in 1870. The initial explanation for the dilated abdominal veins was based on the theory of vasomotor exhaustion where, with progression of injury, the abdominal veins would dilate and accumulate blood taking it away from the periphery and leading to the cold, pale appearance of the patient or experimental animal in shock. Given the experiments suggesting that the vasomotor center was still active in shock, however, blood vessels would be expected to be constricted, as observed in the studies refuting the vasomotor theory of shock.[78,79,95] The concept of abdominal pooling of blood volume persisted. Walter B. Cannon (see **Fig. 4**), a well known physician and physiologist, proposed early in his career that in traumatic shock blood was stagnant in engorged veins between two sets of constricted blood vessels: intestinal arterioles on one side, portal and hepatic vessels of the liver on the other. He also suggested that vasomotor nerves to these constricted vessels were responsible for the pooling of blood. The goal of therapy was to open the constricted vessels or to constrict the dilated vessels holding the trapped blood to move blood back into circulation.[50]

Crile[77] expanded on his idea of intestinal sequestration of blood volume in his 1907 article, "Hemorrhage and Transfusion." This proposed phenomenon, so dominant in the medical literature of the time, however, likely was the unique result of producing shock by manipulating the intestines violently. Henry Janeway's[78] method of inducing experimental shock, although different from Crile's, also caused blood to collect in intestinal veins. Janeway produced shock by placing a band around the inferior vena cava, which backed the blood up into the large veins. In this model, what was interpreted by Janeway as "abdominal vein hemorrhage" causing shock today would be interpreted as reduced return of blood to the heart and a subsequently diminished right heart output. The belief that blood volume pooled in intestinal veins during shock continued to be widespread in the early years of the 20th century.

Frank Charles Mann[96,97] significantly advanced the understanding of shock physiology by suggesting that the blood in the abdominal compartment actually left the veins, oozing into the surrounding tissues. He suggested, "the cause of shock is the tremendous loss of red cells and fluid from the blood, due to the reaction of the great delicate vascular splanchnic area to irritation—an acute inflammation of the peritoneum, due to trauma and exposure to the air and changes of temperature." Mann set out to measure the volume of blood lost from the circulation. To estimate the loss, Mann compared the volume of blood he could drain from the total circulatory system before and after shock induction. In a normal animal, Mann found that he could drain 76% of the blood from the body. He concluded that in normal animals, 24% of the blood was "in the tissues," presumably not subject to draining. But from animals in shock, Mann[98] could drain only 39% of the blood, leaving 61% "in the tissues," not circulating. The difference between 61% and 24% was the volume of blood believed leaked out of the vascular system, which led to shock. This again suggested that blood volume was the crucial determinant of shock.

Crile, Henry Janeway, and Mann all believed that shock occurred as a consequence of blood pooling or sequestration in the abdominal compartment. They each had induced shock (described previously) by manipulating the inferior vena cava or the bowel in a way that may have produced results in the experimental animals that were not reflective of critically ill patients (ie, the abdominal vein blood pooling may have been a phenomenon strictly of the experimental method used and not the true reason for volume loss in shock). During World War I, investigators, such as Wallace,[99] Cannon, and other surgeons, observed that in patients in shock who had abdominal operations, intestinal vein blood pooling and blood extravasation were not found. This observation led Cannon to suggest that fluid must escape from the circulation through the walls of capillaries in a more diffuse manner during shock.[100,101] This theory subsequently led to for a search for a toxic factor as the cause of shock.

Circulating "factors"

The possibility of circulating factors that might adversely affect cardiovascular stability had precedent. The concept of malignant circulating "humors" has existed since the Greek Age[86,102] The concept persisted through the Dark Ages of Europe and into the seventeenth and eighteenth centuries. Benjamin Rush, a signer of the American Declaration of Independence and the foremost North American physician of his day, advocated periodic bleeding to remove these circulating humors for a variety of ailments.[103]

Before World War I, it was known that patients could present in shock after trauma without an obvious loss of blood. At the time, a distinction was made between hemorrhagic shock resulting from obvious loss of blood from a wound and traumatic shock hypotension resulting from injury without obvious loss of blood (wound shock).[99,100] Mapother[104] in 1879 seems to have been the first to suggest that decreased CO in traumatic shock may be caused by intravascular volume loss resulting from extrusion of plasma through the vessel wall from the intravascular space to the interstitium. During the war, Cannon and many other leading physician and physiologists of the day were deployed to the battlefields during the war to study shock and devise medical and surgical therapies for wounded soldiers. As part of the National Research Council's Subcommittee on the Physiology of Shock, Cannon and colleagues produced the first systematic clinical studies of war trauma culminating in release of the monograph, "Traumatic Shock," in 1923.[101] Their studies revealed a greater degree of hemoconcentration in the capillary circulation than the venous circulation in patients in shock compared with patients not in shock. For example, in wounded patients who were not hypotensive, the capillary and venous red cell counts were equal. In patients who had moderate shock (systolic blood pressure of approximately 90 mm Hg), there was a difference of approximately 1 million per microliter and in patients who had severe shock (blood pressure of approximately 70 mm Hg), the difference between the capillary and venous red cell count was 2 to 3 million per microliter.[101,105] This suggested that after major traumatic injury, increased capillary permeability allowed profound extravasation of fluid from the capillaries leading to hypovolemic shock.

Supporting evidence for a toxic factor causing loss of intravascular volume in shock came from experiments in animals. Sir William Bayliss, the brother-in-law of the famous cardiovascular physiologist, Ernest Starling, gained acclaim for his discovery of the first known hormone, secretin (as part of his studies of the pancreas). Although substantially forgotten today, he was also well known at the time for his shock research. Bayliss and colleagues[105,106] hammered the hind limbs of cats, dogs, and rabbits under anesthesia to cause severe crush injuries. These animals developed signs of shock with hypotension, hypovolemia, and hemoconcentration. Shock did not seem to result from local blood loss caused by bruising as the increase in weight of the traumatized limb was only approximately 11% of the animal's blood volume (a small percentage of the volume known to be lost from the animal) as measured by vital red dilution. If the vessels to the traumatized limbs were ligated, then the animals could be protected from shock; alternatively, if the vessels were left open and the traumatized limb massaged, the blood pressure worsened. Extracts of the muscle in the traumatized area could produce a fall in blood pressure if injected intravenously. These observations suggested that there was a toxic factor causing generalized increase capillary permeability with leak of plasma into the interstitium producing hypovolemia and shock. Realizing that intravenous saline would leak out of the capillaries, Bayliss helped develop a new intravenous compound—6% solution of gum acacia in saline (perhaps the first synthetic colloid)—that was used with apparently good results although less than a liter often was given.[105,106]

The next step was to determine the identity of this putative toxic factor. The agent had to result in capillary stasis with hemoconcentration, increased capillary permeability with general extravascular fluid loss, a decrease in blood volume, and a drop in blood pressure. Several potential "toxins" were studied but histamine was foremost among them as it could reproduce many of the required clinical findings, including tissue edema when injected intravenously, and it normally was found in muscle tissue.[105] Dale, Laidlaw, and Richards produced significant support in favor of the concept of histamine as a mediator of shock in the 1910s to 1920s.[107,108]

The concept of toxin-driven generalized increased capillary permeability as the etiologic basis of shock was challenged by several investigators. Blalock,[105,109] in 1930, and others in later years demonstrated that the local edema caused by trauma extends far beyond the immediate area of injury. Cannon and Bayliss measured the volume lost into the lower limb after crushing an animal's leg. They found that although not all the blood volume lost could be recovered in the immediate area of injury, most was accounted for within the limb. This suggested the possibility that earlier studies examining posttraumatic fluid redistribution may have underestimated local fluid extravasation and overestimated distant, presumably toxin-mediated, effects.[105] Blalock found in later studies that if a hindquarter amputation was done in animals that had undergone hindquarter trauma, all the loss of blood volume was accounted for in this hindquarter amputation; generalized capillary leak was not required to account for intravascular fluid loss.[105] In addition, Blalock, Dragstedt, Mead, Code, Macdonald, and Woolfe in the late 1930s and early 1940s found that the histamine content of the blood from injured limbs showed no significant increase over control limbs.[105] Using radioactive tracers in the 1940s, Fine and Seligman showed that the rate of I^{131}-labelled albumin loss from the capillaries in the uninjured parts of shocked animals was the same as the rate of loss in normal animals.[105] A toxic factor responsible for causing shock from trauma has never been found even though a variety of hemodynamically active mediators, including tumor necrosis factor and various eicosanoids, are known to be released.

ORIGINS OF THE MODERN ERA OF SHOCK RESEARCH

Many of the advances in our understanding and treatment of traumatic shock physiology have occurred as a consequence of war. Although physicians such as George Crile and Alfred Blalock asked and answered many important questions, the era of modern shock research begins, in many ways, with the progress made during the 2nd World War when human cardiac catheterization was introduced as research tool for the systematic assessment of critical illness. As a consequence, physicians such as Henry Beecher and Andre Cournand were finally able to definitively demonstrate that hemorrhage and fluid loss was major cause of shock in the battlefield.[22,24,110] Along with Dickinson Richards, Cournand (see **Fig. 2**), a French-born naturalized US citizen, led a team of physicians at the Bellevue Hospital in New York City investigating the use of cardiac catheterization on patients suffering from severe circulatory shock resulting from traumatic injury. In 1943, the Bellvue cardiovascular research group reported their classic study of the circulation in clinical shock.[24] In one of the most comprehensive studies of the physiology of shock ever reported, all the major responses of the systemic circulation during traumatic injury were assessed. The investigators measured intravascular pressures through the femoral artery, median basilic vein and right atrium, cardiac output via the direct Fick technique, and multiple metrics of pulmonary ventilation and respiratory gas exchange. This classic study was based upon 36 cases, 16 of which were patient's suffering from skeletal trauma, four from hemorrhage, four from burns, six with abdominal injury and 6 from head injury. Detailed physiologic measurements of all patient's were undertaken on presentation and the presence or absence of the shock state shock state was characterized for each of the preceding categories and further subdivided into gradations of shock severity. Sequential measurements related to cardiac output, minute ventilation, circulating blood volume and multiple other variables similar to a contemporary ICU flow chart were recorded for all patients. These physiologic measurements of the shock state were recorded throughout the course of resuscitation. Obtaining physiological measurements of cardiopulmonary function in these patients definitively demonstrated the cause of traumatic shock- as decreased circulating intravascular volume resulting in a fall in venous return and cardiac output.[24] As a result of these findings, it was determined that the best treatment for traumatic/hemorrhagic shock was a total blood transfusion rather plasma infusion which had previously been used.

During the second half of the twentieth century, physicians became adept at recognizing and providing immediate treatment to patients who had shock, including aggressive fluid resuscitation, transfusion, operative intervention, antimicrobial therapy, pump failure therapy, and so forth. It has become apparent, however, that patients who have been in shock for a prolonged period of time often develop multi-system organ failure especially when organ support (ie, pressor therapy, mechanical ventilation, or dialysis) is provided to extend life. The concept of multiple organ failure is inextricably linked to that of irreversible shock, as defined by Wiggers.[50] His development of the concept, that shock, if sustained, could lead to irreversible circulatory failure with death as an inevitable outcome, represents the other seminal advance that signaled the start of the modern era of shock research.

The initial studies looking at irreversible shock started in the 1900s and were given increased impetus by the 1st World War.[91] Experiments had been done to determine if there was a relationship between the amount of time an animal was in shock and the severity of the shock on survival. During the 2nd World War, Carl Wiggers,[75,93] one of the foremost physiologists of the past century, performed a series of experiments on dogs varying the blood pressure and the length of time in shock. In a canine model, blood was withdrawn until blood pressure reached a given target (usually mean arterial pressure of 30–65 mm Hg). Animals were left at that blood pressure for a period of time (45 minutes to 5 hours) before shed blood was infused back to the dogs. For a given blood pressure target, prolonged hypotension produced increasingly high mortality. In addition, many dogs recovered from hypotension of 50 mm Hg for 2 to 3.5 hours whereas few dogs survived, even after transfusion of blood back, if the mean arterial pressure had been at 30 to 35 mm Hg for 45 to 60 minutes. At autopsy, Wiggers[92,93] found that the bowel mucosa showed intensive congestion, edema, and hemorrhages with blood or blood-tinged fluid in the lumens of those dogs that failed to survive, whereas the abdominal viscera were pale or pink externally and the mucosa of the intestine appeared normal or only slightly cyanotic and swollen in the dogs that did survive. It was believed that extensive capillary damage occurred only after marked hypotension had existed for a considerable period of time and that the capillary damage was a consequence and not a cause of the hypotension. This was irreversible shock.

At the time, the etiology was believed partly related to bacterial factors.[111,112] In the 1920s, autolysing liver tissue in the abdomen of an experimental animal was believed highly toxic.[105] The basis of this toxicity was hypothesized to be bacteria (such as *Clostridium welchii*), which grew in a state of symbiosis without causing the animal any harm as long as the tissue in which the bacteria were present received an adequate oxygen supply. If the tissue died, the bacteria proliferated and produced toxins, which ultimately killed the animal. The bowel changes seen by Wiggers[92] were believed potentially related to bacteria in the bowel, which released toxins leading to death in the dogs that had irreversible shock. Jacobs and colleagues[113] in 1954 provided some support for the role of bacteria in causing death in irreversible shock by showing that the administration of antibiotics decreased mortality rate (although not totally eliminating it). Other studies suggested a bacterial factor also was associated with irreversibility of endotoxin and bacterial shock.[111] Deriving from his concepts of a toxic factor in irreversible shock, Wiggers[114] initiated the modern search for a myocardial depressant substance in shock, septic or hemorrhagic. This work later was carried forward by others, most notably Lefer and colleagues[115–117] and Parrillo and colleagues.[118]

By the second half of the century, potential irreversibility of shock was well established and formed the theoretic underpinning of concept of the golden hour used for trauma resuscitation, later extended to management of AMI and cardiogenic shock and most recently to therapy of pulmonary embolus or obstructive shock and sepsis or septic shock.[119–123]

Later military conflicts fueled further advances. During the Korean War, the relationship between circulatory shock and risk of acute tubular necrosis and the relationship of survival after trauma with early resuscitation began to be appreciated. During the Vietnam War the dominant shock research concerns became "shock lung" (adult respiratory distress syndrome) and postshock infections.

Septic Shock

Septic shock became recognized as a distinct entity in two different conditions—post-trauma wound injury and nontrauma infection. Wounded soldiers were known to frequently develop gangrene resulting almost uniformly in death; however, the connection between wounds and sepsis or septic shock was not made until the Spanish-American War in 1898 when clinicians recognized the disease progression.[3] Nontraumatic causes of septic shock also were discovered in the late 1800s and early 1900s. One of the earliest descriptions of circulatory failure occurring in the setting of infection was by Laennec[54] in 1831. In 1892, the famous William Osler[124] described a "typhoid state" occurring in patients who developed fatal pyelonephritis. In 1897, Boise[55] made a clear distinction between shock caused by hemorrhage and shock caused by sepsis.

The association of gram-negative bacteremia with sepsis and septic shock became apparent at the turn of the century. In 1909, Jacob[125] reviewed a case series of 39 patients who had *Escherichia coli* septicemia (ie, bacteremia with sepsis), 41% of whom died. He found that the portals of entry into the blood stream were biliary tract, urinary tract, gastrointestinal tract, and female genital tract. In the 1920s to 1940s, it became recognized that intravenous administration of dead bacilli and antigens (eg, typhoid toxin) could produce hypotension (ie, endotoxic shock).[126,127] In the first half of the of the past century, pyrogen (likely endotoxin) derived from *Pseudomonas aeruginosa* was used therapeutically to treat malignant hypertension.[128] In the 1950s, it became clearer that bacteremias by aerobic gram-negative bacilli were the etiologic agent in many cases of septic shock. In a review at the Minneapolis General Hospital[129] (1950–1951), positive blood cultures for aerobic gram-negative bacilli were found more frequently in patients who died of septic shock.

In Laennec's early description of septic shock, the weak heart sounds of circulatory failure were ascribed to heart failure, one of the earliest written suggestions that circulatory shock was manifested by cardiac failure (although the acceptance of the concept in the medical community predated the clinical description by decades).[81] The concept that severe myocardial failure characterized septic shock persisted through the 1800s and well into the second half of the twentieth century. Theodore Janeway[130] in 1907, Atchely[131] in 1930, and Stead and Ebert[132] in 1940 all referred to the "the heart [cardiac] failure" of acute infectious disease and septic conditions.

There were dissenters to the idea that myocardial depression per se dominated circulatory failure associated with infection.[81] Eppinger and Schurmeyer[133] demonstrated that acute infection (sepsis) and traumatic/hemorrhagic shock were associated with decreased plasma volume in 1928. Similarly, Atchely,[131] in 1930, suggested that a "disproportion between blood volume and vascular bed" was common to all forms of shock and that the appropriate treatment should be aimed at increasing blood volume. Warfield[134] in 1934 suggested hemodynamic equivalence between untreated septic and traumatic/hemorrhagic shock and suggested, as therapy, saline infusion of "three to four liters in 24 hours." Moon[135] advanced this idea further, suggesting "a disparity between the volume of blood and the volume-capacity of the vascular system," rather than volume loss alone, was the cause of decreased venous return in septic shock. For the most part, however, the idea that volume loss and venodilatation may have the central role in the hemodynamic collapse of severe infection was not appreciated for decades.

In 1945, Warren and colleagues[136] published one of the earliest studies of "cold" septic shock and demonstrated the potential usefulness of "vigorous anti-shock therapy directed to maintain an adequate circulating blood volume." This concept of "cold" shock in overwhelming infection was expanded on in Waisbren's[129] study (1951–1952) of gram-negative bacteremia. In that study, two clinical pictures of gram-negative bacteremia emerged—a warm and flushed (toxic) state and a cold, shock-like state. The descriptions by Warren and Waisbren of the clinical characteristics of patients who had overwhelming infection likely represent the basis of later descriptions of warm and cold phases of septic shock that dominated the clinical septic shock literature until the 1980s.[137–139]

Waisbren's early description of warm and cold shock was further explored by other investigators. Clowes and colleagues,[137] in a 1966 dye dilution study, sequentially followed 19 patients who had septic shock that resulted from peritonitis. The 12 patients who recovered promptly maintained a cardiac index of greater than 3 L/min/m^2, throughout their illness. Four patients who succumbed within 24 hours experienced a rapid fall in cardiac index between presentation (approximately 4 L/min/m^2) and just before death (approximately 2 L/min/m^2). Three other patients who responded initially but deteriorated and died between 5 and 7 days after presentation had initial low cardiac indices (approximately 2 L/min/m^2) that rose to normal (3–4 L/min/m^2) within days and then fell again preterminally (to approximately 2 L/min/m^2). This view of septic mortality as a biphasic hemodynamic phenomenon was supported by several other early clinical reports that suggested that most cases of septic shock were associated with low CO and increased SVR (for review[139]).[140–142] In 1973, Nishijima and colleagues[138] provided a simple meta-analysis of seven studies performed up to that time correlating survival with cardiac index. A strong association was shown to exist between elevated cardiac index and survival in patients who had sepsis and septic shock. These human studies were supported by animal models using intravenous bolus injections of endotoxin or live organisms.[139,143–147] Almost all of these models produced shock characterized by reduced CO and elevated SVR.

Unfortunately, just as the animal studies were seriously flawed by the assumption that endotoxin or live organism infusion mimics human sepsis, the human studies were undermined by the use of central venous pressure as the best available estimate of left ventricular end diastolic volume (ie, left ventricular preload). Despite this, several studies from that era hinted at the possibility that volume status might be a crucial determinant of cardiac index (and outcome) in sepsis and septic shock. MacLean and colleagues,[148] in 1967, demonstrated that patients who had septic shock could be separated into two groups based on low or normal central venous pressure and CO. The investigators suggested that volume replacement would be the most appropriate therapy for hypovolemic septic patients who had low central venous pressure and decreased CO. In 1970, Blain and colleagues[149] proposed that depletion of circulating volume accounted for decreased CO during human septic shock. Weil and Nifhijima[142] similarly noted a relationship between total blood volume, cardiac index, and survival in patients who had septic shock.

In marked contrast to previous studies, Wilson and colleagues[150] were able, in 1965, to demonstrate that normal or elevated CO usually characterized septic shock in humans. Wilson was among the first to comment specifically on the divergent hemodynamic profile of human septic shock (increased CO and decreased SVR) compared with cardiogenic or hemorrhagic shock. He also noted that this profile was distinct from that of lethal canine endotoxic shock (low CO and high SVR) but that inadvertent administration of small, sublethal amount of endotoxin to humans resulted in an elevated CO and peripheral vasodilatation.[150,151] The work by MacLean, Weil, Blain, and Wilson helped to set the stage for the shock classification systems of shock that followed in a few years. Wilson's view of the hyperdynamic nature of septic shock did not become broadly accepted, however, until the widespread introduction of pulmonary artery catheters with thermodilution CO capacity to critical care units.

Cardiogenic Shock

The history of cardiogenic shock must necessarily focus on the history of coronary artery disease, as AMI is the most common cause of cardiogenic shock. The first recorded description of angina pectoris was by William Heberden,[152] who presented "a disorder of the breast" before the Royal College of Physicians of London in 1768. Most physicians believed that myocardial infarction ("angina pectoris") was a uniformly sudden fatal event; thus, for 125 years, no further progress was made. In 1880, Carl Weigert[153] reported on the pathology of these patients. He noted that many seemed to have coronary thrombosis and atherosclerosis. In 1881, Samuelson[154] first described the clinical manifestations of AMI evolving into cardiac collapse (cardiogenic shock). At the end of the nineteenth century and the beginning of the twentieth century, physicians noted that some patients were surviving this supposedly sudden and fatal event. In 1896, George Dock[155] presented his case series of four patients at the Alumni Association of the Medical Department of the University of Buffalo; one patient survived 1 week after the onset of the attack. In 1910, Obrastzow and Straschesko,[156] from Russia presented two cases of AMI that were diagnosed before death. In 1910, James B. Herrick,[157] who had earlier the same year first described sickle cell disease, suggested that the concept of universal sudden death after AMI was wrong. Efforts were undertaken to determine how to treat these patients and to determine the cause of AMI and cardiogenic shock. The initial treatment of AMI in patients surviving to hospitalization was simple sedation and bedrest.[158] Wearn[159] at the Peter Bent Brigham Hospital in Boston recommended that "every effort [be made] to spare the patient any bodily exertion" to prevent sudden cardiac rupture and death. Early mortality of patients surviving to hospitalization with known AMI was more than 30% in the first decades of the twentieth century.[158]

The care of patients who had AMI improved with advancements in technology. In 1903, Willem Einthoven, a physiology professor in Holland, devised a string galvanometer, which was able to record human electrocardiograms.[160] With this information, physicians learned to recognize patterns suggestive of AMI and learned that the most common reason for sudden death was ventricular arrhythmia. In 1947, Beck and colleagues[161] reported successful open chest cardiac defibrillation on a child who had undergone surgery to correct a defect in the sternum. In 1956, the same group[162] reported open defibrillation in a 65-year-old physician who had fibrillated post AMI. For a time, open thoracotomy, direct cardiac massage, and internal electrical defibrillation became standard management of cardiac arrest.[163] In 1956, Zoll and colleagues[164] developed an external cardiac defibrillator and demonstrated the efficacy of externally applied countershock for therapy of ventricular fibrillation. In 1960, Kouwenhoven and colleagues[165] from John Hopkins Hospital demonstrated the efficacy of sternal compression, external electrical defibrillation, and mouth-to-mouth resuscitation in restoring cardiac function to patients who had suffered a ventricular fibrillation arrest. Also, in the 1960s, Peter J. Safar established public education of cardiopulmonary resuscitation. This, combined with the establishment of coronary care units in 1962 by Meltzer in Philadelphia, Brown in Toronto, and Day in Kansas,[166] led to the identification of more and more patients who developed cardiogenic shock.

In the first half of the past century, significant advances in understanding clinical aspects of AMI and cardiogenic shock were made. The first description of the hemodynamics of cardiogenic shock is credited to Fishberg and colleagues[56] in 1934 when they contrasted the clinical findings of cardiogenic shock from AMI to cardiac dysfunction from mitral stenosis. In 1939, Harrison[167] established cardiogenic shock as a clinical entity distinguished from other forms of shock. Later, Wiggers[168] stated, "myocardial failure is the crux of the circulatory [shock] which follows acute myocardial infarction." In 1952, Agress[169] suggested a definition of cardiogenic shock as "a reduction of approximately 30% in mean systemic arterial pressure, maintenance of this reduction with no upward trend for at least 30 minutes, electrographic evidence of severe ischemia; and the absence of arrhythmias that could account for the arterial pressure reduction." Clinical research in patients initially consisted of descriptive autopsy studies. These studies showed that the location (anterior or posterior) of myocardial necrosis had little relationship to the occurrence of cardiogenic shock but that the size of infarct was crucial.[170–173] Rosenberg and Malach,[174] Walston and colleagues,[171] and Harnarayan and colleagues[175] all found shock more common in patients who had large acute infarcts. Page and colleagues[172] looked at 20 patients who had fatal AMI and shock, 14 patients who had fatal AMI without shock, and 20 patients who had fatal shock but no AMI. Of the 20 patients who had AMI and shock, 19 had lost over 40% of left ventricular myocardium (old and new infarct) and one had lost 35%. Of the 14 patients who had AMI and no shock, 12 had lost less than 30% of left ventricular myocardium, one had lost 35%, and one had lost 40%. Of the 20 patients who had fatal shock but no AMI, all had widespread, microscopic-sized foci of necrosis but no large areas of necrosis. These findings helped provide fairly strong evidence that the amount of myocardium infarcted was important in determining whether or not a patient developed cardiogenic shock.

Initially, the underlying mechanism of cardiogenic shock was not well understood. It was known that the myocardium was nourished from blood that it received via the coronary arteries as opposed to the blood in the ventricular cavities. The favored hypothesis for cardiogenic shock was AMI resulting from coronary occlusion. The many investigators reporting the incidence of coronary thrombosis, however, in patients dying of AMI demonstrated that incidence varied significantly, from 21% to 95%.[176] With such a large range, it was not clear whether or not coronary thrombosis was the cause or a consequence of cardiogenic shock. Some believed that coronary thrombosis was the result of slower blood flow in the coronary circulation associated with cardiogenic shock.[176] Investigators performed experiments on animals, including ligation of different coronary arteries alone or serially; injuring the myocardium by direct trauma, heat, or electricity; and injecting microbeads into the coronaries.[177,178] In general, it was difficult to produce cardiogenic shock as the animals fibrillated with immediate death or recovered quickly without shock. With time, investigators determined that injection of microbeads into the aortic root occluded many small coronary vessels leading to progressive sublethal myocardial injury. By adjusting volume status and peripheral vascular tone, cardiogenic shock could be achieved in animal models. The introduction of selective coronary angiography in 1962 by Mason Sones from the Cleveland Clinic in Ohio[179] eventually allowed investigators to appreciate the importance of coronary occlusion as the primary etiologic agent inciting AMI and cardiogenic shock.

To study the hemodynamic effects of myocardial infarction and cardiogenic shock and to develop methods of treatment, the National Heart, Lung, and Blood Institute funded a group of myocardial infarction research units in the United States in the late 1960s and early 1970s.[166] The relative roles of CO, ventricular filling pressure, and peripheral vascular resistance in producing cardiogenic shock required clarification.

The introduction of the balloon-tipped, thermodilution-capable pulmonary artery catheter in the mid-1970s signaled the ability to systematically assess CO in clinical shock states. With the advent of this device, studies measuring CO and filling pressures with calculation of peripheral vascular resistance could be routinely performed. Kuhn, Gunnar, Loeb, and Rahimtoola performed several clinical hemodynamic studies.[180–182] They noted that increased peripheral vascular tone and supplementation of intravascular volume status could prevent hypotension despite having a low CO. They also were able to make recommendations on the use of vasoactive agents, volume, and other therapies based on hemodynamic parameters leading to modern approach in use today.

Given the understanding that the primary problem leading to cardiogenic shock is AMI resulting from coronary thrombosis, efforts were undertaken to improve coronary perfusion and to support the circulation during the period of shock. Fluids, diuretics, and inotropic agents, including norepinephrine, digitalis, glucagons, and vasodilators, were used to support the circulation during pulmonary edema and cardiogenic shock in the early years. Because the amount of myocardium infracted correlated to the likelihood of cardiogenic shock and cardiogenic shock often is a harbinger of death, efforts were undertaken to limit the infarct size by improving myocardial perfusion. Fletcher and colleagues[183] and Verstraete[184] started the use of thrombolytic therapy into the coronary arteries to dissolve thrombus in the late 1950s and 1960s. The use of intravenous thrombolytic therapy became common in the 1980s after the results of the GISSI[185] and the ISIS-2[186] were published. The intra-aortic balloon pump was first developed for use in humans in 1968 by Kantrowitz and colleagues[187] to improve coronary perfusion and decrease left ventricular afterload. Cardiac surgery began to flourish after the development of the heart-lung machine by John Gibbons in Philadelphia in 1953 but emergency coronary artery bypass surgery to revascularize jeopardized myocardium did not develop until approximately 20 years later.[188]

SUMMARY

This narrative reviews the development of some of the major early ideas regarding the etiology and pathogenesis of shock. Most of the early history of shock has been related primarily to traumatic shock. The more recent history of the shock syndromes centers on differentiation of the clinical syndromes and their individual clinical and pathologic characteristics. Over time, the definitions, classification systems, pathogenic theories, and treatments have evolved. This evolution has been driven by the dedicated physicians and physiologists of the past on whose shoulders current intensivists and shock investigators now stand. The progress made also has been aided by a constant development of improved assessment technologies from the mercury sphygmomanometer, through the balloon-tipped, thermodilution-capable pulmonary artery catheter to current cutting-edge ICU technology that includes 3-D echocardiography and MRI. Today, shock is not a single syndrome and the definition of shock no longer is descriptive in nature. The most accepted current definition involves oxygen supply and demand at the cellular level. This oxygen supply/demand imbalance causing shock also can have various causes—hypovolemia, cardiac dysfunction, vascular failure, or obstructive processes that impair cardiac filling. Today's challenges of adult respiratory distress syndrome, multiple organ failure, and multiresistant infection are different but no less important than those faced by our predecessors who worked to determine the etiology and basic pathogenesis of shock. Hopefully, in the future, our successors will look back on these efforts with the same respect that physicians and investigators of this era hold for the pioneering work of Crile, Blalock, Cannon, Wiggers, and their colleagues in the past.

REFERENCES

1. Silverman ME. William Harvey and the discovery of the circulation of blood. Clin Cardiol 1985;8(4):244–6.
2. Harvey W. Exerciato Anatoica de Motu Cordis at Sanguinis in Animalibus. [translated by Leake CD]. Springfield (IL): Charles C.Thomas; 1970 [Latin].
3. Hardaway RM, Hardaway RM. Wound shock: a history of its study and treatment by military surgeons. Mil Med 2004;169(4):265–9.
4. Guthrie GJ. On gunshot wounds of the extremities. London: Longman; 1815.
5. Morris EA. A practical treatise on shock after operations and injuries. London 1867.
6. Hales S. Statical essays: containing haemastaticks. New York 1733.
7. Mueller RL, Sanborn TA. The history of interventional cardiology: cardiac catheterization, angioplasty and related interventions. Am Heart J 1995;129:146–72.
8. English PE. Shock, physiological surgery, and George Washington Crile: medical innovation in the progressive era. Westport (CT): Greenwood Press; 1980.
9. Major RH. Karl Vierordt. Ann Med Hist 1938;10:463–73.
10. Vierordt K. Die bildliche Darstellung des menschlichen Arterienpulses. Archiv fur physiologische Heilkunde 1854;13:284–7.
11. Von Bashe SS. Uber die Messung des Blutdrucks am Menchen. Zeitschrift 1883; 33:673–5.
12. Riva-Rocci S. Un nuovo sfigmemanometro. Gazetta Medica di Torino 1896;47: 981–6.
13. Lockhart Mummery JP. The physiology and treatment of surgical shock and collapse. i. Lancet 1905;696–703.
14. Crile GW. An experimental research into surgical shock. Philadelphia: Lippincott; 1899.
15. Fulton JF. Harvey Cushing, a biography. Springfield (IL): Charles C.Thomas; 1946.
16. Chauveau JBA, Marey EJ. Determination graphique des rapports de la pulsation cardiaque avec les mouvements do l'oreillette et du ventricule, obtenuse au moyen d'un appareil enregisteur. Cr Soc Biol (Paris) 1861;13:3–11.
17. Chauveau JBA, Marey EJ. Appareils et experiences cardiographiques: demonstration nouvelle du mecanisme des mouvements deu coeur par l'emploi des instruments enregistreurs a indications continues. Mem Acad Med 1863;26: 268–319.
18. Buzzi A. Claude Bernard on cardiac catheterization. Am J Cardiol 1959;4:405–9.
19. Bleichroder F, Unger E, Loeb W. Intra-arterielle therapie. Berlin Clin Woch 1912; 49:1503–5.
20. Forssmann W. The catheterization of the right side of the heart. Klin Wochenschr 1929;8(2085):2087.
21. Forssmann-Falck R. Werner Forssmann: a pioneer of cardiology. Am J Cardiol 1997;79(5):651–60.
22. Franch RH. Andre F. Cournand: father of clinical cardiopulmonary physiology. Clin Cardiol 1986;9(2):82–6.
23. Cournand A, Ranges HA. Catheterization of the right auricle in man. Proc Soc Exp Biol Med 1941;46:462–6.

24. Cournand A, Riley RL, Bradley SE, et al. Studies of the circulation in clinical shock. Surgery 1943;13:964–95.
25. Cournand A, Baldwin JS, Himmelstein A. A cardiac catheterization in congenital heart disease. New York: The Commonwealth Fund; 1949.
26. Bourassa MG. The history of cardiac catheterization. Can J Cardiol 2005;21(12): 1011–4.
27. Fick A. Uber die Messung des Blutquantums in den Heerzventrikeln. Sitz der Physik-Med ges Wurzburg 1870 [German].
28. Grishman A, Master AM. Cardiac output in coronary occlusion studied by the Wezler-Boeger physical method. Proc Soc Exp Biol Med 1941;48:207.
29. Starr I, Wood FC. Studies with ballistocardiograph in acut cardiac infarction and chronic angina pectoris. Am Heart J 1943;25:81.
30. Stewart GN. Researches on the circulation time and on the influences which affect it: IV, the output of the heart. J Physiol 1897;22:159–83.
31. Moore JW, Kinsman JM, Hamilton WE. Studies on the circulation. II Cardiac output determinations; comparison of the injection method with the direct Fick procedure. Am J Phys 1929;89:331–9.
32. Gilbert RP, Aldrich SL, Anderson L. Cardiac output in acute myocardial infarction. J Clin Invest 1951;30:640.
33. Freis ED, Schnaper HW, Johnson RL, et al. Hemodynamic alterations in acute myocardial infarction. J Clin Invest 1951;31:131.
34. Gilbert RP, Honig KP, Adelson BH, et al. The hemodynamics of shock due to infection. J Lab Clin Med 1954;44:801–14.
35. Dotter CT, Lukas DS. Acute cor pulmonale. An experimental study utilizing a special cardiac catheter. Am J Phys 1953;164:254–62.
36. Geddes LA, Geddes LE. The catheter introducers. Chicago: Mobium Press; 1993.
37. Lategola M, Rahn H. A self-guiding catheter for cardiac and pulmonary arterial catheterization and occlusion. Proc Soc Exp Biol Med 1953;84:667–8.
38. Bradley RD. Diagnostic right heart catheterization with miniature catheters in severely ill patients. Lancet 1964;67:941–2.
39. Fegler G. Measurement of cardiac output in anesthetized animals by thermo-dilution method. J Exp Physiol 1954;39:153–63.
40. Branthwaite MA, Bradley RD. Measurement of cardiac ouput by thermal dilution in man. J Appl Phys 1968;24:434–8.
41. Rosengart MR. Critical care medicine: landmarks and legends. Surg Clin North Am 2006;86(6):1305–21.
42. Swan HJ, Ganz W, Forrester J, et al. Catheterization of the heart in man with use of a flow-directed balloon-tipped catheter. N Engl J Med 1970;283(9):447–51.
43. Ganz W, Donoso R, Marcus HS, et al. A new technique for measurement of cardiac output by thermodilution in man. Am J Cardiol 1971;27(4):392–6.
44. Palmieri TL. The inventors of the Swan-Ganz catheter: H.J.C. Swan and William Ganz. Curr Surg 2003;60(3):351–2.
45. Jordan F. Shock after surgical operations and injuries. Br Med J 1867;1:136–9.
46. Warren JC. Surgical pathology and therapeutics. Philadelphia: Saunders; 1895.
47. Gross SD. System of surgery: pathological, diagnostic, therapeutique, and operative, vol 1. 2nd edition. Philadelphia: Blanchard and Lea; 1862.
48. Surgeon General's Office. Medical and surgical history of the war of the rebellion, 3rd surgical volume. Washington: 1883.
49. Blalock A. Acute circulatory failure as exemplified by shock and hemorrhage. Surg Gynecol Obstet 1934;58:551–66.

50. Wiggers CJ. The physiology of shock. Cambridge (MA): Harvard University Press; 1950.
51. Simeone FA. Some issues in problems of shock. Fed Proc 1961;20:3.
52. Kumar A, Parrillo JE. Shock: pathophysiology, classification and approach to management. In: Parrillo JE, Dellinger RP, editors. Critical care medicine: principles of diagnosis and management in the adult. St. Louis (MO): Mosby Publications; 2001. p. 371–420.
53. Baue AE. Physiology of shock and injury. In: Geller ER, editor. Shock and resuscitation. New York: McGraw-Hill Inc.; 1993. p. 67–125.
54. Laennec RTH. Traite de l'uscultation mediate et des maladies des poumons et du coeur. Paris: J.S. Chaude; 1831.
55. Boise E. The differential diagnosis of shock, hemorrhage, and sepsis. Trans Am Assoc Obstet 1897;9:433–8.
56. Fishberg AM, Hitzig WM, King FH. Circulatory dynamics in myocardial infarction. Arch Intern Med 1934;54:997–1019.
57. Chambers NK, Buchman TG, Chambers NK, et al. Shock at the millennium. I. Walter B. Cannon and Alfred Blalock. Shock 2000;13(6):497–504.
58. Blalock A. Shock: further studies with particular reference to the effects of hemorrhage. Arch Surg 1937;29:837–57.
59. Blalock A. Reminiscence: shock after thirty-four years. Rev Surg 1964;21:231–4.
60. Weil MH. Bacterial shock. In: Weil MH, Shubin H, editors. Diagnosis and treatment of shock. Baltimore (MD): Williams and Wilkin Co.; 1967. p. 10.
61. Weil MH. Proposed reclassification of shock states with special reference to distributive defects. Adv Exp Med Biol 1971;23:13–24.
62. Hinshaw LB, Cox BG. The fundamental mechanisms of shock. New York: Plenum Press; 1972.
63. Munford JG. A few hints of the treatment of collapse. Boston Medical and Surgical Journal 1891;125:11–2.
64. Hunter JA. A treatise on the blood, inflammation, and gunshot wounds. Philadelphia: 1817.
65. Cooper A. The principles and practice of surgery. Philadelphia: 1928.
66. Guthrie GJ. A treatise on gunshot wounds, on inflammation, erysipelas, and mortification. London: 1827.
67. Gibson W. The institutes and practice of surgery. Philadelphia: 1824.
68. Ohmsted JMD, Charles Edouard Brown-Sequard. A ninteenth century neurologist and endocrinologist. Baltimore (MD): 1952.
69. Goltz FL. Über reflexionen von and zum Herzwn. Königsberger Medicinische Jahrbucher 1861;3:271–4.
70. Goltz FR. Ueber den Tonus der Gerfaesse und seine Bedeutung fuer die Blutbewegung. Arch F Path Anat U Physiol 1864;29:394–417.
71. Fischer H. Ueber den Shock. Samml klin Vortr, No 10 1870.
72. Mitchell SW, Morehouse GR, Keen WW. Gunshot wounds and other injury of nerves. Philadelphia: 1864.
73. Meltzer SJ. An experimental study of the cause of shock. Proc Soc Exp Biol Med 1903;1:32.
74. Meltzer SJ. The nature of shock. Arch Intern Med 1908;1:571–88.
75. Wiggers CJ. The present status of the shock problem. Physiol Rev 1942;22:74.
76. Paget J. Address in surgery. Thirtieth Annual Meeting of the British Medical Association. Br Med J 1862;2157–8.
77. Crile GW. Hemorrhage and transfusion. Wis Med J 1907;6:191–201.

78. Janeway HH, Ewing EM. The nature of shock. Its relation to acapnia and to changes in the circulation and to exhaustion of the nerve centers. Ann Surg 1914;59:158–75.
79. Seelig MG, Lyon EP. Further experimental data on the vasomotor relations of shock. Surg Gynecol Obstet 1910;11:146–52.
80. Weil MH, MacLean LD, Spink WW, et al. Investigations on the role of the central nervous system in shock produced by endotoxin from gram negative bacteria. J Lab Clin Med 1956;48:661–72.
81. MacKenzie IM. The haemodynamics of human septic shock. Anaesthesia 2001; 56(2):130–44.
82. Latta TA. Relative to the treatment of cholera by the copious injection of aqueous and saline fluids into the veins. Lancet ii (1832). p. 274–7.
83. Landerer A. Ueber transfusion und infusion. Virchow's Archiv 1886;105:351–72.
84. Bischoff JJ. Ein gunstig verlaufner Fall von intraarteriellen Infusion einer alkalischen Kochsalzosung bie drohenden Verblutingstode. Arch Gynakol 1881;23: 545–7.
85. Horrocks P. Intravenous injection of saline solution in cases of severe hemorrhage. Lancet 1893;ii:1390–1.
86. Robertson OH, Bock AV. The use of forced fluids by the alimentary tract in the restoration of blood volume after hemorrhage. J Exp Med 1919;29:155–66.
87. Henderson Y, Barringer TB, Harvey SC. The regulation of venous pressure and its relation to shock. Am J Phys 1908;23:30–1.
88. Keith NM, Rowntree LG, Geraghty JT. A method for the determination of the plasma and blood volume. Arch Intern Med 1915;16:547–76.
89. Keith NM. Blood volume changes in wound shock and primary hemorrhage. [Special report Series No. 27]. London: Medical Research Council; 1919.
90. Robertson OH, Bock AV. Blood volume in wounded soldiers. J Exp Med 1919;29: 139–54.
91. Wiggers CJ. Circulatory failure. The differentiation between that due to shock and that due to other causes. JAMA 1918;70:508–15.
92. Wiggers CJ. Experimental haemorrhage shock. Physiology of shock: The Commonwealth Fund. New York: Harvard University Press; 1950. p. 121–43.
93. Wiggers CJ, Ingraham RC, Dillie J. Hemorrhagic-hypotension shock in locally anesthetized dogs. Am J Phys 1945;143:126–33.
94. Crile GW. The prevention of shock and hemorrhage in surgical practice. JAMA 1905;44:1925–7.
95. Porter WT. The effect of uniform afferent impulses upon the blood pressure at different levels. Am J Phys 1907;20:405–11.
96. Mann FC. The peripheral organs of surgical shock. Johns Hopkins Hospital Bulletin 1914;25:212.
97. Visscher MB. Frank Charles Mann (1887–1962). National Academy of Science Biographical Memories 1965;38:161–204.
98. Mann FC. Shock and hemorrhage. Surg Gynecol Obstet 1915;21:430–41.
99. Wallace C, Fraser J, Drummond H. The distribution of blood in traumatic shock. Lancet 1917;2:727.
100. Cannon W. A consideration of the nature of wound shock. MRC Special Report #25, 1919.
101. Cannon WB. Traumatic shock. New York: Appleton; 1923.
102. Anonymous. The Hippocratic corpus. In: Phillips ED, editor. Greek medicine. London: Thames and Hudson; 1973. p. 48–52.

103. Medical therapy: Benjamin Rush and his therapy. In: Bordley IJ, Harvey AM, editors. Two centuries of American medicine: 1776–1976. Philadelphia: WB Saunders; 1976. p. 37–8.

104. Mapother ED. Shock: its nature, duration, and mode of treatment. Br Med J 1879;2:1023–42.

105. Hunter AR. Old unhappy far off things. Some reflections on the significance of the early work on shock. Ann R Coll Surg Engl 1967;40(5):289–305.

106. Bayliss WM. Intravenous injection in wound shock. Longmans, Green; 1918.

107. Dale HH, Richards AN. The vasodilator action of histamine and of some other substances. J Physiol 1918;52:110–65.

108. Dale HH, Laidlaw PP. Histamine shock. J Physiol 1919;52:355–90.

109. Blalock A. Experimental shock: cause of low blood pressure produced by muscle injury. Arch Surg 1930;20:959–96.

110. Beecher HK, Simeone FA, Burnett CH, et al. The internal state of the severely wounded man on entry to the most forward hospital. Surgery 1947;22:672–711.

111. Lillehei RC, MacLean LD. The intestinal factor in irreversible endotoxin shock. Ann Surg 1958;148:513–9.

112. Lillehei RC, MacLean LD. The intestinal factor in irreversible hemorrhagic shock. Surgery 1958;42:1043–54.

113. Jacobs S, Weizel H, Gordon E, et al. Bacterial action in development of irreversibility to transfusion in hemorrhagic shock in the dog. Am J Phys 1954;179: 523–31.

114. Wiggers CJ. Myocardial depression in shock. A survey of cardiodynamic studies. Am Heart J 1947;33:633–50.

115. Lefer AM, Martin J. Origin of myocardial depressant factor in shock. Am J Phys 1970;218:1423–7.

116. Glenn TM, Lefer AM, Martin JB, et al. Production of a myocardial depressant factor in cardiogenic shock. Am Heart J 1971;82:78–85.

117. Brand ED, Lefer AM. Myocardial depressant factor in plasma from cats in irreversible post-oligemic shock. Proc Soc Exp Biol Med 1966;122:200–3.

118. Parrillo JE, Burch C, Shelhamer JH, et al. A circulating myocardial depressant substance in humans with septic shock. Septic shock patients with a reduced ejection fraction have a circulating factor that depresses in vitro myocardial cell performance. J Clin Invest 1985;76:1539–53.

119. Wood KE. Major pulmonary embolism: review of a pathophysiologic approach to the golden hour of hemodynamically significant pulmonary embolism. Chest 2002;121(3):877–905.

120. Boersma E, Maas AC, Deckers JW, et al. Early thrombolytic treatment in acute myocardial infarction: reappraisal of the golden hour. Lancet 1996;348(9030): 771–5.

121. Blow O, Magliore L, Claridge JA, et al. The golden hour and the silver day: detection and correction of occult hypoperfusion within 24 hours improves outcome from major trauma. Journal of Trauma-Injury Infection & Critical Care 1999;47(5):964–9.

122. Kumar A, Roberts D, Wood KE, et al. Duration of hypotension before initiation of effective antimicrobial therapy is the critical determinant of survival in human septic shock. Crit Care Med 2006;34(6):1589–96.

123. Rivers E, Nguyen B, Havstad S, et al. Early goal-directed therapy in the treatment of severe sepsis and septic shock. N Engl J Med 2001;345(19):1368–77.

124. Osler W. The principles and practice of medicine. New York: Appleton; 1892.

125. Jacob L. Uber allgemein Infecktion durch Bacterium col commune. Dtsch Arch Klin Med 1909;97:307.
126. Scully FJ. The reaction after the intravenous injection of foreign protein. JAMA 1917;69:20.
127. Chasis H, Goldring W, Smith HW. Reduction of blood pressure associated with the pyrogenic reaction in hypersensitive subjects. J Clin Invest 1942;21:369.
128. Page IH, Taylor RD. Pyrogens in the treatment of malignant hypertension. Mod Concepts Cardiovasc Dis 1949;18(10):51.
129. Waisbren BA. Bacteremia due to gram-negative bacilli other than the Salmonella; a clinical and therapeutic study. Arch Intern Med 1951;88:467–88.
130. Janeway TC. Some common misconceptions in the pathological physiology of the circulation and their practical significance. New York Medical Journal 1907;85:193–7.
131. Atchley DM. Medical shock. JAMA 1930;95:385–9.
132. Stead EA, Ebert RV. The peripheral circulation in acute infectious diseases. Med Clin North Am 1940;24:1387–94.
133. Eppinger H, Schurmeyer A. Uber den Kollaps und analoge zustande. Klin Wochenschr 1928;7:777–85.
134. Warfield LM. Treatment of circulatory failure. Ann Intern Med 1934;7:981–90.
135. Moon VH. The shock syndrome in medicine and surgery. Ann Intern Med 1935; 8:1633–48.
136. Warren HD, Balboni VG, Rogliano FT, et al. Shock in acute infections. N Engl J Med 1945;232:671–7.
137. Clowes GHA, Vucinic M, Weidner MG. Circulatory and metabolic alterations associated with survival or death in peritonitis. Ann Surg 1966;163:866–85.
138. Nishijima H, Weil MH, Shubin H, et al. Hemodynamic and metabolic studies on shock associated with gram-negative bacteremia. Medicine (Baltimore) 1973; 52:287–94.
139. Kumar A, Haery C, Parrillo JE. Myocardial dysfunction in septic shock: part I. Clinical manifestation of cardiovascular dysfunction. J Cardiothorac Vasc Anesth 2001;15(3):364–76.
140. Clowes GHA, Farrington GH, Zuschneid W, et al. Circulating factors in the etiology of pulmonary insufficiency and right heart failure accompanying severe sepsis. Ann Surg 1970;171:663–78.
141. Kwaan HM, Weil MH. Differences in the mechanism of shock caused by bacterial infections. Surg Gynecol Obstet 1969;128:37–45.
142. Weil MH, Nishijima H. Cardiac output in bacterial shock. Am J Med 1978;64: 920–2.
143. Weil MH, MacLean LD, Visscher MD, et al. Studies on the circulatory changes in the dog produced by endotoxin from gram-negative microorganisms. J Clin Invest 1956;35:1191–8.
144. Solis RT, Downing SE. Effects of E. coli endotoxemia on ventricular performance. Am J Phys 1966;211:307–13.
145. Postel J, Schloerb PR. Cardiac depression in bacteremia. Ann Surg 1977;186: 74–82.
146. Hinshaw LB. Myocardial function in endotoxin shock. Circ Shock 1979;1(Suppl): 43–51.
147. Lefer AM. Mechanisms of cardiodepression in endotoxin shock. Circ Shock 1979;1(Suppl):1–8.
148. MacLean LD, Mulligan WG, McLean APH, et al. Patterns of septic shock in man: a detailed study of 56 patients. Ann Surg 1967;166:543–62.

149. Blain CM, Anderson TO, Pietras RJ, et al. Immediate hemodynamic effects of gram-negative vs gram-positive bacteremia in man. Arch Intern Med 1970; 126:260–5.
150. Wilson RF, Thal AP, Kindling PH, et al. Hemodynamic measurements in septic shock. Arch Surg 1965;91:121–9.
151. Grollman A. Cardiac output of man in health and disease. Baltimore (MD): Charles C. Thomas; 1932.
152. Heberden W. Some account of a disorder of the breast. Med Trans Coll Physns London 1772;2:59–67.
153. Weigert C. Ueber die pathologiische Gerinnugs-Vorgange. Virchows Arch Pathol Anat Physiol Klin Med 1880;79:87–123.
154. Samuelson B. Ueber den einfluss der coronar-arterien-verschliessung auf die herzaction. Zeit Klin Med 1881;2:12.
155. Dock G. Notes on the coronary arteries. Ann Arbor (MI): Inland Press; 1896.
156. Obrastzow WP, Straschesko ND. Zur Kenntis der Thrombose der Koronararterien des Herzens. Zeitschr fur Lin Med 1910;71:116–32.
157. Herrick JB. Certain popular but erroneous notions concerning angina pectoris. JAMA 1910;55:1424–7.
158. Braunwald E. The Simon Dack lecture. Cardiology: the past, the present, and the future. J Am Coll Cardiol 2003;42(12):2031–41.
159. Wearn JT. Thrombosis of the coronary arteries with infarction of the heart. Am J Med Sci 1923;165:250–76.
160. Braunwald E. Cardiology: how did we get here, where are we today and where are we going? Can J Cardiol 2005;21(12):1015–7.
161. Beck CS, Pritchard WH, Feil HS. Ventricular fibrillation of long duration abolished by electric shock. JAMA 1947;135:985–6.
162. Beck CF, Weckesser EC, Barry FM. Fatal heart attack and successful defibrillation: new concepts in coronary heart disease. JAMA 1956;161:434–6.
163. Day HW. History of coronary care units. Am J Cardiol 1972;30(4):405–7.
164. Zoll PM, Linenthal AJ, Gibson W, et al. Termination of ventricular fibrillation in man by externally applied electric countershock. N Engl J Med 1956;254(16): 727–32.
165. Kouwenhoven WB, Jude JR, Knickerbocker GG. Closed-chest cardiac massage. JAMA 1960;173:1064–7.
166. Khush KK, Rapaport E, Waters D. The history of the coronary care unit. Can J Cardiol 2005;21(12):1041–5.
167. Harrison TR. Failure of the circulation. Baltimore (MD): Williams and Wilkins; 1939.
168. Wiggers CJ. The functional consequences of coronary occlusion. Ann Intern Med 1945;23:158.
169. Agress CM, Rosenberg MJ, Jacobs HI, et al. Protracted shock in the closed-chest dog following coronary embolization with graded microspheres. Am J Phys 1952;170:536.
170. Malach M, Rosenberg BA. Acute myocardial infarction in a city hospital. III. Experience with shock. Am J Cardiol 1960;5:487–92.
171. Walston A, Hackel DB, Estes EH. Acute coronary occlusion and the "power failure" syndrome. Am Heart J 1970;79(5):613–9.
172. Page DL, Caulfield JB, Kastor JA. Myocardial changes associated with cardiogenic shock. N Engl J Med 1971;285:133–7.
173. McQuay NW, Edwards JE, Burchell HB. Types of death in acute myocardial infarction. AMA Arch Intern Med 1955;96(1):1–10.

174. Rosenberg BA, Malach M. Acute myocardial infarction in a city hospital. IV. Clinical-pathologic correlations. Am J Cardiol 1960;6:272–80.

175. Harnarayan C, Bennett MA, Pentecost BL, et al. Quantitative study of infarcted myocardium in cardiogenic shock. Br Heart J 1970;32(6):728–32.

176. Weisse AB. The elusive clot: the controversy over coronary thrombosis in myocardial infarction. J Hist Med Allied Sci 2006;61(1):66–78.

177. Kurland GS, Weingarten C, Pitt B. The relation between the location of coronary occlusions and the occurrence of shock in acute myocardial infarction. Circulation 1965;31:646.

178. Feola M, Glick G. Experimental modesl of cardiogenic shock. In: Gunnar RM, Loeb HS, Rahimtoola SH, editors. Shock in myocardial infarction. New York: Grune and Stratton, Inc.; 1974. p. 23–47.

179. Sones FM Jr. Selective cine coronary arteriography in the diagnosis and evaluation of medical and surgical treatment of coronary atherosclerosis. Nippon Igaku Hoshasen Gakkai Zasshi 1968;28(6):714–9.

180. Kuhn LA. The treatment of cardiogenic shock. II. The use of pressor agents in the treatment of cardiogenic shock. Am Heart J 1967;74(5):725–8.

181. Kuhn LA. The treatment of cardiogenic shock. I. The nature of cardiogenic shock. Am Heart J 1967;74(4):578–81.

182. Loeb HS, Gunnar RM, Rahimtoola SH. Shock in myocardial infarction. New York: Grune & Stratton; 1974.

183. Fletcher AP, Alkjaersig N, Smyrniotis FE, et al. The treatment of patients suffering from early myocardial infarction with massive and prolonged streptokinase therapy. Trans Assoc Am Physicians 1958;71:287–96.

184. Verstraete M. Thrombolytic therapy in recent myocardial infarction. Texbook of coronary care. Amsterdam (The Netherlands): Excerpta Medica; 1972. p. 643–59.

185. Gruppo Italiano per lo Studio della Streptochinasi nell'Infarto Miocardico (GISSI). Effectiveness of intravenous thrombolytic treatment in acute myocardial infarction. Lancet 1986;1(8478):397–402.

186. Randomized trial of intravenous streptokinase, oral aspirin, both, or neither among 17,187 cases of suspected acute myocardial infarction: ISIS-2.ISIS-2 (Second International Study of Infarct Survival) Collaborative Group. J Am Coll Cardiol 1988;12(6 Suppl A):3A–13A.

187. Kantrowitz A, Tjonneland S, Freed PS. Initial clinical experience with intraaortic balloon pumping in cardiogenic shock. JAMA 1968;203:113–8.

188. DeWood MA, Spores J, Berg R Jr, et al. Acute myocardial infarction: a decade of experience with surgical reperfusion in 701 patients. Circulation 1983;68(3 Pt 2): II8–16.

Battlefield Trauma, Traumatic Shock and Consequences: War-Related Advances in Critical Care

Carrie E. Allison, MD*, Donald D. Trunkey, MD, FACS

KEYWORDS

- Trauma • Shock • History • Battlefield • Wound care • War

Over the course of history, while the underlying causes for wars have remained few, mechanisms of inflicting injury and our ability to treat the consequent wounds have dramatically changed. Success rates in treating war-related injuries have improved greatly, although the course of progress has not proceeded linearly. Homer's *Iliad* records the wounds of 147 soldiers with an overall mortality rate of 77.1%.[1] During the Civil War, 14% of soldiers died from their injuries, and that number was down to less than 4% in Vietnam.[2] These significant improvements in mortality, despite a concurrent increase in the lethality of weapons, have occurred primarily as a result of progress in three key areas: management of wounds, treatment of shock, and systems of organization.

WOUND CARE

The anthropologic record illustrates that care of traumatic wounds predated written history. Skulls uncovered in the Tigress-Euphrates Valley, the shores of the Mediterranean, and in meso-America show that trepanation was used to treat skull fractures and possibly epidural hematomas as far back as 10,000 BC.[1] Healing of man-made holes in these specimens suggests that the procedure was performed with some degree of success.[3] Fractures and dislocations were treated with knitting of bones.

The oldest written history referring to surgical treatment of traumatic wounds appeared in 1700 BC in the 282 Laws of King Hammurabi's Code.[4] Written by the Akkadians, the code outlined reimbursement to surgeons for success and punishment for failure. "If a physician make a large incision with an operating knife and cure it, or if

Department of Surgery, Oregon Health & Science University, 3181 SW Sam Jackson Park Road, L223, Portland, OR 97239, USA
* Corresponding author.
E-mail address: hinkc@ohsu.edu (C.E. Allison).

Crit Care Clin 25 (2009) 31–45
doi:10.1016/j.ccc.2008.10.001
0749-0704/08/$ – see front matter © 2009 Elsevier Inc. All rights reserved.

criticalcare.theclinics.com

he open a tumor (over the eye) with an operating knife, and saves the eye, he shall receive ten shekels in money. If a physician make a large incision with the operating knife, and kill him, or open a tumor with the operating knife, and cut out the eye, his hands shall be cut off." There was essentially no understanding of anatomic or physiologic relationships in these times.

Though otherwise extremely diverse, most ancient cultures shared in common the use of poultices to treat wounds and infections using a combination of plant extracts, resins, and spices. While many of these were later found to be active against Staphylococcus and E coli, they were probably chosen primarily for their ability to make the wounds less malodorous.[1] Three ancient medical texts, the Kahun, (1825 BC), Ebers (1550 BC), and Smith Papyri (1600 BC), commonly accepted as the oldest extant medical texts, describe in detail the treatment of wounds. The latter describes 48 surgical cases and includes the use of poultices containing fats and oils, fresh meat, leaves of willow (containing small amounts of aspirin), honey, and "green-pigment" (a copper-containing toxic bactericidal), as well as incantations against pestilence.[5] Abscesses were treated by use of a "fire-drill," a heated metal object that probably provided cautery in addition to draining pus.[1]

A millennium later in Greece, Homer's description of wounds and their treatment in the Iliad and Odyssey (800 BC) showed relatively little change from Egyptian techniques. Homer recorded 147 wounds,[6] mostly treated by human beings, although a few were described as miraculously healed by the gods. Odysseus, when injured, was treated with a bandage and an incantation to stop his bleeding. It is interesting that while the use of cautery is described during Homer's time, the use of such an epaoide (song or charm recited over the wound) for hemostasis was equally as common.[1] The use of tourniquets was condemned as they were believed to make bleeding worse.

Penetrating trauma caused by arrows, swords, maces, and animal bites were well described in Greek literature. Homer details the removal of an arrow from the thigh of Eurypylus by his comrade Patroclus[6] in the Iliad, which was followed by rinsing the wound with warm water, application of an analgesic, and an herbal styptic (contracting agent). Solutions of warm wine and vinegar were commonly used for irrigation and antisepsis. As observed in earlier cultures, Homer also describes blunt injuries treated with reduction of dislocations and setting of fractures.

The era of 450 BC onward in Greece, known as the "Golden Age of Pericles," was a time of great expansion and documentation of medical knowledge. Hippocrates trained in the tradition of the Asclepiea, with knowledge passed down over nearly a millennium.[6] His 72-volume work of medical dicta, later entitled the Corpus Hippocratum, was unprecedented for its scope and volume. Hippocrates outlined the treatment for several types of injuries, including the setting of fractures, draining of abscesses, and trepanning head injuries. In On Head Wounds, Hippocrates described how an injury on one side of the head produced a contralateral deficit, that a brain injury could be localized by questioning of the patient, and that trepanation should occur within 3 days to prevent suppuration.[6] Debridement of bone fragments before setting fractures and tourniquet necrosis to induce autoamputation of severe extremity wounds was suggested. Several of the techniques described, such as mechanisms for reducing dislocations, continue to be used to this day.

However, not all Hippocratic dicta led to the advancement of medical science. While soft tissue abscess drainage and tube thoracostomy for empyema are described,[7] this era also marked the beginning of the theory of "laudable pus," in which suppuration was believed to be required for some types of healing. Pus formation was encouraged by placing items, such as greased wool, into the wound. Paradoxically, it was also understood that some wounds would heal better without suppuration, and antiseptic substances, such as white vinegar, honey, copper oxide, sodium carbonate, and alum were applied to the wound to prevent pus formation.[1] In *On Treating Injuries*, Hippocrates explains, "If the wound is caused by a cut or impact of a sharp weapon, some means is needed to quickly stop the bleeding, as well as preventing pus formation and drying up the wound. If the wound is lacerated or mutilated by the weapon, it must be treated in a way such that makes pus form as quickly as possible."[7] Bloodletting was also encouraged during this time for the treatment of certain types of ailments, including, ironically, bleeding.

Also notable during the time of Hippocrates was the development "humorist" theory of disease, which explained all afflictions as an imbalance of the four humors—yellow bile, black bile, phlegm, and blood—as well as different states (hot and cold, wet and dry, and so forth). For example, it was noted that wounds that contained too much "wet element" would become inflamed and heal poorly. The humorist theory would persist for 2,000 years afterward.

Celsus, born 460 AD in Rome, studied Hippocratic theory and further expanded upon it. In his *De Medicina* Celsus described the four cardinal signs of inflammation—rubor, calor, dolor, and tumor[1]—although this was probably copied either from Greek or Egyptian writings. He also described factors related to the patient, environment, and the wound factors that favored healing.[8] Wound exploration was advocated for treatment of penetrating trauma (**Fig. 1**). While amputation for gangrene was well described by Hippocrates,[9] it was more frequently used in Rome, likely because of improvements in both analgesia and hemostasis. Opium was the primary analgesic agent, although it certainly was not its first use: descriptions and evidence of it appear millennia earlier in China.[7] Celsus' opinion on hemostasis, however, was pioneering. In contrast to the Greeks, Celsus advocated staunching hemorrhage by applying pressure to the wound with lint and ligating blood vessels: "the veins that are pouring out blood are to be seized, and around the wounded spot, they are to be tied in two places."[8]

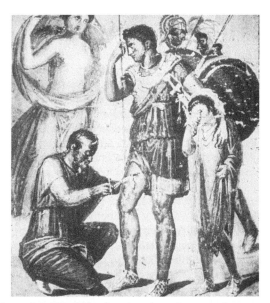

Fig.1. Roman soldier undergoing wound exploration of penetrating wound. (*From* Majno G. The Healing Hand: Man and Wound in the Ancient World. Cambridge, MA: Harvard University Press, 1975.)

Galen,[1] a prolific writer and physician born in 130 AD, treated both gladiators and Roman Emperor Marcus Aurelius. Galen's work using dissection and vivisection to delineate anatomic relationships, such as identifying the nerves responsible for producing the squeal in pigs, was unprecedented. However, Galen was limited by the Roman law against human cadaveric dissection, and consequently may have made several key mistakes in translating the anatomic systems of animals to human beings. Nonetheless, his writings became doctrine for 1,500 years afterward.

Little progress occurred in Western surgical therapy between Roman times and the Renaissance, primarily as a result of a series of ecclesiastic dicta. The Council of Clermont in 1150[7] ruled that priests and monks should no longer practice medicine, in attempt to preserve the monastic lifestyle. Further stunting progress, two doctrines of "Ecclesia Abhorret a Sanguine" ("The Church Abhors Bloodshed") were issued in 1163 and 1215, banning the practice of surgery. While most surgical practice during these years was relegated to practice by quacks and wandering charlatans, parts of the Greek tradition were preserved by Nestorius,[1] who was excommunicated in 431 AD for heresy after refusing to accept the Holy Trinity and the edicts of the Council of Nicaea. He fled to Egypt, where several of his books were burned. His followers ultimately found asylum at Jundi Shapur University in Persia, where his surviving books were translated into Arabic. Eventually, these works were reintroduced into Spain by the Moors via Mecca, Alexandria, and North Africa. Also of note during this era is the work of the Arab physician Rhazes, who described abdominal operations and the use of catgut sutures during the ninth century.[10]

Throughout the Middle Ages, the theory of laudable pus persisted. It was challenged unsuccessfully by Theoderic of Italy in 1267. Henri de Mondeville of France, a student of Theoderic's work, published the surgical textbook *Churugie* in 1320, further supporting the Theoderic concepts, arguing that wounds should have foreign objects removed and then be dressed with clean bandages soaked in warm wine.[11] However, laudable pus was reintroduced only decades later by Mondeville's successor, Guy de Chauliac. Although in this manner de Chauliac regressed the progress of wound care, his *Grande Chirurgie* (Great Surgery), written in 1363, advanced several other concepts, including methods of hemostasis. Listed as possibilities were wound closure, tamponade, vein compression, ligature of an artery, and cauterization,[11] all methods still in use today.

As Europe emerged from the Dark Ages into the Renaissance, two surgeon contemporaries brought dramatic changes to the practice of surgery: Andreas Vesalius and Ambroise Paré. Vesalius, a Belgian anatomist, was a master dissector. In his studies, he found several errors in Galenic anatomy, correcting 200 misconceptions caused by Galen's use of animal rather than human subjects in all, such as the vena cava originating in the liver.[12] His published *Fabrica* was an exhaustive and accurate depiction of human anatomy. More importantly, however, he was perhaps the first to credibly challenge the Galenic dogma that had reigned for 1,300 years.

A second dogmatic theory challenged by Paré was the treatment of patients with gunshot wounds. At the time, it was believed that gunpowder poisoned wounds, and thus they should be treated topically with hot oils. While treating soldiers at the siege of Turin,[10] he noticed that patients treated with a "healing salve" fared much better than those treated by standard methods, and vowed never to inflict such painful treatment again. Paré espoused the virtues of gentle tissue handling and invented several surgical instruments, such as the bec de corbin (crow's beak), the precursor to the modern-day hemostat.[12] Vesalius and Paré once together attended to Henri II of France, who was wounded by a lance blow to the eye in a tournament joust match. Although they were able to correctly discern the extent of his injury, they were unable to save the king, who died 11 days later of an infected subdural hemorrhage.[13]

The nineteenth century brought important change to surgical combat care with two key discoveries, that combined, reduced trauma mortality dramatically: anesthesia and antisepsis. In 1842, Crawford Long introduced ether as a viable anesthetic,[14] confirmed by William Morton in 1846. The following year, James Simpson demonstrated chloroform to be effective.[15] Lack of adequate anesthesia combined with the high mortality rate from infection were the primary limitations for performing advanced surgical procedures, such as abdominal exploration before this era, combined with the high mortality rate from infection. It also limited the ability to humanely perform operations such as amputations. Anesthesia was first used in a military conflict during the Mexican-American War.[16] Edward Barton used chloroform to perform several amputations, with good success. However, it was not well accepted by all. John Porter,[16] an Army surgeon, declared anesthetics to be "universally injurious," and their use was banned. By the American Civil War, anesthetics were back in favor and were used extensively by both the Union and the Confederacy.

Concurrent with the development of anesthetics was the emergence of an equally significant concept—germ theory. Just before its development during the Civil War, the concept of laudable pus still reigned. Wound sepsis was believed to be secondary to "contagions and miasmas" carried in the air. Ventilation was stressed for prevention of infection. Hospital gangrene was rampant.[2] Oral sesqichloride of iron and quinine were given to treat gangrene, and topical agents were used with varying success.[1] Three studies by Union surgeons using bromine, before the work of Joseph Lister, demonstrated that wound sepsis mortality could be reduced from 43.3% to 2.6%.[17,18] Despite the high mortality associated with wounds, more soldiers on both sides died from medical illness rather than wounds as a result of poor sanitary conditions. During the Crimean War,[10] 18,000 of 25,000 soldiers died from cholera, dysentery, or scurvy, prompting the formation of the British Sanitary Commission. Its work, along with the emphasis on sanitation and hygiene by Florence Nightingale and her staff, dramatically reduced mortality from medical illness and set new standards for military hospitals.[19]

Lister,[20] a British Surgeon, questioned the theory of air contamination, postulating that infection instead came through breaks in the skin. His theory gained strength with the results of experiments by Louis Pasteur, demonstrating that fermentation occurs via gas production by small microbes. Lister incorporated Pasteur's findings into his "germ theory," postulating that similar microbes were responsible for infecting wounds. Lister experimented with carbolic acid-soaked dressings with a subsequently dramatic decrease in the incidence of wound sepsis. He would later apply these techniques to wounded soldiers in the Franco-Prussian war with similar results.[21] In 1877 Lister introduced antisepsis to surgery, demonstrating that the once highly mortal open patella repair could be performed with minimal mortality.[21] The combination of the introduction of anesthesia and antiseptic techniques set the stage in the ensuing military conflicts for the development of exploratory abdominal surgery.

Prior to these developments, penetrating abdominal trauma was almost uniformly fatal. During the war of 1812, musket wounds were treated with "simple dressings, warm cataplasms, bleeding, enemas, slight antiphlegistic treatments, cooling diluent drinks."[22] In 1843 Samuel Gross performed experiments on animals treating eviscerated bowel with surgery, and consequently advocated surgical exploration of penetrating abdominal wounds.[23] However, he did not practice this 20 years later during the Civil War. Between 1881 and 1888[2] reports arose of soldiers treated for gunshot wounds to the abdomen, but the results were poor. Wounds were treated with local debridement and were probed directly with fingers or instruments to determine the course of the missile, frequently causing more harm than good. When President

Garfield was shot by Charles Julius Guiteau in 1881,[24] his wound was probed several times by numerous physicians over the course of 2.5 months, ultimately resulting in his slow and painful death following overwhelming systemic sepsis. The introduction of X-rays by Roentgen in 1895[25] obviated the need for wound probing.

Before World War I, laparotomy for penetrating abdominal trauma was reported but associated with high mortality in all but a few exceptions. In the Boer War (1899–1902), a 69% mortality was reported of those who underwent laparotomy, further supporting the continuation of nonoperative management. While the first report of civilian surgeons treating soldiers with gunshot wounds of the abdomen appeared in 1889,[26] the first successful use of therapeutic laparotomy was reported by Russian surgeon and princess Vera Gedroitz during the Russo-Japanese War.[10,27] Her success was attributed in part to her insistence upon operating only on patients injured within 3 hours. Surgeons in World War I also recognized the importance of early operation and observed an associated improvement in mortality. By 1915, laparotomy became the standard of care. In World War II, Major General Ogilvie issued a directive[28] that all patients with penetrating colon injuries must undergo colostomy placement. While this tenet clearly had basis in wartime conditions of constrained time and resources, it persisted in civilian treatment after the war, going unquestioned and untested until recent decades. Modern studies have indicated that most civilian penetrating colon injuries can be treated equally successfully with primary closure,[29] without the associated morbidity of a colostomy. However, in the military setting, with the need for rapid treatment and evacuation, the argument for colostomy may still hold true.[30]

The treatment of contaminated wounds also improved during the World Wars. In 1917, the Inter-Allied Surgical Conference decreed that contaminated wounds should be treated in open fashion.[17] Debridement and delayed primary closure was recommended for large soft tissue defects. These lessons were largely forgotten and had to be relearned in World War II. Major General Kirk issued a directive regarding the treatment of lower extremity injuries, stating that all amputations should be performed in guillotine fashion rather than primarily closed.[1]

In 1928, Fleming discovered penicillin. At the start of World War II, sulfa drugs were available, and by 1945 enough penicillin was available for every Allied soldier.[21] Death from wound sepsis became very uncommon, and mortality associated with penetrating abdominal injury decreased to 9% by the Vietnam conflict.[2] The cause of mortality shifted to late complications, such as multiorgan failure.

Other advances in wound care that have improved outcomes in recent conflicts include the advent of vascular injury repair, decreasing the rate of amputations in Korea,[1] the availability of topical antibiotics for burn care in Vietnam,[10] and the use of negative pressure wound therapy in Iraq and Afghanistan for treatment of large soft-tissue defects (**Fig. 2**).

SHOCK

Until recent history, the concept of shock was poorly understood. Very little description of or reference to shock occurs in the ancient or medieval texts. It was clear from the Smith Papyrus that the Egyptians understood the heart to be the center of circulation, a concept that would be lost for millennia. However, the significance of this fact was not understood. The Romans, as referred to by Pliny in his *Historia Naturalis*, describe the use of "ma huang"[1] or ephedra, which suggests one of the earliest described uses of a vasoconstrictor to treat hemorrhage, as well as the sharing of medical knowledge between the East and West, possibly along the silk road, although the concept of shock per se was not discussed.

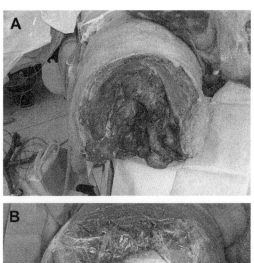

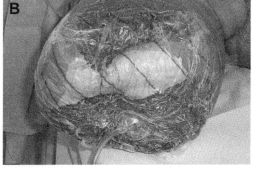

Fig. 2. Soft tissue defect following severe extremity blast injury before (*A*) and after (*B*) negative pressure wound therapy. Landstuhl Regional Medical Center, Landstuhl, Germany. (*Courtesy of* D.D. Trunkey, MD, Portland, OR.)

The works of Galen both furthered and regressed the understanding of the circulation and its role in shock. As mentioned previously, Galen's anatomic work was unprecedented; however, he may have made several key mistakes in translating the anatomic systems of animals to human beings. Much of his work was lost, though, making it uncertain exactly what Galen understood. While surgeon to the gladiators, he treated a number of severe chest wounds, noting that "they died faster if the wound reached into the left cavity. If the wound did not poke through, they could survive for up to 24 hours, and then they died of inflammation."[1] However, despite a thorough understanding of anatomic structures and relationships, he did not appear to understand the significance of the heart as related to the circulation.[31]

Further progress in the understanding and description of shock was not made until several centuries later. William Harvey, in 1628, published "De Motu Cordis,"[32] or "An Anatomic Exercise on the Motion of the Heart and Blood in Living Beings," a seminal work detailing the anatomic relationship between the heart and circulatory system. Harvey described the blood being pumped around the body in a "double circulation" involving the heart and lungs. This was in strong contrast to the Galenic theory that the arterial blood came from the heart while the venous blood came from the liver, and thus understandably met some initial resistance.

French surgeon Henri Francois Le Dran,[33] in 1731, was the first to question why soldiers died from their wounds. He described a "collapse of vital functions" that occurred before death. Later, in 1838, Cooper,[33] describing experiences from the Crimean war, noted that even in the absence of severe pain, serious injury, or a significant loss of blood, many soldiers still died of their wounds. Their death was attributed to shock, a mysterious entity, which was unrelated to hemorrhage. In 1850, Gross,[33] in reference to experiences in the Crimean War, further described shock as "the rude unhinging of the machinery of life."

During the American Civil War, shock was considered as being possibly related to hemorrhage. Surgeon General Joseph Barnes speculated,[34] "It is an open question whether a blow to the abdomen may produce death without an organic lesion. If pain is persistent and radiating from one spot, it may signify internal trouble and if collapse returns a few days after injury, it is supposed to mean internal hemorrhage. The collapse of bleeding, however, resembles syncope as distinguished from shock." His recommendation for the treatment of traumatic shock included "rest in bed, opium, and warm fomentations." At that time, shock was also considered to be related only to immediate trauma. Septic shock was first recognized as a separate entity during the Spanish-American War.[33] The Surgeon General observed that patients who suffered from gas gangrene would also ultimately develop shock. Also during this conflict, the use of crystalloid for shock resuscitation was first described.[33] A soldier who suffered a laceration of the common carotid artery and jugular vein with ensuing massive hemorrhage was given salt solution via enema and subcutaneous clysis. He lived for 16 hours before succumbing to his injuries.

The onset of mass casualties seen in World War I brought major developments in the understanding and treatment of shock. Autologous blood was used for the first time in a major military conflict, with good results. Oswald Robertson built the first donor transfusion service and proved that transfusion worked.[35] Preceding World War I, several theories described the potential physiologic mechanism of shock. This ranged from a paralysis or exhaustion of nerve force (S. Weir Mitchell), fat embolism (William T. Porter), to an imbalance of the excitatory and inhibitory state of the body, "favoring the development of the inhibitory side of all the functions of the body" (Samuel J. Meltzer).[36] "Wound shock" was considered separate from hemorrhage. However, it was observed that shock was associated with a drop in venous blood pressure coupled with an increase in hematocrit. This led observers to speculate that a "toxic factor",[33] arising from injured or dying tissues, led to increased vascular permeability and subsequent escape of the plasma into surrounding tissues. This resulted in a decrease in blood volume, not directly related to blood loss.

In 1930, this idea was "disproved" by Blalock[37] following a series of experiments in dogs. Blalock created severe crush injury to the legs of anesthetized dogs, and by measuring circumference before and after injury, calculated the volume of blood loss. He concluded that the volume of blood loss alone was sufficient to explain the decreased blood pressure, and thus the "toxic factor" did not exist. However, the "toxic factor" continued to be implicated as late as the Korean War, with the development of acute respiratory distress syndrome and multiorgan failure. In fact, modern literature continues to reference the possibility of a "shock toxin," although this concept currently is not widely accepted.

The landmark work of Harvard physiologist Walter B. Cannon, during World War I, into the understanding of shock[38] essentially laid the foundation for our modern concept of this state. In response to the massive numbers of casualties of the war, Cannon was asked by the National Research Council to form a council on shock. Though he never observed shock in a patient until his studies in Europe, after studying casualties for 3 months at Clearing Station 33, he accurately described,[1] "Wound shock occurs as a consequence of physical injury. It is characterized by a low venous pressure, a low or falling arterial pressure, a rapid, thready pulse, a diminished blood volume, a normal or increased erythrocyte count and hemoglobin percentage and peripheral blood nitrogen, a reduced blood alkali, a lowered metabolism, a subnormal temperature, a cold skin with moist sweat, a pallid or grayish or slightly cyanotic appearance, also by this, by shallow and rapid respiration, often by vomiting and restlessness, by anxiety, changing usually to mental dullness, and by lessened sensitivity." In 1923, he published his work *Traumatic Shock*, in which he correctly interpreted shock to be secondary to hemorrhage, recognized the phenomenon of autoregulation, and classified shock into three types: compensated, partially compensated, and uncompensated.

Also in World War I, the importance of maintaining warmth in patients with shock was recognized, and heating chambers and warming blankets were both used. Lyophilized (freeze-dried) plasma was given with good results but later was found to be heavily con-taminated with hepatitis virus,[39] and its use was largely abandoned. Other advances in-cluded the use of vasopressors such as epinephrine,[33] although it was correctly interpreted that while blood pressure would increase, a decrease in blood flow and tis-sue perfusion also occurred, giving a false impression of the adequacy of circulation. This advanced concept was forgotten after WWI, and vasopressors continued to be used for the treatment of hemorrhagic shock, with poor results until 1965.

In World War II, many concepts previously learned were re-learned. In particular, the importance of blood transfusion in treating hemorrhagic shock was a concept that met initial resistance at the beginning of the war. Despite Cannon's work, shock continued to be a problem characterized by low blood pressure and high hematocrit. Thus, it was believed that leakage of plasma into the extravascular space was the source of the problem, and as such, would best be corrected by infusion of plasma. The official opinion of the National Research Council[40] and the Army stated that blood was not recommended for hemorrhagic shock and that plasma was considered adequate. At the start of the war, blood banks did not exist in the military arena. While blood was given occasionally, it was primarily used in small amounts for septic patients.

The United States Surgeon General[40] initially refused to send blood overseas for three reasons: (1) he believed plasma to be adequate for resuscitation; (2) it was logis-tically difficult to send blood farther forward than general hospitals; and (3) shipping space was scarce. However, American surgical consultant Edward Churchill, in the North African-Mediterranean theater, recognized the importance of blood in the resus-citation of wounded soldiers. When his appeals were not addressed, he leaked the story to the *New York Times*[41] at the risk of court-martial. Subsequently, he was given the blood he requested and a system of whole blood distribution was organized, mark-ing one of the major advances in treatment of hemorrhagic shock.

Shock management during the Korean and Vietnam conflicts illustrate the some-times rapidly swinging pendulum of medical dogma. Because of improvements in the efficiency transport systems, many soldiers in Korea who would have succumbed to their injuries in previous wars were reaching treatment facilities alive. Blood was given for resuscitation, replacing blood lost with transfused blood in an equivalent ratio. It was not yet clear that much of the replaced products were lost to the extravas-cular space, resulting in under-resuscitation and consequently high rates of renal fail-ure. The work of Moyer and Butcher[42] and Champion[43] demonstrated that patients in shock lost more extravascular fluid into the intracellular space and confirmed the earlier work of Cannon. In Vietnam, this concept was applied, and aggressive resus-citation with lactated ringers and blood resulted in decreased renal failure. However, over-resuscitation led to the first descriptions of a new condition, Da Nang Lung.[44]

In the current conflicts in Iraq and Afghanistan, research continues to identify the ideal resuscitative fluid type and volume. Interest in the use of easily transportable re-suscitative fluids, such as lyophilized plasma, has resurfaced. The work of Colonel John Holcomb and the United States Army Institute of Surgical Research also continues to bring to the forefront new research in resuscitation, hemostasis, and co-agulation in the setting of the combat theater. While significant progress has been made in the management of hemorrhagic shock, mortality rates from septic shock have changed little over the past 40 years.[33] Current research efforts are aimed at treatment of microvascular thrombosis and maximization of capillary perfusion.

ORGANIZATIONAL SYSTEMS AND TRANSPORT

Organizational systems for the treatment of wounded soldiers in ancient Egypt and early Greece did not exist. Care was primarily given on the field of battle by fellow sol-diers. Occasionally, care was provided by physicians, but they too were fighting on the front lines, many themselves injured. The Greeks ultimately did develop a rudimentary trauma system, with the wounded treated in special barracks or "klisiai."[1]

In the first and second centuries AD, the Romans reintroduced the concept of a trauma system[1,45] in highly organized fashion, typical of the Roman Empire. Special quarters or "valetudenaria" were provided for the sick and wounded who were re-moved from the field of battle. Twenty-five of these quarters have been identified throughout the Roman Empire, including 11 within Roman Britannia, more dedicated trauma facilities than currently exist in this region today (**Fig. 3**). Within the valetudina-ria, patients were triaged according to the severity of their injuries. Open ventilation was stressed, and a variety of surgical instruments and medicinal herbs, such as henbane (scopolamine) and poppies, have been identified.

Little advancement was made in the organization of trauma systems in the ensuing several hundred years. At the start of both the Revolutionary War and the War of

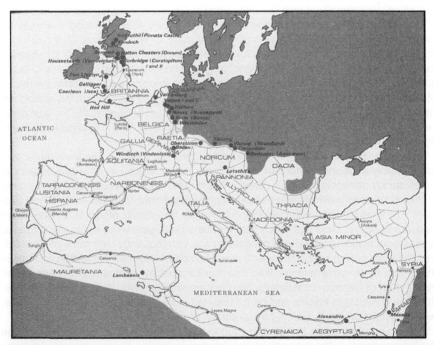

Fig. 3. Map of trauma centers of the Holy Roman Empire. (*From* Majno G. The Healing Hand: Man and Wound in the Ancient World. Cambridge, MA: Harvard University Press, 1975; with permission.)

1812,[39] no formal medical department existed and no organized medical field evacuation took place. The Continental Congress[39] in July 1775 provided for the establishment of "an Hospital" comprised of two surgeons and two surgeons' mates for each regiment. However, this department was disbanded at the conclusion of war, and again for the following war of 1812, the Medical Department had to be recreated from the ground up. This disbanding of the medical service, with the exception of reservists, continued to occur at the conclusion of military conflicts until the Vietnam War.

The Napoleonic Wars of late eighteenth- and early nineteenth-century Europe brought revolutionary change to the organization of military trauma care. Dominique Jean Larrey,[46] a deeply compassionate French doctor, was appalled by the treatment of soldiers who were viewed as problematic and an impediment to the progress of the unit rather than of requiring special attention. Per the contemporary organizational system, injured soldiers were left on the battlefield until 24 to 36 hours after the end of the battle. Assuming victory, they were collected by their regiment in wagons and delivered to *ambulances* or field hospitals. Larrey recognized the inhumanity of this system, as many soldiers suffered greatly before being recovered or simply died prolonged deaths on the battlefield. Larrey conceived a revolutionary concept for transport of the wounded in which medical units called *ambulances volantes* ("flying ambulances") rapidly evacuated wounded soldiers during the battle. The flying ambulance system consisted of a dedicated regiment of men operating a light vehicle, pulled by one or two horses. This in turn carried the men to heavier vehicles for more definitive treatment and evacuation. The speed and agility of this system allowed the regiment to operate essentially on the front lines of battle. This organizational system proved to be very successful, saving the lives of countless French soldiers. Larrey was deeply respected by Napoleon, with whom he spent 18 years of his career. Just before his death, Napoleon said of Larrey, "if the army were to raise a monument to the memory of one man it should be to that of Larrey."[46]

Despite the known success of Larrey's system, organization at the start of the American Civil War was nonexistent. Conditions were unsanitary, there was no evacuation plan, and soldiers were left to die from their wounds on the battlefield. No dedicated field hospitals existed,[10] with the exception of local commandeered buildings, such as churches and homes. The Sanitary Commission,[10] established by President Lincoln in June 1861 before the start of the war and modeled after the British Sanitary Commission, investigated the poor conditions at the Battle of Manassas (Bull Run). Frederick Olmsted, executive secretary of the commission, was the lead investigator. Olmstead proposed several changes, including the organization of an ambulance service, building of dedicated hospitals, provision of medical supplies, and training of physicians and medical personnel, but he met resistance from Surgeon General Finley. After Finley's timely retirement, Olmsted's recommendations were ultimately implemented and the system was developed by Jonathan Letterman.[10,39] In this plan, each regiment was supported by an ambulance corps. Physicians were strategically placed in both the forward setting for wound care and triage, and further back to provide definitive surgical care. An unprecedented component of Letterman's plan called for the evaluation of physicians and only the most skilled and experienced surgeons to perform the major operations.

Further advances included the introduction of formalized nursing care, most notably by Clara Barton.[2] Training was modeled after that outlined by Florence Nightingale during the Crimean War. Additionally, the Union medical division kept meticulous notes regarding the care of the sick and the wounded during the war. At its conclusion, the *Medical and Surgical History of the War of the Rebellion*,[18] credited to Surgeon General William A. Hammond, was published in six volumes. Statistics showed that despite mass casualties from battle wounds, more soldiers actually died from medical than traumatic illness.

With the advent of motorized vehicles, transport time in World Wars I and II from battlefield to definitive care markedly decreased from previous conflicts.[1] However, in WWI, this still could be as long as 12 to 24 hours. By WWII, transport time decreased to less than 4 hours. In the Scudder Oration in 1958,[47] George Curry further stressed the need for and addressed the importance of ambulance service and speedy prehospital transport.

Transport time continued to improve over the course of the following military engagements, with the introduction of helicopter evacuation in the Korean conflict. This decreased transport time to 2 to 4 hours.[1] Also important was the introduction of the forward surgical hospitals (Mobile Army Surgical Hospital). In Vietnam, time to definitive care improved to less than 1 hour.

In the civilian setting, formalized trauma systems did not exist until 1966.[1] In that year the first two United States trauma centers, San Francisco General (under Blaisdell) and Cook County Hospital (under Freeark) were established. Four years later, R. Adams Cowley established the first statewide trauma system in Maryland. In 1976, the American College of Surgeons Committee on Trauma developed a formal outline entitled "Optimal Criteria for Care of the Injured Patient," which continues to be used to this day for establishing state and regional trauma systems.

In the current military conflicts in Iraq and Afghanistan, both immediate and definitive care proceed quickly, with a focus on staged procedures and care occurring in a wide range of locations. Forward surgical teams carry backpacks containing specialized equipment and supplies to rapidly perform procedures, such as intubation and tube thoracostomy, dealing with immediate threats to life in the field. Soldiers are evacuated to a local combat support hospital by air (**Fig. 4**), where damage control procedures are performed if necessary. Transport then proceeds to the regional treatment facility, Landstuhl Regional Medical Center in Germany, where further stabilization and washout is performed as needed. Finally, soldiers are transported in flying intensive care units to Walter Reed Army Medical Center, Bethesda Medical Center, or Brooke Army Medical Center in the United States for definitive care and rehabilitation. Soldiers can be transported 6,500 miles and undergo four operations in 4 to 6 days or less.

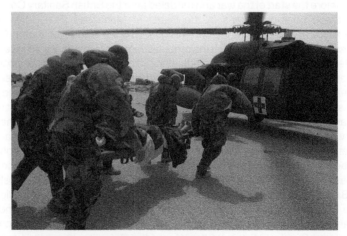

Fig. 4. Air evacuation by the 3rd Infantry Division during Operation Iraqi Freedom March to Baghdad. (*Courtesy of* D.D. Trunkey, MD, Portland, OR.)

CONCLUSION

While progress in the management of battlefield trauma from ancient times to the present has certainly been great, it has not been linear. Several factors have facilitated progress. Knowledge sharing has clearly played a role. Cross-cultural dispersion among geographically related (Egyptians, Greeks, and Romans) or the economically related (Romans and Chinese via the Silk Road) cultures are examples. Dissemination of information across generations, such as seen in the *Asclepiades* of Hippocrates' era, has contributed to this sharing of knowledge as well. Knowledge sharing between the civilian and military sectors has not always occurred seamlessly, but has been invaluable when it has occurred. However, questioning the accepted military and civilian dogma has also played an important a role, with the work of Vesalius as an excellent example.

Other factors that have facilitated progress have been the incorporation of research into the military conflicts, the ability to study large patient populations during mass casualty events, and the incorporation of technologic advances, such as motorized vehicles.

In addition to the obvious regression of progress that occurred as a result of ecclesiastic dicta, the military itself has also at times been a source of stagnation. Many lessons learned in conflicts often were not applied to subsequent engagements. Disbanding of military medical services between conflicts and a lack of research in many conflicts has also limited progress. Military doctrines that dictate a mandatory care protocol often make sense under the circumstances but do not undergo reevaluation when circumstances have changed.

SUMMARY

Evolution and progress in wound care, treatment of shock, and systems of organization are useful areas of study and contemplation. While significant progress has been made, past experiences teach us important lessons for the future, providing both insight for avoiding similar mistakes as well as suggestions as to how we may continue to advance. We should also appreciate the contributions made to our current care of the wounded by the many thoughtful and dedicated scientists and surgeons over the past millennia.

REFERENCES

1. Trunkey D. Trauma care and trauma systems: past, present, and future. In: Meredith JW, Flint L, Schwab C, editors. Trauma: contemporary principles and therapy. Philadelphia: Lippincott Williams & Wilkins; 2007. p. 1–28.
2. Trunkey DD. History and development of trauma care in the United States. Clin Orthop Relat Res 2000;374:36–46.
3. Andrushko VA, Verano JW. Prehistoric trepanation in the Cuzco region of Peru: a view into an ancient Andean practice. Am J Phys Anthropol 2008;137:4–13.
4. King L. The code of Hammurabi. Whitefish (MT): Kessinger Publishing; 2004. p. 22.
5. Atta HM. Edwin Smith Surgical Papyrus: the oldest known surgical treatise. Am Surg 1999;65(12):1190–2.
6. Pikoulis EA, Petropoulos JS, Tsigris C, et al. Trauma management in ancient Greece: value of surgical principles through the years. World J Surg 2004; 28(4):425–30.
7. Haeger K. The illustrated history of surgery. 1988. New York: Bell Publishing Company.

8. Broughton G II, Janis JE, Attinger CE. A brief history of wound care. Plast Reconstr Surg 2006;117(Suppl 7):6S–11S.
9. Stansbury LG, Branstetter JG, Lalliss SJ. Amputation in military trauma surgery. J Trauma 2007;63(4):940–4.
10. Pruitt BA Jr. Combat casualty care and surgical progress. Ann Surg 2006;243(6): 715–29.
11. Pilcher JE. Guy de Chauliac and Henri de Mondeville: a surgical retrospect. Ann Surg 1895;21(1):84–102.
12. Menzoian JO. Presidential Address. Lest we forget: the contributions of Andreas Vesalius and Ambroise Pare to my surgical practice. Am J Surg 1999;178(2): 85–91.
13. Martin G. The death of Henry II of France: a sporting death and post-mortem. ANZ J Surg 2001;71(5):318–20.
14. Hammonds WD, Steinhaus JE, Crawford W. Long: pioneer physician in anesthesia. J Clin Anesth 1993;5(2):163–7.
15. Dunn PM. Sir James Young Simpson (1811–1870) and obstetric anaesthesia. Arch Dis Child Fetal Neonatal Ed 2002;86(3):F207–9.
16. Aldrete JA, Marron GM, Wright AJ. The first administration of anesthesia in military surgery: on occasion of the Mexican-American War. Anesthesiology 1984; 61(5):585–8.
17. Wangensteen OH, Wangensteen SD. The rise of surgery: from empiric craft to scientific discipline. Minneapolis (MN): University of Minnesota Press; 1978.
18. Woodward J. The medical and surgical history of the War of the Rebellion, vol. 1. Washington, DC: Government Printing Office; 1875.
19. Rutkow I. Surgery: an illustrated history. The eighteenth century. St. Louis (MO): CV Mosby; 1993. p. 312–15.
20. Cope Z. Joseph Lister, 1827–1912. Br Med J 1967;2(5543):7–8.
21. Rosengart MR. Critical care medicine: landmarks and legends. Surg Clin North Am 2006;86(6):1305–21.
22. Loria F. Historical aspects of abdominal injuries. Gunpowder and the development of firearms. Springfield (IL): Charles C. Thomas; 1968.
23. Mullins RJ, Trunkey DD, Samuel D. Gross: pioneer academic trauma surgeon of 19th century America. J Trauma 1990;30(5):528–38.
24. Trunkey D, Farjah F. Medical and surgical care of our four assassinated presidents. J Am Coll Surg 2005;201(6):976–89.
25. Glasser O. WC Roentgen and the discovery of the Roentgen rays. AJR Am J Roentgenol 1995;165(5):1033–40.
26. Trunkey DD. Doctor George Goodfellow, the first civilian trauma surgeon. Surg Gynecol Obstet 1975;141(1):97–104.
27. Bennett JD. Princess Vera Gedroits: military surgeon, poet, and author. BMJ 1992;305(6868):1532–4.
28. Ogilvie W. Abdominal wounds in the Western desert. Surg Gynecol Obstet 1944; 78:225–38.
29. Nelson R, Singer M. Primary repair for penetrating colon injuries. Cochrane Database Syst Rev 2003;(3):CD002247.
30. Duncan JE, Corwin CH, Sweeney WB, et al. Management of colorectal injuries during Operation Iraqi Freedom: patterns of stoma usage. J Trauma 2008; 64(4):1043–7.
31. Bylebyl JJ, Pagel W. The chequered career of Galen's doctrine on the pulmonary veins. Med Hist 1971;15(3):211–29.

32. Harvey W. On the motion of the heart and blood in animals. London: George Bell and Sons; 1889.
33. Hardaway RM. Wound shock: a history of its study and treatment by military surgeons. Mil Med 2004;169(4):265–9.
34. Barnes J. Medical and surgical history of the War of the Rebellion, Part 2, vol. 11. Washington, DC: US Army; 1876. p. 15.
35. Hess JR, Schmidt PJ. The first blood banker: Oswald Hope Robertson. Transfusion 2000;40(1):110–3.
36. Benison S, Barger AC, Wolfe EL, et al. Cannon and the mystery of shock: a study of Anglo-American co-operation in World War I. Med Hist 1991;35(2):216–49.
37. Blalock A. Experimental shock: cause of the low blood pressure produced by muscle injury. Arch Surg 1930;20:959–96.
38. Cannon W. Traumatic shock. In: DA Co, editor. A conception of the nature of shock. New York: Appleton & Co.; 1923. p. 160–7.
39. Hardaway RM. 200 years of military surgery. Injury 1999;30(6):387–97.
40. Hardaway RM III. The army at Pearl Harbor. J Am Coll Surg 2000;190(5):593–600.
41. Churchill E. Surgeon to soldiers. Wound shock and blood transfusion. Philadelphia: JB Lippincott Co; 1972.
42. Broido PW, Butcher HR Jr, Moyer CA. A bioassay of treatment of hemorrhagic shock. II. The expansion of the volume distribution of extracellular ions during hemorrhagic hypotension and its possible relationship to change in the physical-chemical properties of extravascular-extracellular tissue. Arch Surg 1966; 93(4):556–61.
43. Champion HR, Sturdivan L, Nolan J, et al. A mathematical model for volume replacement in bleeding patients. J Surg Res 1975;19(5):297–302.
44. Pearce FJ, Lyons WS. Logistics of parenteral fluids in battlefield resuscitation. Mil Med 1999;164(9):653–5.
45. Cilliers L, Retief FP. Medical practice in Graeco-Roman antiquity. Curationis 2006; 29(2):34–40.
46. Skandalakis PN, Lainas P, Zoras O, et al. "To afford the wounded speedy assistance": Dominique Jean Larrey and Napoleon. World J Surg 2006;30(8):1392–9.
47. Curry GJ. The immediate care and transportation of the injured. Bull Am Coll Surg 1959;44(1):32–4.

Preparedness Lessons from Modern Disasters and Wars

Saqib I. Dara, MD, FCCP[a], J. Christopher Farmer, MD, FCCM[b,c,d],*

KEYWORDS

- Disaster medicine • Critical care • Disaster planning
- Intensive care • Disasters • Chernobyl nuclear accident

> In life, unlike chess, the game continues after checkmate.
>
> Isaac Asimov, 1920–1992

In 2003, the severe acute respiratory syndrome (SARS) outbreak unmasked the vulnerability of health care professionals caring for these contagious patients.[1,2] In some countries, 50% of the SARS casualties were health care workers.[3] A tsunami in 2004 killed an estimated 230,000 people, mostly in Indonesia.[4] In 2005, Hurricane Katrina struck the United States, an industrialized nation with enormous resources. Despite the presence of a substantial response infrastructure in the United States, news images revealed an initial paralytic aftermath with individuals "dying in the streets" and stranded critically ill patients in the shells of hospitals. Ensuing floods rendered intensive care units (ICUs) nonfunctional.[5,6] News headlines in 2008 estimated that more than 100,000 people died in Myanmar[7] as a consequence of cyclone Nargis and almost 70,000 people died following earthquakes in China last spring.[8]

Fortunately, in the wake of these events, medical response to disasters significantly evolved.[9–11] Most recent disasters around the world have witnessed brisk execution of well-structured, integrated response, albeit with occasional operational flaws.[12,13] Much of this progress has occurred as a result of governmental policy shifts that followed disasters.[14] In the United States, for instance, there has been a clear increase in focus on disaster preparedness since the events of September 11, 2001.[15]

---

[a] Critical Care Medicine, Al Rahba Hospital—Johns Hopkins International, Abu Dhabi, United Arab Emirates
[b] Critical Care Medicine, Mayo School of Graduate Medical Education, Mayo Clinic College of Medicine, Rochester, MN, USA
[c] Department of Medicine, Mayo Clinic College of Medicine, Rochester, MN, USA
[d] Program in Translational Immunovirology and Biodefense, Mayo Clinic College of Medicine, Rochester, MN, USA
* Corresponding author. Department of Medicine, Mayo Clinic College of Medicine, 200 First Street SW, Old Marian Hall, OL2-115, Rochester, MN 55905.
E-mail address: farmer.j@mayo.edu (J.C. Farmer).

Crit Care Clin 25 (2009) 47–65
doi:10.1016/j.ccc.2008.10.005
0749-0704/08/$ – see front matter © 2009 Elsevier Inc. All rights reserved.

At the government level, we witnessed the creation of the Department of Homeland Security to streamline and improve the efficiency of multiple response agencies.[16] In addition, the ongoing scientific,[17,18] technical,[19–21] and educational advances[22–24] and their integration with disaster medicine[25,26] have advanced our ability to respond to disasters. For example, we have increased capability of transporting very sick patients,[27,28] improved early detection of unusual and previously unidentified microbes,[29] and enhanced our ability to rapidly acquire information from disaster scenes through mobile telecommunications systems, global positioning, and telemedicine technologies.[30]

What lessons can we learn from these events and from other disasters over the last many decades? Despite the varied nature of these catastrophes, many critical care themes are common to all:

Planning matters—a lot![12,31,32]

The absence of sufficient training and education equals confusion, uncertainty, and increased secondary casualties (including injuries and fatalities to health care professionals).[33]

The provision of critical care must include "portability," defined as the ability to provide credible, sustainable, sophisticated care outside of the normal confines of an ICU.[9,34–36]

Dispelling myths: It's too many casualties, so what possible impact would a (relative) "handful" of resources mean to this many patients?

To address these issues, we need to identify simple, broadly available technologies that can be universally employed.[28,37]

What follows is a representative, but not exhaustive, list of representative disasters that have occurred over the last few decades, with a summary of each disaster, as well as specific clinical lessons learned. Finally, we offer suggestions regarding how each of these disaster events should influence our current critical care preparedness planning.

EVENT: CHERNOBYL NUCLEAR DISASTER
Summary

On April 26, 1986, a large-scale nuclear disaster occurred at Chernobyl, a small town in Ukraine, which was a part of the Soviet Union.[38,39] Compared with other large-scale disasters, such as the nuclear bomb detonations in Hiroshima and Nagasaki and exposure to cesium-127 in Brazil,[40] this is the worst nuclear disaster in history. It resulted from overheating of a reactor core, while testing a safety procedure. An estimated 56 deaths occurred, including 28 radiation deaths among reactor operators and firefighters.[41] Additionally, it is estimated that there may be have been hundreds of subsequent cancer occurrences among the adjacent population, as well as among the 6 million people who lived within the radiation fallout plume.[42]

Relevance to Today and Clinical Teaching Points

The medical literature contains little about the immediate response to the Chernobyl disaster. Even so, lessons can be learned about the gaps in reporting and communication and the secrecy of the authorities at the time. This failure to inform generated fear, rumors, and uncertainty.[39]

There could be very high rates of posttraumatic stress disorder after a major radiation exposure. Groups particularly at risk include children, pregnant women, mothers of young children, and emergency workers. Prevention is essential through openness and communication.[43]

Another important lesson from Chernobyl is that a major radiation incident also results in thermal and radiation burns, wounds, fractures, and other trauma injuries, thus adversely affecting the prognosis of the patient. The immune function may become compromised, predisposing patients to sepsis. Compromised immune function was observed for Chernobyl firefighters and should be a treatment priority.[44]

These lessons have assumed greater significance in the context of the current geopolitical realities. The ongoing oil crisis makes it likely that there will be more reliance on nuclear production of energy. Although global nuclear war may be less likely than in the past, terrorist use of radiologic weapons is an increasing threat.[45]

Lessons for Critical Care

- We often overlook the need to provide surveillance for posttraumatic stress disorder in our critical care health care professionals, as well as follow-up for patients and family members. Posttraumatic stress disorder may have more significant longer-term negative ramifications than we earlier believed.[46]
- It is anticipated that in the event of a nuclear disaster, a casualty stream would include significant numbers of patients with both traumatic injuries and radioactive contamination. Critical care preparedness should include provisions (ie, decontamination access) to deal with both problems.[40]
- Potassium iodide is touted as an "antidote" to "radiation poisoning." Remember, however, that this is protective only to the thyroid gland.
- Complete critical care planning includes a triage plan for radiation-exposure victims. This plan should incorporate a predictive matrix that projects severity of illness and probability of survival (based on probable radiation-dose exposure). **Table 1** offers an example. Others employ more complicated methodologies, such as rate of lymphocyte depletion.
- The secondary radiation risk to health care workers from exposure to contaminated casualties (or their excreta, body fluids) is limited.[41]

EVENT: BHOPAL DISASTER
Summary

One of the worst chemical disasters in history occurred on December 2, 1984, in Bhopal, Madhya Pradesh, India.[47] At a Union Carbide plant, a faulty valve allowed 1 ton of water for cleaning internal pipes to mix with 40 tons of methyl isocyanate.[47] Pressure and heat from the reaction in the tank continued to build. As a safety valve

---

Table 1
Predicting radiation-dose exposure by using time to onset of vomiting

Time from Exposure to Onset of Vomiting	Estimated Dose	Predicted Mortality
<10 min	>8 Gy	100%
10–30 min	6–8 Gy	100%
31–59 min	4–6 Gy	100%
1–2 h	2–4 Gy	>50%
>2 h	<2 Gy	>50%

Adapted from Radiation Emergency Assistance Center - Training site (REACTS) and International Atomic Energy Agency (IAEA). (Other sources quote different times, but trend is similar.)

gave way, a plume of methyl isocyanate gas escaped, killing around 4000 people immediately.[47] The injured soon overwhelmed the local hospitals, a crisis deepened by a lack of knowledge of exactly what gas was involved.[47]

The number of people killed in the first few days are estimated at 10,000.[47] At least 200,000[48] and, according to some reports, more than 500,000 people were exposed to the gas. These data are, however, likely to underrepresent the true extent of adverse events as many exposed individuals left Bhopal immediately following the disaster and were lost to follow-up.[47]

Relevance to Today and Clinical Teaching Points

These mass casualty incidents pose an overwhelming demand on hospital resources because of the need to decontaminate and manage a large number of critically ill patients. Following the initial release of methyl isocyanate, an estimated 200,000 people sought medical care.[49] The city had four major hospitals but there was a shortage of physicians and hospital beds and no mass casualty emergency response system was in place in the city.[49]

The greatest numbers of patients seeking care in such disasters are often those who perceive they have been poisoned, but do not exhibit obvious signs or symptoms of poisoning.[50] Many of these patients may have no exposure, and are merely worried.[51] Demands from these anxious people decrease the ability of the medical system to effectively triage and identify the most critically ill patients.[49] This event can be circumvented by planning for treatment of thousands of patients at the same time.[52]

This event in Bhopal dramatically highlighted the threat to the first responder, as was proven later in the sarin incident in Tokyo where almost 10% of the 1364 first responders sustained injured.[53] These injuries to first responders were related to inadequate training and preparation.[54]

The events in Bhopal revealed the disastrous consequences of expanding industrialization in developing countries without simultaneous investment in safety regulations.[55] Accidents involving hazardous toxic materials are predicted to occur predominantly in developing countries.[56] However, the sarin poisoning incident in Japan revealed that developed nations may be equally vulnerable.[57]

The danger to communities from hazardous materials accidents is continuously on the rise. Of the 70,000 chemicals used industrially in the United Kingdom, more than 2000 are considered harmful and 200,000 tons are transported daily.[50] In the United States, 15 events of gas release exceeding the Bhopal incident in quantity and toxicity occurred during the 1980s.[49] Over 80,000 chemical agents commonly produced, transported, or used in the United States are toxic enough to rapidly produce life-threatening conditions.[49] Even so, a survey conducted in 2003 revealed gross underpreparation.[58] With the heightened threat of deliberate offensive use of chemical warfare agents, it is imperative that hospitals be adequately prepared to handle such large-scale disasters[59] through an effective response strategy,[60] drawn on basic toxicologic principles.[49]

Lessons for Critical Care

- A mass casualty incident involving a toxic plume of gas may generate a significant number of casualties with impending or actual acute respiratory failure.
- Do you know if there is a hazardous materials route through your region/city/town that carries these sorts of materials? Do you currently have a critical care–specific triage plan that includes the procurement and allocation of mechanical ventilators?[61]

- Do you have an education plan in place that instructs critical care personnel in self-protection from contamination?[50,62]
- A lot can be learned from the evolution of the chemical disaster response system in Japan over the last decade.[57]
- Rescue workers and medical personnel must be trained to operate under the threat of chemical contamination.[52]

EVENT: OKLAHOMA CITY BOMBING
Summary

On April 19, 1995, a truck carrying a mixture of ammonium nitrate fertilizer, nitro meth-ane, and diesel fuel exploded near the Alfred P. Murrah Federal Building in downtown Oklahoma City, Oklahoma. This terrorist attack destroyed one third of that building and damaged numerous other buildings in a 16-block radius. Of the 361 persons who were in the federal building, 319 were injured, of whom 163 died, including 19 chil-dren. The most frequent cause of death was multiple injuries. Among survivors, mus-culoskeletal and head injuries were most common.[63]

Relevance to Today and Clinical Teaching Points

The most important lesson learned from the events of Oklahoma was that terrorists could wage their war on American soil.[54]

The second most important lesson—and one that is more sobering—is how easily explosives can be assembled. The bomb used by the Oklahoma bombers was prim-itive and assembled from easily available material.

Members of the hospital staffs at the receiving hospitals, such as the Columbia Presbyterian Hospital, have written of the valuable lessons about managing a sudden increase in activity, equipment and supplies, and staffing resources.[64] One of the most significant problems was maintaining adequate communications. Even the hospital emergency administrative radio system was operational in only 3 of the 15 hospitals that handled patients.[65] We need to have alternative back-up plans tested and in place now, before any event.

We also learned that structural collapse is the most important risk factor for fatality in a building bombing. Better building designs might make structural collapse less likely. Evacuation drills might reduce potential fatalities.[66]

Lessons for Critical Care

- Do you have a communications plan in place that will allow you to mobilize and augment critical staffing on extremely short notice? Can this plan be executed if usual telephone (including cell phone) access is overloaded?
- Posttraumatic stress disorder in health care workers is significant and must be treated early and effectively.[67]
- This does not require terrorists to make these a reality…what about a large-scale conventional explosion at a factory? Are you ready? Does your ICU have a plan?

EVENT: SEPTEMBER 11, 2001
Summary

On September 11, 2001, terrorists hijacked four passenger planes and crashed two of these planes against the World Trade Center towers in New York City.[68] This was the largest terrorist attack ever on United States soil. At the time, approximately 60,000 people worked and an estimated 90,000 more people visited the buildings each day. A total of 2726 persons were killed.[68] In Washington, D.C., a hijacked jet was flown into the Pentagon building. The crash and fire killed almost 200 people and injured an additional 500.[69]

Relevance to Today and Clinical Teaching Points

Preparedness

The city of New York was prepared adequately at multiple levels. St. Vincent's Hospital was one of the main receiving hospitals and performed well to avoid over-triage[70] and kept a balance between early treatment of the critically ill patients while catering to a large number of minimally injured patients.[71] The most important factor in enhancing the hospital's preparedness for this event was the prior involvement in caring for the 1993 World Trade Center bombing victims. As a result of that event, the hospital had developed a more detailed disaster plan and conducted a series of drills.

At the city level, New York had the Metropolitan Medical Response System, a well-developed system that made for smooth coordination with regional response networks and quick distribution of the National Emergency Stockpile assets.[54]

Lateral thinking

However, there were instances of flawed communications and inefficient sharing of information in the wake of the September 11 tragedy.[72] These problems stemmed from the vertical hold some agencies and organizations had on decision-making capacity.[73] All large-scale mass casualty events require decision-making capacities that are lateral in nature as no one organization has the expertise needed to make all vital decisions.[74]

Poor awareness of secondary contamination

A number of health care providers were sent to Ground Zero without taking precautions for possible involvement of nuclear, biologic, or chemical weapons, or even for the toxic productions of combustion. This put them at great risk for significant illness.[71]

Logistical problems

Several logistic problems made an impact on treatment efforts. Within hours of the disaster, electricity and phone services were lost, cellular communications were not operative, and computer communication lines failed. The use of two-way radios by key hospital personnel served to minimize the disruption in intrahospital communications.[71] These problems illustrate the need for systems that simultaneously use several communication alternatives, all of which may be deployed on handheld computers.[75]

Lessons for Critical Care

- Even though the September 11 attack involved conventional explosives, critical care specialists must be prepared to deal with contaminated casualties as a secondary complication.[76]
- Communications, communications, communications…
- Clinical volunteers may not be who they claim to be. Credentials must be verified.
- We are critical care specialists, not first responders. We are not trained to recognize danger at the incident site (eg, live electrical wires, unstable building structures, toxic substances). Stay in the hospital.
- Doctors can be trained in such skills as extrication, triage, and transport.[77]
- Hospitals are only a small part of an overall disaster response plan. The primary function of an incident response plan is not only to evacuate casualties, but also to protect the uninjured.

EVENT: OUTBREAK OF SEVERE ACUTE RESPIRATORY SYNDROME
Summary

In 2003, an infectious disease outbreak began in China. Initially involving animal-to-human transmission of a coronavirus that caused a severe and even fatal acute respiratory illness, this outbreak originated with food handlers in the "wet" markets of Southern China, rapidly spread to Hong Kong, to other parts of Asia, and then to other parts of the world over the ensuing weeks to months.[78] The rapid worldwide transmission of this disease reflects our current global mobility via commercial air travel.[79] Ultimately, SARS killed approximately 800 people and infected over 8000 others in almost 30 countries on every continent.

Relevance to Today and Clinical Teaching Points

Notably, a startlingly high percentage of the patients were health care workers.[80] These cases illustrated how insufficient infection control practices can be lethal And also raised important questions about how people react to such an outbreak: Who will show up for work in the hospital? How will people respond if their workplace (ie, the ICU) significantly places them at risk for contracting a life-threatening illness?[81]

The SARS epidemic has better prepared the world's public health authorities for a major influenza or other pandemic.[81] While there are differences, many of these same issues are applicable to pandemic influenza or a bioterrorism event.[82] In fact, many authorities remain concerned that a pandemic influenza outbreak (such as an avian influenza outbreak) would be orders of magnitude greater in scope than SARS and the goal to minimize damage from such an event has become a global health priority.[83] Therefore, infection control and other preventative measures are of major importance,[84] but so will be triage and allocation of mechanical ventilators and other life-support measures.[85]

Furthermore, education and training of ICU personnel in the assiduous practices of self-protective measures will also be key to ensuring that absenteeism does not become a problem (ie, not coming to work because of concerns related to contracting the disease).[86] Finally, no plan equals chaos. To ensure that the appropriate education and training occur, and to establish effective triage strategies/algorithms for your hospital,[87] advance work to achieve leadership consensus should happen now, not after a disaster begins.

One of the key lessons is that we are vulnerable to events far away.[81]

Lessons for Critical Care

- What percent of your ICU personnel are current for fit-testing of N-95% masks? If your hospital is typical, that number is perhaps 50%. And if we can keep up with this simple requirement, then what of more advanced vital skills, like flawless (error-free) donning and doffing of personal protective equipment?[88]
- Do you have a ventilator triage plan?[89]
- Do you have a pandemic influenza plan that includes your ICU?[90] Does it work? Has it been exercised or practiced in some measurable capacity?
- Do you have a plan to prevent bronchoscope-associated infection?[91]

EVENT: TSUNAMI
Summary

On December 26, 2004, an earthquake beneath the Indian Ocean triggered a large tsunami that struck in Indonesia, Sri Lanka, India, Somalia, and Thailand.[92] This 9.2-magnitude earthquake and the ensuing tsunami led to the death of an estimated

225,000 people in at least 11 countries and the displacement of over 1 million people. In terms of deaths and population displacement, this tsunami was among the most devastating in human history. Between 30% and 40% of the total number killed were children. The medical infrastructure in most of the coastal region was destroyed in these countries,[93] and there was no secure (uncontaminated) water source.[92] Consequently, many people had little or no access to medical care for trauma injuries, infections, and subsequent public health–related outbreaks, such as cholera and malaria.[94] There were also very high rates of posttraumatic stress disorder among survivors.[95]

Relevance to Today and Clinical Teaching Points

The clinical teaching points from the tsunami disaster were best described by Claude de Ville de Goyet, MD,[93] retired director of the Emergency Preparedness Program of the Pan-American Health Organization (PAHO), and others[96] in detail. One of the essential flaws was a gaping gulf between the needs of the local communities as they perceived them and the needs assessment performed by the aiding agencies.[93] World response to the event included over $13 billion in aid.[93] However, many donations from industrialized countries included aid items that were not germane to postdisaster needs of casualties. Nevertheless, these items required the same logistical support to unload or store, thus redirecting time and energy away from important relief efforts to things that were not as helpful.[97] A hasty response that is not based on familiarity with local conditions contributes to more chaos. It is prudent to wait until real needs have been assessed.[98]

False alarms were raised about the probability of more deaths from secondary epidemics than from the tsunami itself.[93] These "overly alarmist announcements" related to problems that did not materialize provide valuable lessons in appropriate and responsible disaster communication.

Foreign mobile hospitals rarely arrived in time for immediate trauma care, leaving local, sometimes damaged facilities to provide immediate, life-saving care.[93] In many instances, immediate assistance to the injured was provided by uninjured survivors with whatever basic first aid they knew without any tools or resuscitation equipment.[99] This experience supports proposals for teaching life-supporting first aid courses to the public.[100]

A lot has been written about the dynamics of assistance during disasters. In general, however, as depicted in **Fig. 1**, human nature dictates an initial outpouring of generosity as attention focuses on the first news of the disaster. This widespread generosity falls off quickly over time, leaving committed responders behind to carry the burden of responsibility for aid. The response to the tsunami followed this pattern.

Lessons for Critical Care

- History keeps repeating itself: In the wake of a large-scale disaster that creates an austere care environment, systems are needed for rapidly deploying portable, sophisticated care, but such systems are rarely in place.
- Critical care doctors must be prepared to perform in surroundings with suboptimal public health structure in the wake of a disaster.[101,102]
- Flexibility to adapt to local circumstances and fit in the local incident command system is essential for doctors helping in foreign disasters.[93]

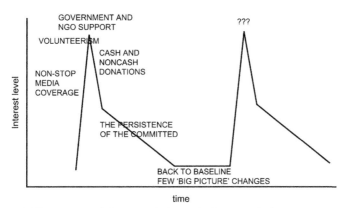

time

Fig. 1. Rise and fall over time of desire to "help" with disaster relief, NGO, nongovernmental organization.

EVENT: HURRICANE KATRINA
Summary

In August 2005, Hurricane Katrina caused the rupture of levees protecting New Orleans, Louisiana, leading to devastating flooding and the destruction of much of the city's infrastructure. This resulted in a public health emergency that displaced more than 4400 physicians in the greater New Orleans area and led to the closure of 13 of 16 hospitals. This caused widespread destruction, reducing hospital capacity by 80% and clinic capacity by 75% in New Orleans.[103]

Relevance to Today and Clinical Teaching Points

As we look at the big picture, it appears that the poor outcome in this disaster was not the result of lack of knowledge, but rather the result of inaction[103] and poor implementation[104] of the necessary measures.[105]

We witnessed the impact of a complete loss of critical care capability on the general population. Specifically, there were numerous secondary casualties—patients with chronic critical illnesses who lost access to care rapidly became ill.[106] These patients consumed a significant amount of the available rescue medical care.[107]

A number of lessons pertinent to critical care were (re)learned at a very high cost.[108] The foremost was how much the delivery of critical care services depends on support services, such as water and electricity. The worst hit hospital in New Orleans was Charity Hospital. Rising floodwaters submerged the hospital's emergency electrical generators. This left no reliable electrical power for life-support systems, such as mechanical ventilators, suction machines, bedside monitors, intravenous fluid pumps, and dialysis machines. Even air conditioning was lost.[109] Radiology and laboratory capability became extinct. Patients who required positive-pressure ventilation had to be hand ventilated with bag-valve devices in total darkness.[6]

Lesson in evacuation surge capacity

Many hospitals were incapacitated simultaneously.[110] This left the option to either deploy field hospitals or to evacuate. Unfortunately, portable critical care exists only at certain facilities and is generally not developed as a deployable asset. Therefore, all hospitals in general and especially those located in regions subject to hurricanes and earthquakes should make extraordinary investments to develop coalition partners and to ensure portability of sophisticated care.[111] A reasonable solution would be collaboration across regions to enable long-distance patient and staff transfer during emergencies.[112] Adequate knowledge of the operational status of surrounding facilities expedites such transfer. The Department of Health and Human Services Critical Infrastructure Data System was employed to track the local, state, and national availability of medical care for hurricane victims following Hurricane Rita in 2005. A means of rapidly assessing the needs of the affected area would allow proper resource deployment and use.[113]

Field hospitals
Significant experience was gained in the deployment and management of field hospitals. A prominent example is the Carolinas Med-1.[114] This mobile hospital consisted of two 53-ft tractor-trailers. One served as an equipment storage unit and the other as the patient care facility.[114] Up to 130 beds, including emergency room beds, ICU beds, and surgical suites, could be accommodated. It also provided diagnostic radiology and point-of-care laboratory services. During the 6-week deployment, more than 7400 patients were evaluated and treated at this mobile facility by integrating seamlessly into the existing local, state, and federal facilities.[114]

Staffing issues
Out-of-state physician volunteers who responded to this were practicing medicine without a license, potentially placing them at risk for penalties. Louisiana Governor Kathleen Blanco issued an executive order that suspended regular licensing procedures. However, the policies of each state regarding physician licensure during disasters ought to be determined.[115]

Lessons for Critical Care

- What happens if you suffer a power outage in your ICU, and the generators fail to work? It happens…sometimes even without a natural disaster[5,116]
- If you had to completely evacuate your ICU out of the building, including even the sickest patients, could you do it safely?[117] How? Where would you go? What is the plan?[118]
- Under extreme circumstances, would you come to work?[119] Think about it…
- Do you have a plan for regional cooperation between hospitals and ICUs?[120] Have you ever conducted an exercise around this premise?[111]
- Chronic illnesses will coexist and may aggravate management of acute illness.[121–123]
- Responsible crisis communication is essential to prevent avoidable secondary complications.[124]

EVENT: OPERATION IRAQI FREEDOM AND OPERATION ENDURING FREEDOM
Summary

Operation Enduring Freedom (OEF) was the coordinated military operation that started in October 2001 in Afghanistan to oust the Taliban from power. In Operation Iraqi Freedom (OIF), the United States–led coalition forces entered into armed conflict with Iraq on March 19, 2003, and by May 1, 2003, active hostilities were declared over.[125] According to the US Department of Defense online data of American military casualties (the number of wounded or dead) from OIF/OEF, the operations led to the deaths of 4733 American servicemen as of September 3, 2008.[126]

Traditional battlefield medicine has focused on providing "definitive" trauma casualty care within the theater of operations. Injured soldiers were then transported back to their home country when they became "stable." This translated to 15 to 45 days in-theater before evacuation to hospitals in their home countries. In addition, because moving unstable casualties (who now require advanced ICU care) rearward after surgery is so difficult and unreliable, moving trauma surgical care closer to the point of injury was generally not done. So historically, casualties had to survive until they were evacuated back to an echelon where surgical care became available.

During these most recent conflicts in Iraq and Afghanistan, a concept of portable critical care has been employed with great success and has proven to be an advancement over the traditional methods of battlefield medicine.[127,128] A casualty receives "damage control" (targeted, limited, life-saving) surgery as soon as possible after the injury and as close as possible to the battlefield location of injury.[20] Then, critical care teams are used to evacuate these patients rearward.[129] Along the way, subsequent additional "damage control" procedures may be required. Today, from time of injury a casualty is typically evacuated back to the United States within 72 to 96 hours, and may have had several incremental surgical procedures performed along the way.[130] This approach has resulted in the lowest died-of-wounds rate in the history of warfare.[131]

These critical care teams were developed and are maintained by the U.S. Air Force. They are part of the Critical Care Aeromedical Transport Team program.[132] These teams are capable of providing all aspects of critical care, including advanced mechanical ventilatory support; invasive cardiovascular monitoring; pharmacologic support, diagnosis, and treatment of sepsis or other forms of shock; limited laboratory assessment; portable ultrasound; portable bronchoscopy; and even extracorporeal support in limited circumstances.[133] Much of this occurs in austere settings, such as the back of an Air Force cargo plane during flights from the Middle East to Germany, and again across the Atlantic Ocean.[134,135]

Relevance to Today and Clinical Teaching Points

Provision of critical care in a transport setting imposes unique challenges, particularly when the duration of patient transfer is prolonged.[9,136] As a simple example, monitoring technologies must overcome limitations imposed by noise. Automated blood pressure monitors, measurement of oxygen saturation, and end-tidal carbon dioxide with limited electrocardiography may represent the only available cardiopulmonary monitoring. Ventilators must offer a range of tidal volumes, but a limited number of modes may be available. Variable minute ventilation must be provided over a wide range of barometric pressure conditions. Infusion devices must be compact and robust with extended battery life and pressure-activated occlusion alarms. Only point-of-care laboratory testing may be available in remote settings and in the transport environment. Finally, a limited drug list must be developed to include provision for analgesia and sedation, and to accommodate the need for vasoconstriction, inotropic support, or vasodilatation with various shock states.

Beyond its use by the Critical Care Aeromedical Transport Team, this approach to critical care may be adapted for a significant potential role in disaster response medicine. An aeromedical transport system adapted for civilian use could go a long way toward addressing many of the issues raised in this article, including (1) the transport of ICU patients when a hospital is rendered unusable or the number of critically ill or injured casualties exceeds local/regional capability, (2) a surge of patients with chronic critical illnesses who lose access to ongoing support following a disaster (and who significantly tax other disaster-response assets), and (3) the overall need to extend critical care capability within the disaster response locale (eg, expanding hospital ICU capability to non-ICU areas of the facility).

Lessons for Critical Care

- "Portable" critical care is a necessary component of any robust disaster medical response capability. Without this, we do not have an effective answer for the needs articulated in this article.
- Interagency collaboration and communication assumes even greater importance during complex humanitarian emergencies, such as wars.[125]
- Opportunities for collaboration exist between military and civilian response systems to translate shared expertise into benefits for all critically ill patients, whether in a roadside accident or on the battlefield.[25]

SUMMARY

This effort represents our attempts to review a cross-section of representative disasters that illustrate recurring, important themes related to critical care and hospital disaster response. It is by no means comprehensive; unfortunately disasters that impact large numbers of patients, and require critical care resources occur commonly. We selected disasters for discussions that illustrate core principles relevant to critical care practitioners. To summarize these "lessons learned" include:

1. *Disaster preparation typically focuses all pre-hospital care requirements, and often neglects the needs of the hospital, and especially intensive care units.* This impacts ICU response in several ways including sufficiency of space, equipment and supplies, triage protocols, and so forth.
2. *A burgeoning number of non-hospitalized individuals with chronic critical illness.* When a disaster occurs that limits access to advanced medical care, these patients rapidly decompensate, and in many circumstances utilize/consume more disaster response resources than primary casualties.
3. *Following a disaster, existing critical care resources may be insufficient to meet demand for services.* Developing a deliberate plan (5) that pre-identifies alternative care sites for ICU patients is essential. This must include access to sufficient quantities of 50 psi oxygen, suctioning, medical devices, and necessary pharmacy support.
4. *Following a disaster of sufficient magnitude, non-critical care hospital personnel will be called to assist with the care of ICU patients.* It is important to know, in advance what will be the scope of practice of these individuals, what education is needed to ensure that this care is efficient and of reliable quality, and who will provide supervision and assistance for these activities.
5. *Following a disaster, it is vitally important to ensure the protection of ICU personnel from communicable diseases/outbreaks, as well as physical harm.* This requires a plan, practice, and proper education of staff.
6. *When a large scale disaster occurs, medical care processes quickly migrate below usual standards of care due to resource limitations.* This degradation of care should be planned and not haphazard. This can also be pre-planned as it relates to access to mechanical ventilation, staffing ratios, aggressiveness of resuscitation based on probability of survival, etc. The goal is to predictably orchestrate transition from "standard of care" to "sufficiency of care."

Except for individuals who volunteer their time or who are engaged in disaster preparedness, there is generally a limited willingness by health care professionals to accept that these concerns as relevant to their daily professional lives. Furthermore, in a cost-constrained hospital, these low probability but high consequence needs do not compete favorably with more tangible, other needs (eg, purchasing a new CT scanner).

But as with everything else ...
Those who cannot learn from history are doomed to repeat it.
—George Santayana.

REFERENCES

1. Avendano M, Derkach P, Swan S. Clinical course and management of SARS in health care workers in Toronto: a case series. CMAJ 2003;168(13):1649–60.
2. Scales DC, Green K, Chan AK, et al. Illness in intensive care staff after brief exposure to severe acute respiratory syndrome. Emerg Infect Dis 2003;9(10): 1205–10.
3. Fowler RA, Guest CB, Lapinsky SE, et al. Transmission of severe acute respiratory syndrome during intubation and mechanical ventilation. Am J Respir Crit Care Med 2004;169(11):1198–202.
4. Gautschi OP, Cadosch D, Rajan G, et al. Earthquakes and trauma: review of triage and injury-specific, immediate care. Prehospital Disaster Med 2008;23(2): 195–201.
5. Dr Okie S. Pou and the hurricane—implications for patient care during disasters. N Engl J Med 2008;358(1):1–5.
6. deBoisblanc BP. Black Hawk, please come down: reflections on a hospital's struggle to survive in the wake of Hurricane Katrina. Am J Respir Crit Care Med 2005;172(10):1239–40.
7. Myae K. Six days in the delta. CMAJ 2008;179(1):30.
8. Chan EYT. The untold story of the Sichvan earthquake. The Lancet 2008;372: 359–62.
9. Grissom TE, Farmer JC. The provision of sophisticated critical care beyond the hospital: lessons from physiology and military experiences that apply to civil disaster medical response. Crit Care Med 2005;33(1 Suppl):S13–21.
10. Dara SI, Ashton RW, Farmer JC, et al. Worldwide disaster medical response: an historical perspective. Crit Care Med 2005;33(1 Suppl):S2–6.
11. Noji EK. Disasters: introduction and state of the art. Epidemiol Rev 2005;27:3–8.
12. Dara SI, Ashton RW, Farmer JC. Engendering enthusiasm for sustainable disaster critical care response: Why this is of consequence to critical care professionals? Crit Care. 2005;9(2):125–7.
13. Pou AM. Hurricane Katrina and disaster preparedness. N Engl J Med 2008; 358(14):1524.
14. Noji EK. Creating a health care agenda for the Department of Homeland Security. Manag Care 2003;12(11 Suppl):7–12.
15. Michael WS, Julia AM. Chemical–biological terrorism and its impact on children. Pediatrics 2006;118(3):1267–78.
16. About FEMA. Available at: http://www.fema.gov/about/index.shtm. Accessed September 6, 2008.
17. Handler JA, Gillam M, Kirsch TD, et al. Metrics in the science of surge. Acad Emerg Med 2006;13(11):1173–8.
18. Kanter RK, Moran JR. Pediatric hospital and intensive care unit capacity in regional disasters: expanding capacity by altering standards of care. Pediatrics 2007;119(1):94–100.
19. Ksiazek TG, Erdman D, Goldsmith CS, et al. A novel coronavirus associated with severe acute respiratory syndrome. N Engl J Med 2003;348(20):1953–66.

20. Blackbourne LH. Combat damage control surgery. Crit Care Med 2008; 36(Suppl 7):S304–10.
21. Beekley AC. Damage control resuscitation: a sensible approach to the exsanguinating surgical patient. Crit Care Med 2008;36(7 Suppl):S267–74.
22. Birnbaum ML. Times have changed. Prehospital Disaster Med 2003;18(4):276–7.
23. Frykberg ER. Disaster and mass casualty management: a commentary on the American College of Surgeons position statement. J Am Coll Surg 2003; 197(5):857–9.
24. Waeckerle JF, Seamans S, Whiteside M, et al. Executive summary: developing objectives, content, and competencies for the training of emergency medical technicians, emergency physicians, and emergency nurses to care for casualties resulting from nuclear, biological, or chemical incidents. Ann Emerg Med 2001;37(6):587–601.
25. Moore EE, Knudson MM, Schwab CW, et al. Military-civilian collaboration in trauma care and the senior visiting surgeon program. N Engl J Med 2007; 357(26):2723–7.
26. Collins ST. Emergency medical support units to critical care transport teams in Iraq. Crit Care Nurs Clin North Am 2008;20(1):1–11, v.
27. Carlton PK Jr, Jenkins DH. The mobile patient. Crit Care Med 2008;36(7 Suppl): S255–7.
28. Grathwohl KW, Venticinque SG, Blackbourne LH, et al. The evolution of military trauma and critical care medicine: applications for civilian medical care systems. Crit Care Med 2008;36(Suppl 7):S253–4.
29. Drosten C, Gunther S, Preiser W, et al. Identification of a novel coronavirus in patients with severe acute respiratory syndrome. N Engl J Med 2003;348(20): 1967–76.
30. Teich JM, Wagner MM, Mackenzie CF, et al. The informatics response in disaster, terrorism, and war. J Am Med Inform Assoc 2002;9(2):97–104.
31. Auf der Heide E. The importance of evidence-based disaster planning. Ann Emerg Med 2006;47(1):34–49.
32. Baker MS. Creating order from chaos: part I: triage, initial care, and tactical considerations in mass casualty and disaster response. Mil Med 2007;172(3): 232–6.
33. Seynaeve G, Archer F, Fisher J, et al. International standards and guidelines on education and training for the multi-disciplinary health response to major events that threaten the health status of a community. Prehospital Disaster Med 2004; 19(2):S17–30.
34. Farmer JC. Respiratory issues in aeromedical patient transport. Respir Care Clin N Am 1996;2(3):391–400.
35. Szalados JE. Critical care teams managing floor patients: the continuing evolution of hospitals into intensive care units? [comment]. Crit Care Med 2004;32(4): 1071–2.
36. Kvetan V. Intensive care in a field hospital in an urban disaster area: Are we ready? Crit Care Med 2003;31(5):1589–90.
37. Hick JL, Hanfling D, Burstein JL, et al. Health care facility and community strategies for patient care surge capacity. Ann Emerg Med 2004;44(3):253–61.
38. Hatch M, Ron E, Bouville A, et al. The Chernobyl disaster: cancer following the accident at the Chernobyl nuclear power plant. Epidemiol Rev 2005;27:56–66.
39. Rahu M. Health effects of the Chernobyl accident: fears, rumours and the truth. Eur J Cancer 2003;39(3):295–9.
40. Radiation disasters and children. Pediatrics 2003;111(6 Pt 1):1455–66.

41. Turai I, Veress K, Gunalp B, et al. Medical response to radiation incidents and radionuclear threats [see comment]. BMJ 2004;328(7439):568–72.

42. Bar Joseph N, Reisfeld D, Tirosh E, et al. Neurobehavioral and cognitive performances of children exposed to low-dose radiation in the Chernobyl accident: the Israeli Chernobyl Health Effects Study. Am J Epidemiol 2004;160(5):453–9.

43. Mettler FA Jr, Voelz GL. Major radiation exposure—what to expect and how to respond. N Engl J Med 2002;346(20):1554–61.

44. Burnham JW, Franco J. Radiation. Crit Care Clin 2005;21(4):785–813, vii–viii.

45. Koenig KL, Goans RE, Hatchett RJ, et al. Medical treatment of radiological casualties: current concepts. Ann Emerg Med 2005;45(6):643–52.

46. Hammond J, Brooks J. The World Trade Center attack. Helping the helpers: the role of critical incident stress management. Crit Care 2001;5(6):315–7.

47. Broughton E. The Bhopal disaster and its aftermath: a review. Environ Health 2005;4(1):6.

48. Ranjan N, Sarangi S, Padmanabhan VT, et al. Methyl isocyanate exposure and growth patterns of adolescents in Bhopal. JAMA 2003;290(14):1856–7.

49. Kirk MA, Deaton ML. Bringing order out of chaos: effective strategies for medical response to mass chemical exposure. Emerg Med Clin North Am 2007;25(2):527–48 [Abstract xi].

50. Clarke SF, Chilcott RP, Wilson JC, et al. Decontamination of multiple casualties who are chemically contaminated: a challenge for acute hospitals. Prehospital Disaster Med 2008;23(2):175–81.

51. Baker DJ. Critical care requirements after mass toxic agent release. Crit Care Med 2005;33(1 Suppl):S66–74.

52. Lorin HG, Kulling PE. The Bhopal tragedy—What has Swedish disaster medicine planning learned from it? J Emerg Med 1986;4(4):311–6.

53. Tucker JB. National health and medical services response to incidents of chemical and biological terrorism. JAMA 1997;278(5):362–8.

54. Johannigman JA. Disaster preparedness: It's all about me. Crit Care Med 2005;33(1 Suppl):S22–8.

55. Varma R, Varma DR. The Bhopal disaster of 1984. Bull Sci Technol Soc 2005;25(1):37–45.

56. Arnold JL. Disaster medicine in the 21st century: future hazards, vulnerabilities, and risk. Prehospital Disaster Med 2002;17(1):3–11.

57. Okumura T, Ninomiya N, Ohta M. The chemical disaster response system in Japan. Prehospital Disaster Med 2003;18(3):189–92.

58. Keim ME, Pesik N, Twum-Danso NA. Lack of hospital preparedness for chemical terrorism in a major US city: 1996–2000. Prehospital Disaster Med 2003;18(3):193–9.

59. Tur-Kaspa I, Lev EI, Hendler I, et al. Preparing hospitals for toxicological mass casualties events. Crit Care Med 1999;27(5):1004–8.

60. Farmer JC, Carlton PK Jr. Who is 9-1-1 to the 9-1-1? Crit Care Med 2002;30(10):2397–8.

61. Devereaux AV, Dichter JR, Christian MD, et al. Definitive care for the critically ill during a disaster: a framework for allocation of scarce resources in mass critical care: from a Task Force for Mass Critical Care summit meeting, January 26–27, 2007, Chicago, IL. Chest 2008;133(5 Suppl):51S–66S.

62. Okumura S, Okumura T, Ishimatsu S, et al. Clinical review: Tokyo—protecting the health care worker during a chemical mass casualty event: an important issue of continuing relevance. Crit Care 2005;9(4):397–400.

63. Mallonee S, Shariat S, Stennies G, et al. Physical injuries and fatalities resulting from the Oklahoma City bombing. JAMA 1996;276(5):382–7.

64. Anteau CM, Williams LA. The Oklahoma bombing. Lessons learned. Crit Care Nurs Clin North Am 1997;9(2):231–6.
65. Maningas PA, Robison M, Mallonee S. The EMS response to the Oklahoma City bombing. Prehospital Disaster Med 1997;12(2):80–5.
66. Glenshaw MT, Vernick JS, Li G, et al. Preventing fatalities in building bombings: What can we learn from the Oklahoma City bombing? Disaster Med Public Health Prep 2007;1(1):27–31.
67. Rhoads J, Pearman T, Rick S. PTSD: therapeutic interventions post-Katrina. Crit Care Nurs Clin North Am 2008;20(1):73–81, vii.
68. Cruz MA, Burger R, Keim M. The first 24 hours of the World Trade Center attacks of 2001—the Centers for Disease Control and Prevention emergency phase response. Prehospital Disaster Med 2007;22(6):473–7.
69. Wang D, Sava J, Sample G, et al. The Pentagon and 9/11. Crit Care Med 2005; 33(1 Suppl):S42–7.
70. Roccaforte JD, Cushman JG. Disaster preparedness, triage, and surge capacity for hospital definitive care areas: optimizing outcomes when demands exceed resources. Anesthesiol Clin 2007;25(1):161–77, xi.
71. Kirschenbaum L, Keene A, O'Neill P, et al. The experience at St. Vincent's Hospital, Manhattan, on September 11, 2001: preparedness, response, and lessons learned. Crit Care Med 2005;33(1 Suppl):S48–52.
72. Roccaforte JD. The World Trade Center attack. Observations from New York's Bellevue Hospital. Crit Care 2001;5(6):307–9.
73. Burkle FM Jr. Integrating international responses to complex emergencies, unconventional war, and terrorism. Crit Care Med 2005;33(1 Suppl):S7–12.
74. Burkle FM Jr, Hayden R. The concept of assisted management of large-scale disasters by horizontal organizations. Prehospital Disaster Med 2001;16(3): 128–37.
75. Grasso MA. Handheld computer application for medical disaster management. AMIA Annu Symp Proc 2006;932.
76. Shamir MY, Rivkind A, Weissman C, et al. Conventional terrorist bomb incidents and the intensive care unit. Curr Opin Crit Care 2005;11(6):580–4.
77. Ryan J, Montgomery H. The London attacks—preparedness: terrorism and the medical response. N Engl J Med 2005;353(6):543–5.
78. Weinstein RA. Planning for epidemics—the lessons of SARS. N Engl J Med 2004;350(23):2332–4.
79. Diaz JH. Global climate changes, natural disasters, and travel health risks. J Travel Med 2006;13(6):361–72.
80. Ho AS, Sung JJ, Chan-Yeung M. An outbreak of severe acute respiratory syndrome among hospital workers in a community hospital in Hong Kong. Ann Intern Med 2003;139(7):564–7.
81. Emanuel EJ. The lessons of SARS. Ann Intern Med 2003;139(7):589–91.
82. Varkey P, Poland GA, Cockerill FR 3rd, et al. Confronting bioterrorism: physicians on the front line. Mayo Clin Proc 2002;77(7):661–72.
83. Ferguson NM, Cummings DA, Fraser C, et al. Strategies for mitigating an influenza pandemic. Nature 2006;442(7101):448–52.
84. Gomersall CD, Joynt GM, Ho OM, et al. Transmission of SARS to healthcare workers. The experience of a Hong Kong ICU. Intensive Care Med 2006; 32(4):564–9.
85. Christian MD, Hawryluck L, Wax RS, et al. Development of a triage protocol for critical care during an influenza pandemic. CMAJ 2006;175(11):1377–81.

86. Ruderman C, Tracy CS, Bensimon CM, et al. On pandemics and the duty to care: Whose duty? Who cares? BMC Med Ethics 2006;7:E5.
87. Challen K, Bentley A, Bright J, et al. Clinical review: mass casualty triage—pandemic influenza and critical care. Crit Care 2007;11(2):212.
88. Loutfy MR, Wallington T, Rutledge T, et al. Hospital preparedness and SARS. Emerg Infect Dis 2004;10(5):771–6.
89. Hick JL, O'Laughlin DT. Concept of operations for triage of mechanical ventilation in an epidemic. Acad Emerg Med 2006;13(2):223–9.
90. Gomersall CD, Loo S, Joynt GM, et al. Pandemic preparedness. Curr Opin Crit Care 2007;13(6):742–7.
91. Mehta AC, Prakash UB, Garland R, et al. American College of Chest Physicians and American Association for Bronchology [corrected] consensus statement: prevention of flexible bronchoscopy–associated infection. Chest 2005;128(3):1742–55.
92. Kohl PA, O'Rourke AP, Schmidman DL, et al. The Sumatra-Andaman earthquake and tsunami of 2004: the hazards, events, and damage. Prehospital Disaster Med 2005;20(6):355–63.
93. de Ville de Goyet C. Health lessons learned from the recent earthquakes and tsunami in Asia. Prehospital Disaster Med 2007;22(1):15–21.
94. Cranmer HH. The public health emergency in Indonesia—one patient at a time. N Engl J Med 2005;352(10):965.
95. Lamberg L. As tsunami recovery proceeds, experts ponder lessons for future disasters. JAMA 2005;294(8):889–90.
96. Kapila M, McGarry N, Emerson E, et al. Health aspects of the tsunami disaster in Asia. Prehospital Disaster Med 2005;20(6):368–77.
97. Kripalani M. India pulls together amid disaster 2005. Available at: http://meaindia. nic.in/bestoftheweb/2005/01/11bw01.htm. Accessed Sep 6, 2008.
98. de Ville de Goyet C. Stop propagating disaster myths. Lancet 2000;356(9231): 762–4.
99. Smith J, Fink S, Hansch S, et al. Session 1.4: health services delivery: a critical review of experience. Prehospital Disaster Med 2005;20(6):389–92.
100. Crippen D. The World Trade Center attack. Similarities to the 1988 earthquake in Armenia: time to teach the public life-supporting first aid? Crit Care 2001;5(6): 312–4.
101. Cranmer HH. Hurricane Katrina. Volunteer work—logistics first. N Engl J Med 2005;353(15):1541–4.
102. Noji EK. Public health in the aftermath of disasters. BMJ 2005;330(7504): 1379–81.
103. Lambrew JM, Shalala DE. Federal health policy response to Hurricane Katrina: What it was and what it could have been. JAMA 2006;296(11):1394–7.
104. Gheytanchi A, Joseph L, Gierlach E, et al. The dirty dozen: twelve failures of the Hurricane Katrina response and how psychology can help. Am Psychol 2007; 62(2):118–30.
105. Nates JL, Moyer VA. Lessons from Hurricane Katrina, tsunamis, and other disasters. Lancet 2005;366(9492):1144–6.
106. Kessler RC. Hurricane Katrina's impact on the care of survivors with chronic medical conditions. J Gen Intern Med 2007;22(9):1225–30.
107. Miller AC, Arquilla B. Chronic diseases and natural hazards: impact of disasters on diabetic, renal, and cardiac patients. Prehospital Disaster Med 2008;23(2):185–94.
108. Curiel TJ. Murder or mercy? Hurricane Katrina and the need for disaster training. N Engl J Med 2006;355(20):2067–9.

109. Barry M, Hughes JM. Talking dirty—the politics of clean water and sanitation. N Engl J Med 2008;359(8):784–7.
110. Bonnett CJ, Peery BN, Cantrill SV, et al. Surge capacity: a proposed conceptual framework. Am J Emerg Med 2007;25(3):297–306.
111. Devereaux A, Christian MD, Dichter JR, et al. Summary of suggestions from the Task Force for Mass Critical Care summit, January 26–27, 2007. Chest 2008; 133(5 Suppl):1S–7S.
112. Sternberg E, Lee GC, Huard D. Counting crises: US hospital evacuations, 1971–1999. Prehospital Disaster Med 2004;19(2):150–7.
113. Shatz DV, Wolcott K, Fairburn JB. Response to hurricane disasters. Surg Clin North Am 2006;86(3):545–55.
114. Blackwell T, Bosse M. Use of an innovative design mobile hospital in the medical response to Hurricane Katrina. Ann Emerg Med 2007;49(5):580–8.
115. Boyajian-O'Neill LA, Gronewold LM, Glaros AG, et al. Physician licensure during disasters: a National Survey of State Medical Boards. JAMA 2008;299(2):169–71.
116. Nates JL. Combined external and internal hospital disaster: impact and response in a Houston trauma center intensive care unit. Crit Care Med 2004; 32(3):686–90.
117. Schultz CH, Koenig KL, Lewis RJ. Implications of hospital evacuation after the Northridge, California, earthquake. N Engl J Med 2003;348(14):1349–55.
118. Schultz CH, Koenig KL, Auf der Heide E, et al. Benchmarking for hospital evacuation: a critical data collection tool. Prehospital Disaster Med 2005;20(5): 331–42.
119. Hawryluck L, Lapinsky SE, Stewart TE. Clinical review: SARS—lessons in disaster management. Crit Care 2005;9(4):384–9.
120. Mattox KL. Hurricanes Katrina and Rita: role of individuals and collaborative networks in mobilizing/coordinating societal and professional resources for major disasters. Crit Care 2006;10(1):205.
121. Greenough PG, Lappi MD, Hsu EB, et al. Burden of disease and health status among Hurricane Katrina–displaced persons in shelters: a population-based cluster sample. Ann Emerg Med 2008;51(4):426–32.
122. Vest JR, Valadez AM. Health conditions and risk factors of sheltered persons displaced by Hurricane Katrina. Prehospital Disaster Med 2006;21(2 Suppl 2): 55–8.
123. Howe E, Victor D, Price EG. Chief complaints, diagnoses, and medications prescribed seven weeks post-Katrina in New Orleans. Prehospital Disaster Med 2008;23(1):41–7.
124. Arnold JL. Disaster myths and Hurricane Katrina 2005: Can public officials and the media learn to provide responsible crisis communication during disasters? Prehospital Disaster Med 2006;21(1):1–3.
125. Burkle FM Jr, Noji EK. Health and politics in the 2003 war with Iraq: lessons learned. Lancet 2004;364(9442):1371–5.
126. Department of Defense. U.S. casualty status 2008. Available at: http://www.defenselink.mil/news/casualty.pdf. Accessed Sep 6, 2008.
127. Grathwohl KW, Venticinque SG. Organizational characteristics of the austere intensive care unit: the evolution of military trauma and critical care medicine; applications for civilian medical care systems. Crit Care Med 2008;36 (Suppl 7):S275–83.
128. Venticinque SG, Grathwohl KW. Critical care in the austere environment: providing exceptional care in unusual places. Crit Care Med 2008;36(Suppl 7): S284–92.

129. Johannigman JA. Maintaining the continuum of en route care. Crit Care Med 2008;36(Suppl 7):S377-82.
130. Gawande A. Casualties of war—military care for the wounded from Iraq and Afghanistan. N Engl J Med 2004;351(24):2471-5.
131. Roudebush JG. Today's commitment: Transforming military medicine. Air Force Defense Strategy and Transformation Seminar Series. Washington, DC; November 15, 2006.
132. Beninati W, Meyer MT, Carter TE. The critical care air transport program. Crit Care Med 2008;36(7 Suppl):S370-6.
133. Rice DH, Kotti G, Beninati W. Clinical review: critical care transport and austere critical care. Crit Care 2008;12(2):207.
134. Fang R, Pruitt VM, Dorlac GR, et al. Critical care at Landstuhl Regional Medical Center. Crit Care Med 2008;36(Suppl 7):S383-7.
135. Colombo CJ, Mount CA, Popa CA. Critical care medicine at Walter Reed Army Medical Center in support of the global war on terrorism. Crit Care Med 2008; 36(Suppl 7):S388-94.
136. Kashani KB, Farmer JC. The support of severe respiratory failure beyond the hospital and during transportation. Curr Opin Crit Care 2006;12(1):43-9.

Plagues in the ICU: A Brief History of Community-Acquired Epidemic and Endemic Transmissible Infections Leading to Intensive Care Admission

R. Bruce Light, MD

KEYWORDS

- Infectious diseases in the ICU
- History of intensive care medicine
- Epidemic infectious diseases

From its very inception Intensive Care Medicine has been plagued by plagues. Indeed, infection is such a common and diverse theme in everyday ICU work that any article about the history of the problem must be somewhat selective. This article highlights eight different infection syndromes acquired in the community, that is, primarily transmissible from loci in the environment or from other people. All are serious infections frequently leading to ICU admission for shock, respiratory failure, or both. The short historical vignettes in this article are aimed at giving younger members of our specialty, who will not have personal memories of all of these events (as, unfortunately, some of us do) some sense of the variety and difficulty of the challenges posed by new infectious diseases, and examples of how, in each case, the scientific and critical care communities rose to those challenges. Each documented outbreak of disease was a surprise (and often a mystery) and the source of much public consternation, and each has taught us valuable lessons in improving the diagnosis, treatment, and prevention of infectious disease.

St. Boniface General Hospital, 409 Tache Avenue, Winnipeg, Manitoba R2H 2A6, Canada
E-mail address: blight@sbgh.mb.ca

Crit Care Clin 25 (2009) 67–81
doi:10.1016/j.ccc.2008.11.002
0749-0704/08/$ – see front matter © 2009 Elsevier Inc. All rights reserved.

POLIOMYELITIS

Intensive care, the epitome of the application of modern technology to medicine, arguably began as a response to the increasing numbers of older children and young adults developing paralytic polio during the early 1950s. Severe paralytic polio itself turns out to have been among the products of increasing modernity in the Western world.

Clinical recognition of the syndromes associated with the polio virus date back about 200 years. The fact that the disease was caused by a transmissible viral particle was demonstrated by 1908. Until early in the twentieth century the virus was readily transmitted throughout the population almost continuously by personal contact and by the fecal–oral route via water. The result was that most people's first exposure to the virus occurred in infancy. At this age most infections resulted in a clinically unapparent infection, in part due to partial protection by maternal antibody, after which lifelong immunity was established. Only a few suffered a paralytic episode with the infection, at the time termed "infantile paralysis."[1]

As hygienic standards of the advanced economy nations rose throughout the first half of the century, early childhood exposure to the virus declined. An increasing fraction of the population had their first exposure in late childhood or during young adulthood. In these age groups the likelihood that the infection will cause a paralytic syndrome is greatly increased, so both the incidence of clinically recognized infection and that of paralysis rose. By the early 1950s clinically recognized cases had reached 15–25 annually for every 100,000 people in the United States, making it a major public health concern and a source of a great deal of fear in the general populace.[2]

More than 90% of polio virus infections are asymptomatic. However, at the more severe end of the clinical spectrum are the paralytic syndromes which range from paralysis of one or more limbs ("spinal polio") to syndromes with respiratory muscle or bulbar paralysis ("respiratory polio" or "bulbospinal polio") with loss of respiratory or upper airway muscle function or both. These more severe outcomes rise in incidence from about 0.1% in infants to more than 1% in older children and adults.

In the early part of the century development of polio with bulbar involvement was associated with a death rate of greater than 90%, generally from respiratory failure. Use of a mechanical respirator to try to avert death was first attempted at the Children's Hospital in Boston in 1928, using an "iron lung."[3] The machine was basically a sealed box with a hole at one end for the patient's head to protrude, attached to two vacuum cleaners. The motors were then cycled to alternately create vacuum inside the box, expanding the patient's chest and causing the patient to inhale through the mouth (outside the box), then allowing air back into the box to permit exhalation. The design was further improved in 1931, and the machines came into increasingly broad use throughout North America and Europe during the severe outbreaks of the 1930s. Adoption of this therapy resulted in a significant reduction in mortality during these years.

Iron lungs, however, were cumbersome, difficult to use when trying to provide nursing care, and expensive. A more cost-effective and user-friendly approach to providing respiratory support was clearly needed. This finally came by bringing the positive pressure ventilation (PPV) concept out of the operating room. PPV was first used for respiratory support for polio victims at Blegdam Hospital in Copenhagen, Denmark, an innovation attributable to Danish anesthetist Bjorn Ibsen.[4] During this large outbreak in 1952, some 200 medical students were put to work hand-ventilating dozens of patients through tracheostomies until the worst of the paralytic phase of the illness had passed, often several weeks. The concept quickly spread elsewhere and was widely adopted, yielding substantial reductions in mortality. For reasons of efficiency and convenience, patients needing respiratory support were often grouped in a single location where the necessary expertise and equipment were available. The introduction of PPV into a defined area of the hospital used to support respiratory failure was the genesis of the modern ICU and represents a signal event in the development of the field of Critical Care Medicine.

The introduction of effective vaccines, the Salk (inactivated) vaccine in 1952 and later the Sabin (live attenuated oral) vaccine in 1962, immediately and dramatically reduced the incidence of polio to less than one per 100,000 population by the early 1960s and the incidence continued to fall thereafter. The last case of wild strain polio in North America was reported in 1979, and since that time the only cases of paralytic polio have been rare instances of disease due to variants of the live oral vaccine strain.

Polio does, however, still contribute to illnesses that may require intensive care in the form of the "post-polio syndrome." This occurs in patients who survived paralytic polio decades ago and who, over the years, develop a gradual decline in function in the originally affected nerves and muscles which can years later once again threaten them with disability and, in some cases, respiratory failure requiring intensive care.[5]

LEGIONNAIRE'S DISEASE

In July 1976, American Legion members attending a convention at a hotel in Philadelphia suddenly began falling ill with an acute febrile illness with pneumonia, often associated with extrapulmonary symptoms such as myalgia or diarrhea.[6] Many developed acute respiratory failure requiring mechanical ventilatory support in ICU. Over 200 were affected and 34 died, an alarming mortality rate, especially since physicians caring for the patients had no idea what was causing the illness. Conventional microbiologic investigations yielded no convincing pathogens despite intensive investigation for the usual bacteria and viruses and other potential pathogens. Epidemiologic and various biologic investigations were quickly implemented by local health authorities and by the Centers for Disease Control and Prevention (CDC). These showed that the disease was likely airborne and that it occurred more frequently in older individuals who had underlying lung disease, smoked, or were relatively immunocompromised. Analysis of the likelihood of death revealed that those who received tetracyclines or macrolide antibiotics were more likely to survive than those who received only beta-lactams. However, no causal agent was uncovered, though many potential causes were excluded—most known bacteria and viruses, many biologic toxins and many environmental agents such as toxic chemicals and metals.

In 1977, Joseph McDade and Charles Shepard of the CDC reported the isolation of a novel fastidious gram-negative bacillus from the available clinical specimens.[7] They named it *Legionella pneumophila.* This discovery was quickly followed by an explosion of knowledge about the organism and its ecology, antimicrobial susceptibility, and of other bacteria within the genus. Over time, demonstration that it was a widely occurring colonizer of brackish water, particularly in air conditioners, cooling towers, and water heaters and pipes, led to the implication of these reservoirs in several hundred outbreaks of the disease worldwide, especially in hospitals and other public health institutions, and hotels. Thus began widespread development of regulations and guidelines for limiting the degree of colonization of these water sources by *Legionella*, resulting in a reduction in the size, number, and scope of subsequent outbreaks.

Since the initial description of the disease, *Legionella* has, of course, been shown to be one of the major causes of community-acquired pneumonia (CAP), particularly in the more severe subset requiring ICU care; this fact underlies the major lesson from the outbreak—the nearly universal recommendation for inclusion of antimicrobial therapy for Legionell spp in any treatment regimen for severe CAP without another obvious cause. Although we now know that no amount of continuing effort can completely eliminate this organism from our environment, and that we will continue to see endemic cases, we also know that clusters of cases should trigger an investigation into finding the point source of the outbreak, a situation that continues to occur several times a year somewhere in the world.

In addition, the 1976 Philadelphia outbreak that defined "Legionnaire's Disease" was the first in the modern ICU era to demonstrate that major unknown infectious disease syndromes of severe consequence still exist, presaging the new infectious disease syndromes to be discovered in the years that followed.

STAPHYLOCOCCAL TOXIC SHOCK SYNDROME

In the late 1970s, emergency rooms and ICUs throughout North America began to see an increasing number of young menstruating women presenting with a previously little-known syndrome characterized by sudden onset of a high fever, often associated with vomiting and diarrhea, quickly followed by severe hypotension. Early in the course most patients developed a diffuse macular rash, often with mucous membrane inflammation, with subsequent desquamation during convalescence. Patients frequently required massive fluid resuscitation because of systemic capillary leak, as well as vasopressor support, mechanical ventilation for adult respiratory distress syndrome, and even renal replacement therapy for acute renal failure, complicating the shock episode. One of the early clusters of observed cases was reported in 1978, and the term "toxic shock syndrome" was coined based on the isolation of an exotoxin-producing Staphylococcus aureus from mucosal surfaces or the site of a minor infection in the absence of bacteremia.[8]

As the case numbers rapidly increased case definitions for the syndrome were formulated and epidemiologic studies mounted. By 1980, over 1000 cases had been formally reported to the CDC.[9] The case fatality rate was reported to be as high as 15% in the more severe cases included in the earliest reports, falling to about 3%–5% as recognition of the syndrome improved. By this time there were clear epidemiologic links between the syndrome and menstrual use of high-absorbency tampons which were often left in place longer than less absorbent products. Colonization of the tampon with Staphylococcus aureus was also implicated, consistent with the postulated toxin-mediated disease mechanism.[10] Within months of these revelations the main manufacturer of the implicated tampons withdrew them from the market and women began changing tampons with greater frequency or stopped using them at the urging of public health authorities. The incidence of the syndrome immediately began to fall and within a few years, with the changing of use patterns of tampons and changes in their manufacture, toxic shock syndrome disappeared, for the most part, but not entirely, from the ICU.

Even at the height of TSS incidence in the United States, about 6% of the cases reported were nonmenstrual and 4% were in males.[11] Subsequent development of the knowledge that the clinical syndrome was due to strains of Staphylococcus aureus that secrete a particular toxin (Toxic shock syndrome toxin 1, or TSST-1), which is both absorbable from mucosal surfaces and capable of producing a profound shock syndrome even in the absence of significant invasive infection, soon led to the more widespread recognition of the nonmenstrual toxic shock syndrome. This syndrome, which was almost certainly extant before but little-recognized, was perhaps the main lesson from the outbreak: even trivial staphylococcal skin or wound infections or mucosal surface colonization in the presence of a foreign body such as a nasal pack for nosebleed can lead to a severe shock syndrome if the organism is present and produces this toxin or one of several related ones. The recognition of the staphylococcal toxic shock syndrome also led to increasing understanding of the role of "superantigens" as a mechanism of disease—bacterial toxins capable of activating a large fraction (up to 20%) of the total T-lymphocyte population. Such superantigens have since been implicated in a number of other disease syndromes, among them the streptococcal toxic shock syndrome (see below).

Over the past two decades, the incidence of menstrual and nonmenstrual staphylococcal TSS has been about one per 100,000 population in most areas. Busy ICUs will, therefore, continue to see occasional cases. However, there is some recent evidence that case numbers may be on the rise again in at least some areas, possibly because of a resurgence in the prevalence of toxin-producing strains in the community.[12]

PNEUMOCYSTIS JIROVICII (FORMERLY CARINII)

In 1980, physicians working in infectious diseases and critical care medicine thought they knew all about Pneumocystosis. The organism, then thought to be a protozoon, had been first described in 1909 by Carlos Chagas in Brazil, and since then had been clearly implicated as a cause of interstitial pneumonia in debilitated and malnourished children (in the aftermath of World War II) and, later, a cause of severe opportunistic pneumonia in immunocompromised patients, usually those being treated with high-dose corticosteroids for connective tissue diseases or lymphoreticular neoplasms.[13] In these patients it caused an impressively aggressive bilateral pneumonia leading to acute respiratory failure. This pneumonia was notoriously difficult to definitively diagnose, requiring bronchoscopy or open lung biopsy to demonstrate the small numbers of characteristic Pneumocystis organisms on special silver stains of clinical specimens. The mainstay of treatment at that time was pentamidine, generally given intramuscularly, giving way to trimethoprim/sulfamethoxazole after the publication in 1978 of a randomized clinical trial showing that it was at least as effective and generally better tolerated.[14]

In the early 1980s, a new form of the infection began to be seen with regularity. Young men began to present to hospital with a rather more indolent diffuse bilateral pneumonia that nevertheless went on to cause respiratory failure and which, when investigated, proved to be due to Pneumocystis.[15] The course of the disease was quite different from what physicians had been used to up to then. It began more gradually, progressed at a slower pace and was associated with a much lesser systemic inflammatory response. Microscopy of respiratory specimens revealed exponentially more organisms than previously seen, such that many patients could be diagnosed from sputum specimens rather than bronchoscopy, and biopsy was virtually never needed. Nobody had any idea why this was happening, although it quickly became apparent that the underlying cause of the infection was a new form of severe deficiency of cell-mediated immunity.

Epidemiologic investigations were soon underway. Patterns began to emerge. Many of the young men were Haitian or had been to Haiti. Many were homosexual, bisexual, or had worked in the sex trade; others had abused intravenous drugs. The many fewer women with the disease had similar exposures. Theories proliferated. Was it immunologic exhaustion from exposure to too many microbial stresses? Toxins? Drugs used in the sex trade? Multiple and synergistic viral infections?

Through the early 1980s, the case load grew. ICUs throughout North America and, later, in Europe and elsewhere, saw increasing numbers of young people, mainly men, with severe respiratory failure due to Pneumocystis pneumonia. By 1981 they were being called patients with acquired immunodeficiency syndrome (AIDS) on the basis of demonstration of low numbers of CD4 lymphocytes in the blood, but the cause remained unclear. Then, in 1984, Montagnier and Barre-Sinoussi at the Pasteur Institute in France isolated a viral pathogen that they named Lymphadenopathy-Associated Virus (LAV). At the National Institutes of Health in the United States, Gallo demonstrated that the virus (which he referred to as Human T-cell Leukemia Virus III, based on an unproven relationship to other viruses he had previously discovered) definitively caused AIDS. The virus, now called human immunodeficiency virus (HIV)-1 was isolated and described and the first diagnostic kits devised, resolving the mystery of causation. Montagnier and Barre-Sinoussi would eventually win the Nobel Prize in Medicine in 2008 for their contribution.

During the 1980s, patients continued to present with severe pneumonia requiring respiratory support and intensive antimicrobial therapy, often with less than satisfactory results. As knowledge progressed, HIV-associated Pneumocystis infection in the ICU changed its face several times over the years. At the beginning of the epidemic, most patients presenting for care with HIV/AIDS and Pneumocystosis were severely ill with diffuse pneumonia and hypoxemic respiratory failure and many died, 80%–90% in most centers, prompting widespread debate about whether such patients should even be admitted to ICU for mechanical ventilatory support. However, as experience with the disease developed it became clear that an early and aggressive approach could improve prognosis. It was found that in the AIDS population even minor respiratory symptoms with few or no abnormalities on chest radiograph could be due to Pneumocystis infection in the earlier stages, and that even modest degrees of arterial oxygen desaturation signaled impending respiratory failure. Earlier bronchoscopy for diagnosis followed by prompt antimicrobial therapy, with pentamidine predominantly in the early 80s and later primarily with trimethoprim/sulfamethoxazole, led to overall mortality rates falling to the 50%–60% range by the middle of the decade.

The advent of systemic corticosteroids therapy for early respiratory failure in AIDS-associated Pneumocystosis was then shown to further reduce the numbers of patients progressing to advanced respiratory failure, leading to reductions in the numbers of cases needing ICU admission and further reducing overall mortality rates to the 15%–20% range.[16] But for patients requiring ICU care mortality rates were as high as before the use of steroids and often higher, likely related to the fact that most patients developing respiratory failure had already failed to improve or had progressed despite intensive antimicrobial and corticosteroid therapy.[17]

Along with these developments in management of the disease, progress was being made on HIV itself. Following identification of the virus in 1984, there soon followed increasingly reliable diagnostic tests for the infection, leading to earlier identification of cases and monitoring of CD4 lymphocyte counts. By the early 1990s, studies supporting widespread use of chemoprophylaxis against Pneumocystis in all patients with CD4 counts <200/mm³ were available and became standard public health agency recommendations. Pneumocystosis, which in the 1980s and 1990s was one of the principal causes of hypoxemic respiratory failure in many ICUs in North America and western Europe, began to decline rapidly in incidence, becoming relatively uncommon even before the widespread adoption of highly active antiretroviral therapy, which has, since the mid-1990s, caused the disease to all but disappear from our ICUs.

Although many lessons can be drawn from the battle against AIDS-related pneumoncystis pneumonia during the 1980s and 1990s, for ICU and infectious diseases practitioners one of the main ones comes from the sad fact that once patients had developed full-blown hypoxemic respiratory failure even the best intensive care could only deliver 20% survival rates. The really large gains in survival came not from better ICU technology but from pre-empting the disease on multiple fronts, including earlier diagnosis of HIV infection, early diagnosis and antimicrobial treatment of pneumonia, steroid treatment of early respiratory failure, antimicrobial prophylactic regimens and, later, effective antiretroviral therapy.

HANTAVIRUS PULMONARY SYNDROME

Until 1993, the only members of the Bunyaviridae family of viruses known to cause disease in North America were members of the genus *Bunyavirus*, all causing mosquito-borne viral encephalitis, mainly in children (California encephalitis). Other members of the family were known to cause serious febrile illnesses, encephalitides and hemorrhagic-fevers in Africa and Asia (Rift Valley Fever, Crimean-Congo Hemorrhagic Fever, Hemorrhagic Fever with Renal Syndrome). However, in the spring of 1993 wetter-than-usual conditions in the American Southwest led to increased availability of food for deer mice, leading to a population explosion and increasing movement of rodents into human-occupied spaces, increasing the chance that humans might be exposed to the rodents and their excreta.

In rapid succession, several previously healthy young people, mainly Navajos, presented to health care institutions in the Four Corners area of the Southwestern United States, all with fulminant illnesses leading to shock and acute respiratory failure requiring ICU care. By early June that year, 24 cases had been identified and 12 had died.[18] In most cases the illness had started with fever and widespread myalgia, soon followed by cough, then by cardiovascular collapse due to a severe systemic capillary leak syndrome and by acute respiratory failure due to low-pressure pulmonary edema. In some cases the time from onset to ICU or death was as little as 24 hours, in others a few days.[19]

Remarkably, although no pathogen was initially identified from blood or tissues, in less than a month after the first report of a possible outbreak, serologic testing had demonstrated antibody cross-reactivity with a range of known pathogens of the Hantavirus group, suggesting that the disease was due to a previously unknown member of this group. Shortly thereafter exposure to deer mice and their excreta was implicated as the likely source of the infection.

The mortality rate for the early cases of hantavirus pulmonary syndrome (HPS) was extremely high—80% in the initially reported group of patients—mostly due to intractable shock and unsupportable hypoxemic respiratory failure due to acute respiratory distress syndrome (ARDS). However, this improved with clinical experience as it became evident that administration of large amounts of intravenous fluids in the face of profound capillary leak only resulted in much worse generalized and pulmonary edema, with little improvement in the shock state and only worsening of the respiratory failure. Management changed to an approach limiting the amount of fluid administered early in the course together with earlier institution of inotropic support, resulting in a much improved survival rate of about 60%, generally with minimal or no long-term sequelae in survivors.[20]

In subsequent years development of increasingly specific serologic and virologic testing has demonstrated that this disease had been present but unrecognized throughout North and South America long before this outbreak, and that there are several related viruses, each associated with a particular rodent, causing endemic disease and the occasional outbreak. By the mid-1990s, over 150 cases were reported in 25 states, mainly in the Southwest, and cases have since been reported in small numbers in most other states, Canada, Mexico, and South America, where several outbreaks have occurred. Whereas occasional cases continue to be seen in ICUs in all these areas, no further major outbreaks have yet occurred in the United States or Canada, though clearly remaining a threat under the right conditions; the only currently available preventive measure is avoiding rodent contact.[21]

Steven Simpson, MD, one of the intensivists at the Health Sciences Center in Albuquerque, New Mexico, who was closely involved in the initial Four Corners outbreak, points out that the event highlights several trends in subsequent disease outbreaks in North America. One is the extreme rapidity with which novel pathogens and potential pharmacotherapeutic agents can now be identified. Whereas the pathogen in the Legionnaire's outbreak took almost a year to identify, researchers identified the HPS pathogen and its source in just months. Computerized access to data and data analysis along with virtually instantaneous electronic transmission of information plays a central role in this development.

The initial HPS outbreak has several ICU-related lessons to teach us. While the aforementioned treatment strategies effective in a systemic capillary leak syndrome have been absorbed by the critical care community, it appears that one lesson taken to heart by the local ICU teams failed to disseminate to the broader ICU community. The initial outbreak was accompanied by a marked element of fear and concern among health care workers, including those in the ICU, and a significant level of panic in the local community; a combination of this fear, the requirement for rigorous quarantine precautions, and a marked increase in transfers to the ICU of any severely ill patients with symptoms remotely compatible with HPS resulted in some compromise of ICU operations, due to being completely overwhelmed. This might potentially have been avoided by an awareness that for an effective epidemic response, it is essential to include both hospital and ICU operations in each locale.

The outbreak also reinforces the principle that nearly all old and most new epidemic infectious diseases have their origin in close contact between humans and other species of animal, both wild and domestic, and new kinds and quantities of such contact are likely to cause new, or newly recognized, disease syndromes.

STREPTOCOCCAL TOXIC SHOCK SYNDROME AND NECROTIZING FASCIITIS

Streptococcus pyogenes was one of the first bacteria ever to be conclusively linked to human disease (puerperal infection associated with childbirth). However, over the past 125 years the nature of the diseases stemming from it has changed dramatically on several occasions. At the turn of the last century, it was well known as a cause of streptococcal pharyngitis, erysipelas, and wound infections. It also caused severe septicemic illnesses that frequently led to death. Osler[22] knew *Streptococcus pyogenes* as a principal cause of thoracic empyema following pneumonia or severe cases of scarlet fever, and also as a major cause of primary bacteremia with sepsis. These more severe manifestations of streptococcal infection became increasingly uncommon as the twentieth century progressed, particularly after the arrival of antibiotics mid-century.

Notably, Osler did not mention Streptococcus as a cause of necrotizing fasciitis or being associated with soft tissue necrosis in wound infections. This syndrome was first described by Meleney in 1924;[23] at that time, it was characteristically a slowly evolving gangrenous infection, usually of surgical wounds, which often responded well to debridement and was associated with a mortality rate of only 20%.[24]

For over a generation after the advent of the modern antibiotic era, *Streptococcus pyogenes* was seldom a problem that led to critical illness — soft tissue infections and the occasional bacteremia were generally very amenable to treatment; extensive surgery or drainage was seldom required, and cases requiring ICU support for shock or respiratory failure were rare. Beginning in the mid-1980s, medical practitioners in centers across North America and Europe began seeing previously unknown forms of severe streptococcal disease, soon labeled Streptococcal necrotizing fasciitis and Streptococcal toxic shock syndrome.[25]

Streptococcal toxic shock syndrome (Strep TSS) is any infection with *Streptococcus pyogenes* that is associated with a rapidly progressing systemic toxic response characterized by early onset of high fever and myalgia, often with prominent gastrointestinal symptoms, and by rapid progression to hypotension and multiple organ system failure. The illness usually requires ICU support for massive fluid resuscitation, vasopressor and inotropic support and mechanical ventilation. Although some cases have primary bacteremia, many others have a localized focus of infection, most often in soft tissues, that only becomes clinically apparent after the onset of shock.

Streptococcal necrotizing fasciitis is often associated with Strep TSS and, as mentioned, is often only correctly diagnosed after the onset of shock. The most characteristic story is presentation to a physician or an emergency room with abrupt onset of severe pain, often in an extremity with minimal or no evidence of cutaneous injury. At this stage severe systemic toxicity is usually not present and, since examination of the painful site is also at this stage quite unremarkable, patients are frequently sent home with analgesics and reassurance. Over the next 4–48 hours pain at the site of infection continues to increase, soft tissue swelling and redness appear above the deeper tissues that are undergoing ongoing necrotizing infection, eventually resulting in full-thickness necrosis evidenced by ecchymosis, cutaneous necrosis, and bullae formation.[26] Early or later in this course Strep TSS frequently occurs.

When these cases first began to appear, clinicians' approach to both the sepsis and the tissue necrosis was essentially the same as that used for apparently similar syndromes caused by other bacteria. A broad spectrum antimicrobial was started, fluid resuscitation begun and imaging studies ordered to better define the source of infection causing pain or localized swelling. Imaging frequently demonstrated only soft tissue swelling consistent with cellulitis, so surgery was often deferred until superficial signs of tissue necrosis became obvious, and then when surgery was done it was often performed using the conventional approach of trying to conserve as much tissue as possible. The result was that treatment was often too little and too late, with mortality rates exceeding 70% in many reported series.

With the realization that treatment, to be successful, must be swift and aggressive, approaches to therapy changed. Emergency physicians were increasingly alerted to the fact that severe pain at any body site, even with relatively minimal localized physical findings and particularly if accompanied by signs of systemic inflammation, could represent necrotizing fasciitis. Surgeons began to be consulted much earlier, and any localized pain with swelling more often led to diagnostic surgical exploration rather than imaging and waiting. Antimicrobial strategies changed. Addition of clindamycin to the usual penicillin or other beta-lactam therapy was advocated and widely adopted, based on results from animal models of the syndrome and on pharmacologic and physiologic considerations, including its ability to inhibit bacterial protein (ie, toxin) synthesis, penetrate necrotic tissues, and inhibit inflammatory cytokine synthesis.[27] Toxin neutralization using pooled intravenous gamma globulin was also advocated with the support of primarily historical case–control studies.[28] In most centers, implementation of these approaches has led to dramatic reductions in mortality rates to about 20%–30% although, in the absence of any adequate controlled trials, it remains unclear what the relative contribution of each of these measures has been to the improved outcome.

Unlike several of the other "plagues" discussed above, this is one that is still very much with us. The *Streptococcus pyogenes* strains most strongly associated with severe invasive disease (M-protein types 1 and 3) have increasingly been supplanting those associated with less severe disease resulting in an endemic sporadic case-rate for severe disease of one to 20 cases/100,000 population yearly, with intermittent larger-scale community outbreaks, both of which will continue to require vigilance and an aggressive therapeutic stance from the critical care community.[29]

SEVERE ACUTE RESPIRATORY SYNDROME

The first case of this apparently novel severe viral respiratory infection occurred in Guangdong Province in southern China in November 2002. The victim, a farmer, died of an undiagnosed "atypical pneumonia." Over the ensuing weeks several more cases of severe respiratory syndromes began to appear in the region, also undiagnosed. By the end of November there had been enough such cases to generate considerable alarm among the medical community in China, generating Internet communications between institutions which were picked up by international monitoring agencies. This led to a request from the World Health Organization (WHO) for information about the outbreak, but no information was forthcoming from Chinese authorities. The first official report about the outbreak was made to public health authorities in Guangdong in early January 2003, with a later report to the WHO in February that, in retrospect, did not fully make clear either the nature or the scale of the problem.[30]

Transmission of the disease within China continued to occur, leading to rapidly increasing numbers of cases in South China, then throughout the country and to the capitol Beijing (where one of the largest outbreaks occurred). Exposure of Chinese travelers and visitors to the country was inevitable, given the scale of the outbreak. One exposed individual was a physician from mainland China who, incubating the disease during his travel, stayed at the Metropole hotel in Hong Kong in early March. Later investigations showed that he transmitted the virus to at least 16 other guests at the hotel, who then carried it by international air travel to Taiwan, Singapore, Vietnam, and Canada.

One of these contact cases was an American businessman headed for Singapore. Becoming ill while in transit, he stopped in Hanoi where he was admitted to hospital with a severe pneumonia, to which he eventually succumbed. Soon after, a number of health care workers who had been in contact with him also became acutely ill. Fortunately for the course of the outbreak, one of the consultants on the case was an Italian physician working with the WHO in Vietnam, Dr. Carlo Urbani. He immediately recognized that this was a previously unknown severe atypical pneumonia that was relatively easily transmissible and reported it to the WHO; this led to immediate mobilization of investigative efforts and worldwide alerts about the threat.[31] Unfortunately, in the course of caring for the victims of the disease in Hanoi, Dr. Urbani himself contracted the infection and died of it later.

As information from China became more available, it became clear that by this time there had already been hundreds of cases and numerous deaths. The majority of the initial wave of cases were noted to have occurred primarily in farmers and food handlers, particularly those working in food markets where live wild animals were kept and sold for food. The second large wave of those affected were health care workers exposed in hospital to patients with the disease. The illness was characterized by fever and myalgia with gastrointestinal symptoms in the initial phase, occurring an average of 5 days after exposure (range 2–10 days). Many cases got no worse than this, but others went on to develop dyspnea associated with radiographic evidence of a diffuse, patchy pneumonitis which, in some, progressed to ARDS. An average of

15% required mechanical ventilatory support, and when the data were all in from later phases of the outbreak, mortality rates averaged about 10% overall, worse in the aged and debilitated, lower in the young and healthy.

The largest outbreak outside Asia occurred in Toronto, Canada. The index case, a visitor to China, returned to Canada and died of pneumonia at home, undiagnosed, in early March 2003. Shortly thereafter, one of his sons was admitted to hospital with a severe respiratory illness and died a few days later. By this time, four other family members had become ill and had been admitted to hospital; the first cases of affected health care workers appeared soon after among those who had cared for the dying son of the index case. Within days, other instances of transmission from undiagnosed contacts of the initial cases in hospitals, doctors' offices, emergency rooms, and at social events were leading to admission of cases to several hospitals throughout Toronto. The response of the public health authorities, beginning soon after the WHO global alert and coincident with the recognition of the first local cases, was quick and vigorous, including closure of the main affected hospital, intensive follow-up of probable contacts, quarantine of suspected cases based on a fairly inclusive case definition and strict institution of barrier contact protection for health care workers.[32] By mid-April the number of new cases was rapidly declining, although there was one cluster of late cases related to exposure of a large number of health care workers during the resuscitation and difficult intubation of a critically ill patient. A later cluster of cases also occurred in a rehabilitation hospital, where it appeared that unrecognized contacts from the first phase of the outbreak had been transferred and transmitted the disease to other patients and staff.

The worldwide outbreak was essentially over by July 2003. There were a total of 8098 reported cases from 26 countries, with 774 deaths.

Intensive epidemiologic and laboratory study of the disease by investigators and laboratories worldwide led to unprecedented rapid growth in knowledge about the causative agent. The virus, more or less simultaneously characterized at a number of laboratories around the world, proved to be a previously unknown coronavirus (severe acute respiratory syndrome [SARS]-CoV) with capacity to infect and spread from a variety of wild animals to humans. Epidemiologic, serologic, and virologic evidence was developed linking human cases to exposure to infected wild animals, including masked palm civets, raccoon dogs, ferrets and ferret badgers, all being sold for human consumption in markets in China.[33] Control of their transport and sale and exposures to humans by Chinese health authorities was probably one of the major factors in bringing the first outbreak under control, the partial failure of which later led to a second, much smaller outbreak late in 2004. Although the initial speculation was that one or more of these wild animals were the reservoir in nature for the infection, it now appears more likely that the viral reservoir is actually bats, with cross-transmission of the virus between bats, food animals, and humans in crowded markets leading to development of strains with the capacity to transmit between humans.[34]

Public health authorities worldwide learned much from SARS about the importance of effective international communication in developing a rapid and effective response to outbreaks of novel viruses, and more about how to go about containing such infections within communities and hospitals. Several intensivists involved in the outbreak credit e-mail communications from other international outbreak sites for effective advice on critical elements of disease protection (eg, Powered Air Purifying Respirators and full contact rather than droplet precautions) and therapy. For the critical care community, perhaps one main lesson was the importance of "super-spreading incidents" in propagating the disease in hospitals. Many of these occurred in critically ill patients undergoing resuscitation with difficult or traumatic intubation, generating aerosols in closed spaces which contained many superfluous and inadequately protected health care workers. Handling these situations safely depends crucially on identifying the potential risk and undertaking the resuscitation and intubation using the most experienced operators available, adequately protected with basic barrier precautions (eye protection, gloves and surgical face-masks), using sedation or paralysis as necessary to minimize trauma and aerosol generation, and with only essential and adequately protected staff in the room.[35] This likely applies to many other situations with potential for disease transmission to health care workers.

Unfortunately, this epidemic again points out the primary lesson that was not absorbed from the earlier HPS outbreak, namely, the need for detailed preplanning and preparation for a major infectious disease epidemic that is inclusive of hospital and ICU operations in each locale. According to participants, the SARS outbreak demonstrated many of the same early ICU operational problems that plagued the HPS outbreak albeit on a larger scale.

INFLUENZA

In the ICU era, there has yet to occur a true influenza pandemic with a high attack rate in all age groups and associated high hospitalization and mortality rates, as was seen in the great 1918 pandemic. In that worldwide disaster, it is estimated that 30% of all people became ill with the virus and an estimated 50–100 million died.[36] Minor recent pandemics in 1968 and 1977 had less than one twentieth of the impact of the 1918 influenza, not greatly different from the yearly interpandemic influenza the world has been experiencing in the 30 years since.

Interpandemic influenza epidemics since 1977 have been caused primarily by H3N2 and H1N1 influenza viruses, to which most of the population has developed some degree of immunity from prior infection or vaccination. The result is what public health authorities have become used to seeing: each year a slightly different influenza A appears in Asia with minor antigenic changes in the HA or NA surface proteins (termed *drift*), making it infectious once again for humans whose immune systems have yet to be exposed to the new variant, and a new epidemic is launched. When the "flu" arrives in an area, cases begin to appear suddenly and there is rapid spread in the population, usually with 20%–30% becoming infected over a 6-week period with a peak in case numbers at week two or three. About half of those infected will seek medical attention, many more than once, and one to about 25 per thousand infected will be admitted to hospital with a respiratory syndrome such as pneumonia, chronic obstructive pulmonary disease exacerbation, asthmatic attack, or cardiac failure, the rate depending on age and underlying comorbidities. Overall, about 0.1% of those infected die, with mortality rates among those with major comorbidities up to 5%. These latter cases constitute most of the increase in the ICU case load which most units experience every winter. The load is sometimes taxing but usually not overwhelming.

A true pandemic is unlikely to play out this way. How different it would be depends on a number of factors: the antigenic difference in the new Influenza virus compared with the old (ie, the antigenic "shift" to a different one of 15 HA or 9 NA protein subtypes due to introduction of a variant from another influenza-susceptible species), how transmissible the new virus is, how virulent it is, how susceptible it is to antiviral drugs, and whether the world is prepared for it with drug availability and vaccines.

The prototype severe pandemic was the Spanish influenza of 1918, an H1N1 virus. The most recent circulating influenza virus just before that time was an H3N8 that had arrived in 1901. Current evidence suggests that an avian influenza virus underwent a period of evolutionary adaptation, possibly in another susceptible species such as swine, fitting it for transmission to humans, which it then did.[36,37] This H1N1 virus had not been previously experienced by any segment of the population except the very old, so nearly everyone, particularly non-elderly adults and children, was without immunity and was at risk of severe infection. Attack rates, as noted earlier, were extremely high everywhere as were rates of primary influenza pneumonia, complicating bacterial pneumonia, and death. In the United States, death rates were more than 20-fold higher than in any influenza pandemic since. An outbreak of influenza on this scale, if unchecked by effective antiviral therapy or vaccines, would render ICU care such as mechanical ventilatory support for respiratory failure irrelevant. Even today, with maximal respiratory support, most patients with diffuse primary viral pneumonia complicated by respiratory failure cannot be saved, and the numbers presenting for such care in a short space of time, if comparable to the 1918 pandemic, would overwhelm our current ICU capacity within days.

Currently the main apparent threat of a new pandemic comes in the form of the H5N1 influenza virus. This virus is now present nearly worldwide in migratory and, intermittently, domestic bird populations. From time to time, transmission of the virus from birds to humans occurs, generally from close contact situations. WHO data indicate that there have been 387 laboratory-confirmed cases of such transmission from 2003 to mid-2008.[38] The mortality rate has exceeded 60%, although it is likely that many less severe cases do not come to medical attention and are therefore not counted as confirmed case survivors. To date no instances of transmission to humans by humans or other mammals has been documented. However, the threat remains that if this virus were to become capable of human-to-human transmission by adaptation in another susceptible mammalian host such as swine, a pandemic on the order of the 1918 event could occur.

With no true pandemic for over 30 years, including all of the ICU era, health authorities worldwide are deeply engaged in trying to learn the lesson of this new "plague" before it actually occurs. It is clear that we will need excellent international communication, rapidly enactable containment and quarantine plans and, if possible, effective antivirals and vaccines to deal with the H5N1 virus. If it evolves as feared and becomes easily transmissible while retaining its current virulence; modern life-sustaining technology alone will be no shield at all.

The last 60 years have seen remarkable advances in the ability to diagnose and treat infectious diseases and handle infectious disease outbreaks. For the most part, the major plagues of antiquity remain historical footnotes. However, despite these advances, there is clear evidence that major pandemic illness is always just one outbreak away. In addition to the HIV pandemic, the smaller epidemic outbreaks of Legionnaire's disease, hantavirus pulmonary syndrome, and SARS, among many others, points out the potential risk associated with a lack of preplanning and preparedness. Although pandemic influenza is at the top of the list when discussing possible future major infectious disease outbreaks, the truth is that the identity of the next major pandemic pathogen cannot be predicted with any accuracy. We can only hope that general preparedness and the lessons learned from previous outbreaks suffice.

REFERENCES

1. Paul JR. A history of poliomyelitis. New Haven (CT): Yale University Press; 1971.
2. Oshinsky DM. Polio: an American story. New York: Oxford University Press; 2005.
3. Drinker P, Shaw LA. An apparatus for the prolonged administration of artificial respiration. J Clin Invest 1929;7:229–47.

4. West JB. The physiologic challenges of the 1952 Copenhagen poliomyelitis epidemic and a renaissance in clinical respiratory physiology. J Appl Physiol 2005;99:424–32.

5. Trojan D, Cashman N. Post-poliomyelitis syndrome. Muscle Nerve 2005;31:6–19.

6. Fraser DW, Tsai TB, Orenstein W, et al. Legionnaire's disease: description of an epidemic of pneumonia. N Engl J Med 1977;297:1189–97.

7. McDade JE, Shepard CC, Fraser DW, et al. Legionnaire's disease: isolation of a bacterium and demonstration of its role in other respiratory diseases. N Engl J Med 1977;297:1197–203.

8. Todd J, Fishout M, Kapral F, et al. Toxic-shock syndrome associated with phage-group-1 staphylococci. Lancet 1978;2(8100):1116–8.

9. Centers for Disease Control. Toxic-shock syndrome – United States. MMWR Morb Mortal Wkly Rep 1980;29:229–30.

10. Shands KN, Schmid GB, Dan BB, et al. Toxic-shock syndrome in menstruating women: association with tampon use and Staphylococcus aureus and clinical features in 52 cases. N Engl J Med 1980;303:1436–42.

11. Centers for Disease Control. Epidemiologic notes and reports, toxic-shock syndrome, United States. MMWR Morb Mortal Wkly Rep 1982;31:201–4.

12. Schlievert PM, Tripp TJ, Peterson ML. Reemergence of staphylococcal toxic-shock syndrome in Minneapolis- St. Paul, Minnesota, during the 2000–2003 surveillance period. J Clin Microbiol 2004;42:2875–6.

13. Hughes WT, Feldman S, Aur RJ, et al. Intensity of immunosuppression and the incidence of Pneumocystis carinii pneumonia. Cancer 1975;36:2004–9.

14. Hughes WT, Feldman S, Chaudharg SC, et al. Comparison of pentamadine iso-thionate and trimethoprim/sulfamethoxazole in the treatment of Pneumocystis carinii pneumonia. J Pediatr 1978;92:285–91.

15. Centers for Disease Control. Pneumocystis pneumonia – Los Angeles. MMWR Morb Mortal Wkly Rep 1981;30:250–2.

16. Bozette SA, Sattler FR, Chiu J, et al. A controlled trial of early adjunctive treatment with corticosteroids for PCP in AIDS. N Engl J Med 1990;323:1451–7.

17. Azoulay E, Parrot A, Flahault HA, et al. AIDS-related pneumonia in the era of adjunctive steroids. Am J Respir Crit Care Med 1999;160:493–9.

18. Centers for Disease Control. Outbreak of acute illness – southwestern United States, 1993. MMWR Morb Mortal Wkly Rep 1993;42:421–4.

19. Duchin JS, Koster FT, Peters CJ, et al. Hantavirus pulmonary syndrome: a clinical description of 17 patients with a newly recognized disease. N Engl J Med 1994; 330:949–55.

20. Halin GW, Simpson SQ, Crowell RE, et al. Cardiopulmonary manifestations of Hantavirus pulmonary syndrome. Crit Care Med 1996;24:252–8.

21. Centers for Disease Control. Hantavirus pulmonary syndrome – United States: updated recommendations for risk reduction. MMWR Morb Mortal Wkly Rep 2002;51:1–12.

22. Osler W. The principles and practice of medicine. New York: D. Appleton and Company; 1892. p. 110–8.

23. Meleney FL. Hemolytic streptococcus gangrene. Arch Surg 1924;9:317–64.

24. Meleney FL. Hemolytic streptococcal gangrene: the importance of early diagnosis and operation. JAMA 1929;92:2009–12.

25. Cone LA, Woodward DR, Schlievert PM, et al. Clinical and bacteriological observations of a toxic-shock-like syndrome due to Streptococcus pyogenes. N Engl J Med 1987;317:146–9.

26. Barker FG, Leppard BJ, Seal DV. Streptococcal necrotizing fasciitis: comparison between histological and clinical features. J Clin Pathol 1987;40:335–41.

27. Stevens DL, Bryant AE, Hackett SP. Antibiotic effects on bacterial viability, toxin production and host response. Clin Infect Dis 1995;20(Suppl 2):S154–7.

28. Kaul R, McGeer A, Norrby-Teglund A, et al. Intravenous immunoglobulin therapy for streptococcal toxic-shock syndrome – a comparative observational study. The Canadian Streptococcal Study Group. Clin Infect Dis 1999;28:800–7.

29. Johnson DR, Stevens DL, Kaplan EL. Epidemiologic analysis of group A streptococcal serotypes associated with severe systemic infections, rheumatic fever, or uncomplicated pharyngitis. J Infect Dis 1992;166:374–82.

30. WHO – Epidemic and Pandemic Alert and Response (EPR). Acute respiratory syndrome in China. Available at: http://www.who.int/csr/don/2003_02_11/en/index.html. Accessed January 8, 2009.

31. WHO – Epidemic and Pandemic Alert and Response (EPR). Acute respiratory syndrome in Hong Kong special administrative region of China/Vietnam. Available at: http://www.who.int/csr/don/2003_03_12/en/index.html.

32. Svoboda T, Henry B, Shulman L, et al. Public health measures to control the spread of the severe acute respiratory syndrome during the outbreak in Toronto. N Engl J Med 2004;350:2352–61.

33. Guan Y, Zhang BJ, He YQ, et al. Isolation and characterization of viruses related to the SARS coronavirus from animals in southern China. Science 2003;302:276–8.

34. Li W, Shi Z. Bats are natural reservoirs of SARS-like coronaviruses. Science 2005;310:676–9.

35. Fowler RA, Lapinsky SE, Hallett D, et al. Critically ill patients with severe acute respiratory syndrome. JAMA 2003;290:367–73.

36. Taubenberger JK, Morens DM. 1918 Influenza: the mother of all pandemics. Available at: http://www.cdc.gov/eid/index.htm. Emerging Infect Dis 2006;12:15–22.

37. Ito T, Couceiro JN, Kelm S, et al. Molecular basis for the generation in pigs of Influenza A viruses with pandemic potential. J Virol 1998;92:7367–73.

38. WHO-epidemic and pandemic alert and response (EPR). Available at: http://www.who.int/csr/disease/avian_influenza/country/cases_table_2008_09_10/en/index.html.

Sepsis and Septic Shock: A History

Duane J. Funk, MD, FRCP(C)[a], Joseph E. Parrillo, MD[b], Anand Kumar, MD[c,d,]*

KEYWORDS

• Sepsis • Septic shock • History • Endotoxin • Cytokines
• Coagulaiton • Nitric oxide • Sepsis hemodynamics

Infectious disease has been a leading cause of death in humans since the first recorded tabulations. For example, available evidenced suggests that one third to one half of the entire population of Europe and Asia were wiped out in the Black Death Plague of the early fifteenth century. Evidence for the presence of sepsis in humans stretches into antiquity. Emperor Shen Nung's 2375 BC treatise on the treatment of fever using the herb, ch'ang shan, is one of earliest known written references to pharmacological therapeutics. From Hippocrates and Galen, to Lister, Fleming and Semmelweiss, this article reviews the notable historical figures of sepsis research. The early descriptions and theories about the etiology (microbial pathogens), pathogenesis (toxins and mediators), and treatment of sepsis-associated disease are also discussed.

SEPSIS AND THE ANCIENT GREEKS AND ROMANS

The word "sepsis" derives from the Greek "σηψιζ" which refers to the "decomposition of animal, or vegetable or organic matter in the presence of bacteria."[1] The first use of "sepsis" in the medical context occurred over 2700 years ago in the poems of Homer. In this use, the term "sepsis" derives directly from the word "sepo" (σηπω), which means "I rot." The term is also found in the writings of the great physician and philosopher Hippocrates (circa 400 BC) in his Corpus Hippocraticum. Hippocrates is well known for the introduction of the concept of dysregulated body humors (the bodily fluids of blood, yellow bile, black bile, and phlegm) as a cause of disease. Hippocrates viewed sepsis as the dangerous, odiferous, biological decay that could

[a] Anesthesiology and Critical Care, University of Manitoba, Manitoba, Canada
[b] Department of Medicine, Robert Wood Johnson Medical School, University of Medicine and Dentistry of New Jersey, Cooper Heart Institute, Cooper University Hospital, Camden, NJ, USA
[c] Section of Critical Care Medicine, Section of Infectious Diseases, Medical Microbiology and Pharmacology/Therapeutics, University of Manitoba, Manitoba, Canada
[d] Section of Critical Care Medicine, Section of Infectious Diseases, Robert Wood Johnson Medical School, University of Medicine and Dentistry of New Jersey, Camden, NJ, USA
* Corresponding author.
E-mail address: akumar61@yahoo.com (A. Kumar).

Crit Care Clin 25 (2009) 83–101
doi:10.1016/j.ccc.2008.12.003
0749-0704/08/$ – see front matter © 2009 Elsevier Inc. All rights reserved.

criticalcare.theclinics.com

occur in the body. It was further believed that this biological decay occurred in the colon and released "dangerous principles" that could cause "auto-intoxication." Hippocrates was one of the first to examine antisepsis properties of potential medicinal compounds including alcohol in wine and vinegar.

Galen (129–199 AD) was a prominent Roman physician and philosopher of Greek origin. Galen was also a well-revered historical figure in the study of the theories of sepsis. Based of his keen powers of observation, he was considered an authority on medicine. His initial writings and theories on medicine remained largely unchallenged until some 1500 years later.

Galen's practice was devoted to blood letting and the drainage of abscesses, but it was the use of medications to treat disease that was his passion. His collection of medicinals ("apotheca") was the forerunner of today's apothecary (pharmacy). One of his most popular medicinal creations was theriac, a mixture of over 70 substances.[2] It was used for everything including the treatment of venomous bites, inflammation and to ward off the Black Death. No doubt theriac's popularity stemmed from one of its main ingredients: opium.

It was Galen who first described that wounds healed by secondary intention. He also theorized that the formation of pus (he described it as "laudable pus") was critical to the healing of injured tissues. This theory remained unchallenged until Leonardo DaVinci and Andreas Vesalius in the fifteenth century questioned the purported benefit of wound suppuration.

Further building on the putrefaction theories of the Greeks, the early Romans were convinced that within swamps, sepsis resulted from the production of invisible creatures that emitted putrid fumes called "miasma" or "miasmata." The theory that these harmful organisms spontaneously generated formed the basis of the public health initiatives of the Romans. To the Romans, health and hygiene were paramount. Thus, early health initiatives were directed at eliminating these swamps and the creation of safe and elaborate water delivery systems and communal baths. Unfortunately, early Roman physicians did not develop the theory of infectious disease transmission by contact and preventive measures to reduce transmission were never implemented.

EARLY WORK ON THE TRANSMISSION OF INFECTIOUS DISEASE AND THE DISCOVERY OF "ANIMACULES"

Marcus Terentius Varro, in "De re rustica libri III" (three books on agriculture circa 100 BC), was the first to articulate the notion of contagion. He suggested, "small creatures invisible to the eye, fill the atmosphere, and breathed through the nose cause dangerous diseases." In the millennia since his insightful analysis, major pandemics of bubonic and pneumonic plague, cholera, smallpox, measles, tuberculosis, syphilis, gonorrhea and influenza have devastated the human population.

In "De contagione et contagiosis morbis" (1546), Hieronymus Fracastorius wrote of "contagium virum," the first clear suggestion of what has become to be know as the "germ theory."[2] In his treatise, three forms of contagion were described. He theorized that that the transmission of infections was either by direct contact, indirectly through infected articles (foments), or by transmission from a distance (airborne). He further proposed that the transmission of infection was due to tiny bodies that had the power to self-replicate and multiply. His theories bore a superficial but notable resemblance to Koch's postulates that came some 300 years later.

It wasn't until 1684 that the theory of spontaneous generation of infection began to be refuted. Francisco Redi (1626–1697) conducted experiments on the putrefaction of meat.[3] In an ingenious yet simple experiment, he placed meat in pots and covered it with either mesh gauze or an airtight seal. For a "control group" he left one container of meat open to air.

He discovered that when the meat was left open to air, flies landed on the meat and it was soon covered with maggots. In the meat that was in the gauze covered pot, maggots were only present on the gauze but not on the meat itself. Meat that was in the pot covered with the airtight material had no maggots on it whatsoever. This led Redi to conclude that rather than the meat generating the "spontaneous" organisms, it seemed that the flies were attracted to the meat and laid eggs on it, thus creating the maggots.

This compelling experiment challenged the spontaneous generation dogma expounded by Galen. Ironically, the contemporaneous development of the microscope was used to refute Redi's experimental results. The microscope allowed visualization of "tiny animals" and was used as proof that putrefaction could spontaneously generate these organisms.

Galileo was the first to develop a compound microscope that was essentially a modification of his telescope. Because of technical problems, however, the images created by his microscope were blurry and had poor resolution. Therefore, despite Fracastorius' theorizing about the transmission of infectious agents, little work was initially carried out to discover or describe potential pathogenic agents.

It wasn't until several hundred years later that the resolution of the microscopes improved and allowed scientists to study life at a cellular level. Anthony van Leeuwenhoek (1632–1723) had no scientific background or medical training, yet he was able to build his own compound microscope and made a number of significant discoveries to advance the study of infectious disease.[4] Leeuwenhoek's first description and drawings of "animacules" in 1674, including spheres, rods and spirals (ie, cocci, bacilli and spirochetes), paved the way for other scientists to further develop germ theory (**Fig. 1**).

THE GOLDEN AGE OF GERM THEORY: SEMMELWEISS, LISTER, KOCH AND PASTEUR

The nineteenth century ushered in an era of exponential growth in the knowledge of the origin and transmission of infectious disease. Joseph Lister, Ignaz Semmelweiss Louis Pasteur, and Robert Koch were all physicians in the nineteenth century who contributed seminal advancements in the origin of sepsis.

The earliest of these men, Ignaz Semmelweiss (1818–1865) was a physician in Vienna, Austria. In 1841, he worked on a maternity ward in a hospital and noticed that there was a high rate of death from childbed fever, also called puerperal sepsis.[5] Semmelweiss further observed that women whose deliveries were assisted by midwives had a significantly lower rate of infections than those who were assisted by medical students (2% versus 16%). At the time, medical student's practice was to perform autopsies on the women that had died the previous day, and then without hand washing, proceed to perform deliveries later in the day.

It wasn't until one of his colleagues died of an infection (acquired after cutting himself accidentally during an autopsy) that Semmelweiss made the connection between the medical student deliveries, autopsies, and puerperal sepsis. Semmelweiss commented: "The fingers and hands of students and doctors, soiled by recent dissections, carry those death-dealing cadaver's poisons into the genital organs of women in childbirth."[6]

Semmelweiss then instituted a hand washing policy in his maternity ward before patient contact and he saw the rates of puerperal sepsis drop to less than 3%. Despite these impressive results, the concept of hand washing was not met with great enthusiasm by the medical establishment of the day. Semmelweiss was told that "Doctors

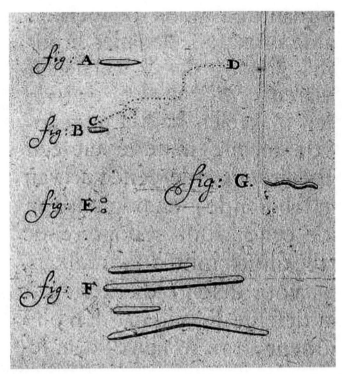

Fig. 1. Leeuwenhoek's first drawings of "animacules" including spheres, rods and spirals (ie, cocci, bacilli and spirochetes).

are gentlemen, and gentlemen's hands are clean." He was fired from his position in the hospital and later died in an insane asylum of an infection he acquired after a finger laceration. Ironically the infection was probably due to either *Staphylococcus* or *Streptococcus*, and thus bore a striking resemblance to puerperal sepsis. It is also somewhat ironic that 160 years after his discovery of hand hygiene as an important tool in infection control, many medical professionals still fail to utilize this key preventative measure on a routine basis.

The mid-nineteenth century also saw the exponential growth of surgical procedures. The development of anesthetics reduced the fear and pain associated with surgery. However, the incidence of infection and resultant death from postoperative sepsis paralleled the rise in the number of surgical procedures performed.

Joseph Lister (1827–1912) **(Fig. 2)** was born in England shortly before Semmelweiss' observations on the cause of puerperal sepsis were published. He was born to parents with scientific interest; his father was a member of the Royal Society of Fellows. At the age of 17, Lister entered University College of London and subsequently graduated from medical school in 1852. He accepted a surgical internship at the Edinburgh Royal infirmary, and it was here that he challenged the perceived etiology of wound suppuration that was widely held at that time.[7] Despite the findings of Redi and Leeuwenhoek and the early bacterial classification system developed by Christian Ehrenberg (circa 1838), it was still widely believed that wound sepsis was due to contagions in the air. Lister astutely observed that wound sepsis occurred in patients who had open wounds and theorized that the infectious agents gained access to the body through breaks in the skin. Lister eventually accepted a position

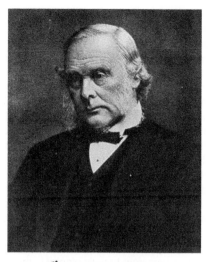

Fig. 2. Portrait of Joseph Lister (1827–1912).

as Professor of Surgery in Glasgow. He was placed in charge of a new facility whose mandate was to reduce the deaths from postoperative sepsis. His early efforts in this regard were disastrous as 45%–50% of patients died of infections.[8]

Around the same time, Louis Pasteur (1822–1895) was conducting his experiments on the germ theory of disease. Pasteur boiled broth (to sterilize it) in flasks that had swan shaped, curved necks. He allowed the flasks to remain open to air. Microbes invariably were present in the neck of the flask but were not in contact with the broth. In the flasks where the broth did not contact the microbes that accumulated on the neck of the flask, no growth occurred and the broth remained clear. Pasteur tipped some of the flasks so that the broth was in contact with the neck of the flask, and the microbes from the air. Those flasks that were tipped consistently demonstrated a change in the broth from transparent to opaque, indicating bacterial growth. Pasteur thus clearly demonstrated that putrefaction required living organisms and finally disproved the spontaneous generation theory of disease transmission.[3,6]

Eventually, Pasteur formally proposed "Germ Theory" to the French Academy of Medicine in 1878. Later he presented data demonstrating streptococci as the cause of puerperal sepsis.

News of Pasteur's experiments found its way to Lister in England. This news led to the formalization of Lister's own thoughts regarding germ theory as it related to wound sepsis. Lister hypothesized that the fermentation that Pasteur demonstrated was the same process that Lister observed in his patients with infected wounds. Lister then emulated the approach of an acquaintance, an engineer who was able to eliminate the odor from sewage with the use of carbolic acid. By the addition of carbolic acid to wound dressings, Lister was able to significantly reduce the rate of wound sepsis and death in his hospital.

In 1867, Lister presented his research to the British Medical Association demonstrating his wards at the Royal Glasgow infirmary were free of infections for 9 months. The same year, *The Lancet* published his seminal paper "On a New Method of treating

Compound Fracture, Abscess, etc., with Observations on the Conditions of Suppuration," Lister's first paper on antisepsis.

Despite the impressiveness of his results, the medical community at large was slow to accept his findings, and this frustrated Lister. He wrote: "but the carrying out of this rule implies a conviction of the truth of the germ theory of putrefaction, which, unfortunately, is in this country the subject of doubts such as I confess surprise me, considering the character of the evidence which has been adduced in support of it."[6]

In 1877, as Chair of Clinical Surgery in King's College, Lister introduced his theory of antisepsis to the department. He all but eliminated the smell of wound sepsis on the wards. That same year, under aseptic technique, he performed an open patellar repair that was successful and did not result in postoperative sepsis. This was remarkable at the time, as this operation was associated with a high rate of death. News of his success was widely publicized and resulted in a paradigm shift in the surgical community and resulted in the reduction of postoperative infectious complications.

Lister further revolutionized the field of antisepsis by discovering that sutures soaked in carbolic acid and cut short further reduced wound infections. Interestingly, in the 15th and sixteenth century, gunshot wounds were thought to be poisoned. For that reason, a suture (or seton) was intentionally placed in the wound and left to suppurate to facilitate healing.

Like many scientists of his day, Lister conducted experiments using himself as a subject. He worked on trying to find the right concentration of carbolic acid in dressings that provided an adequate amount of antisepsis, without being caustic to skin, a problem that affected both wounds and surgeons' hands.

During the same era as Lister and Pasteur, Robert Koch (1843–1910), who would eventually be recognized as one of the fathers of modern microbiology, was also working on the germ theory of disease. Koch was able to demonstrate that sheep infected with anthrax had tiny rod shaped organisms growing in their blood. He was able to culture and grow this agent with nutrient gelatin that he created. Inoculating healthy sheep with the cultured material also led to the development of anthrax. Koch then formulated his famous postulates on the identification of infectious agents. Koch said that in order to establish an agent as the cause of disease: (1) the agent must be isolated from the diseased animal; (2) the agent must be grown in culture; (3) infection of a healthy host with the culture must produce the disease; and finally, (4) the same organism must be recovered from the newly infected animal. Koch, along with his partner Julius Petri (who created the eponymous plate), were instrumental in developing modern microbiological techniques that allowed the furthering of the germ theory of disease.[3,6] Koch is also credited with the demonstration that steam could sterilize instruments with greater efficacy than the chemical disinfectants of the day. This led to the first surgical autoclaves by Ernst von Bergmann and Curt Schimmelbusch in 1885, a seminal event in the development of modern aseptic surgery.

MAGIC BULLETS AND EARLY ANTIBIOTICS

The use of agents to treat infection and sepsis goes back at least to the time of Hippocrates who used myrrh, wine, and inorganic salts to treat wounds. The Chinese utilized moldy soybean curd to treat carbuncles, boils and other infections some 2500 years ago. Up until the germ theory became accepted, therapy for infections remained strictly empiric. With the germ theory fully entrenched in the medical community, attention then turned to the targeted eradication of these newly discovered infectious organisms.

The development of modern antibiotics is often credited to Alexander Fleming's discovery of penicillin. However, it was Paul Erlich (1845–1915) who first theorized about the existence of compounds that might kill these newly discovered causative agents of infection and sepsis. Erlich's early work focused on the identification and staining of bacteria. Erlich theorized that if bacteria were able to selectively take up dye, then perhaps this property would allow the creation of a "magic bullet," as he called it, to kill the bacteria. The discovery of *Treponema pallidum* as the causative agent of syphilis in 1905 set Erlich out to discover a compound that killed the bacterium but didn't harm the host. After many unsuccessful attempts, Erlich finally discovered his magic bullet after more than 600 other compounds failed. The compound he created was called "salvarsan" and contained arsenic. It soon became the standard treatment of syphilis.[2]

Thirty years later, the discovery of sulfa drugs as viable antimicrobial agents was directly attributable to Erlich's work. Gerhard Domagk (1895–1964) in 1935 showed that when prontosil red (a dye commonly used to stain bacteria) was injected into mice, they seemed to be protected from developing sepsis when infected with streptococci. It was later realized that the dye was converted in the body to sulfanilamide. Several compounds were then created that had increased effectiveness against bacteria. For his work, Domagk was awarded the Nobel Prize in 1939.[9]

Sir Alexander Fleming (1881–1955) was born in England and, at the suggestion of his brother, became a doctor. His initial posting was at the St. Mary's hospital where he was an assistant bacteriologist. He served during World War I and saw many soldiers die from overwhelming infection and sepsis. This observation fueled his interest in discovering a cure for infections.[10]

Fleming's discovery of penicillin, like other great scientific discoveries, was serendipitous. While working on the properties of staphylococci, Fleming discovered that some of his culture plates had been contaminated with a spore of the blue mold *Penicillum notatum* from a neighboring mycology lab. Fleming noticed that there was an area around the mold where bacteria didn't grow, and he was able to identify the substance that caused the bacterial inhibition. He called the substance "penicillin" and published his work in 1929 (**Fig. 3**). Fleming had difficulty purifying the substance,

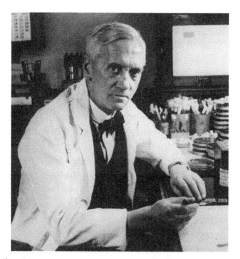

Fig. 3. Sir Alexander Fleming.

and didn't think, at the time, that it would be an important contribution to the treatment of infections.

Ernest Chain, a chemist, and Howard Florey, a pathologist, studied Fleming's work while they were both at Oxford. They were able to deduce the structure of penicillin and then developed the process to purify and mass-produce it. Fortuitously, their discovery came in time for the Second World War, a development that doubt saved tens of thousands of soldiers from a septic death.

Despite Fleming's initial skepticism about the utility of penicillin, he made several important observations about bacterial resistance. He noted that bacteria became resistant to the effects of penicillin if they were exposed to too little concentration of the drug or for too short a duration. Fleming also was an accomplished painter and used bacterial culture as his paint. He used *Serratia* for red, different species of *Micrococcus* for yellow, red and pink, and *Bacillus* for purple.[8]

The work of Fleming, Florey and Chain opened the floodgates of antimicrobial development and ushered in the golden era of antibiotics. For their combined work, they were awarded the Nobel Prize in 1945. Streptomycin, the first aminoglycoside antibiotic, was developed the same year they were awarded the prize.

THE DISCOVERY OF THE ROLE OF ENDOTOXIN

Very early in the descriptions of infectious diseases, there was controversy as to the mechanistic cause of death. The debate as to whether contagion or 'miasmata' ultimately resulted in death dates back to the time of Galen and Hippocrates.

Early physicians recognized that the malodorous smell emanating from patients with the plague bore a similarity to that found in swamps and marshes. This observation led the early physicians to conclude that there was some decay or putrefaction process that was going on in the patients that was similar to what was occurring in the swamps. The reasoning was then extended, and the thought of the miasma or miasmata (from the Greek meaning to "pollute") as the cause of the disease was postulated. The rapid spread of diseases, such as the plague through the air, was used as proof of this theory. However, the common practice at the time was to isolate patients for 40 days to quarantine them. The reason that this seemed to decrease the spread of the disease could not be adequately explained by these early physicians. The remnants of this historical concept of miasma as cause of disease persist today in the term "malaria", literally bad air, used to name the parasitic disease.

The alternative belief was that a poisonous material that was created by the putrefaction process caused disease. In distinction to the miasma hypothesis, those that subscribed to the contagion (from the Latin contigere, to touch) view of infectious disease thought that direct contact between an infected and susceptible individual was necessary to transmit infectious disease.

One flaw in the contagionist's reasoning was that a single contact with a sick person could transmit so much poison that it would be fatal for the affected person and potentially thousands of others. It was the hypothesis of Jacob Henle (1809–1885) that the contagion could reproduce in the body of the susceptible host and lead to further infection.[11] The implication of this conjecture was that the contagion had to be a living organism in order to reproduce. Henle later went on to become one of Robert Koch's teachers and his early postulates on the transmission of infectious disease clearly influenced Koch later work.

With these theories in mind, the search began for the mechanism of action of these poisons. It seemed unusual that infective material could have such serious consequences for a host organism. It appeared that a remarkably small amount of infectious particles caused serious toxicity and even death, which seemed out of proportion to the apparent inoculum size.

The heat sensitive toxins isolated by Ludwig Brieger (1849–1919) in the culture supernatant of diphtheria were the first true exotoxins to be discovered.[11] These toxins were noted to be produced during the life of the parent microorganisms. Other organisms studied also seemed to have these heat labile toxins that acted as mediators of disease.

Richard Pfeiffer (1858–1955) (**Fig. 4**) was researching the mechanism of cholera pathogenesis using *Vibrio cholerae* but could not find the typical exotoxin that had been described in other organisms. Pfeiffer inoculated guinea pigs with *V cholerae* that had either been actively or passively immunized. Much to his surprise, the animals still died, but no organism was found in their abdominal cavity. It appeared that the bacteria had undergone lysis and a toxic intracellular factor had been released. Pfeiffer then showed that the toxic factor was not destroyed by heat like the typical exotoxin. It was, thus, not a classic heat sensitive exotoxin protein generated during bacterial growth that caused the guinea pigs to die. His experiments led him to conclude that there was a heat stable substance in the bacterial cell wall released with cell death that was responsible for the toxic effects of *V cholerae.* He named this substance "endotoxin" (because it came from inside the cell) and went on to discover this substance in several other bacterial species.[11]

Later, Italian pathologist Eugenio Centanni discovered the relationship between Pfeiffer's endotoxin and the ability of bacteria to cause fever. He found that these substances were chemically inseparable from the bacterial cell wall and he named the material pyrotoxin, from the Greek meaning fire.

Further work in the twentieth century by Osborn and Nikaido has demonstrated the numerous bacterial species that use endotoxin as a pathogenic mediator. They are also largely responsible for determining the chemical composition of the substance including the O antigen, core region and lipid A components of endotoxin.

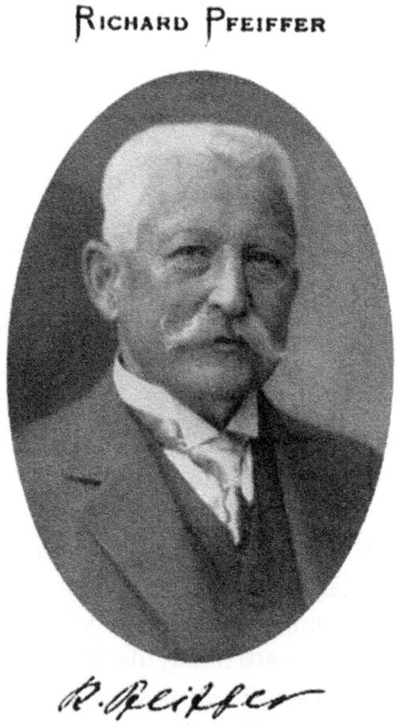

RICHARD PFEIFFER

R. Pfeiffer

Fig. 4. Richard Pfeiffer (1858–1955), discoverer of endotoxin.

THE COAGULATION SYSTEM

The coagulation cascade is well preserved throughout phylogeny. Even primitive organisms without an organized circulatory system have a rudimentary coagulation system.[12] It is thought that this system was developed to isolate invasive microbes and prevent them from gaining access to the whole organism.[13] In retrospect, the involvement of the coagulation system in overwhelming infection is reflected in history in the purpura associated with plague and other overwhelming "pestilent fevers" of antiquity. Hornung recognized a form of febrile purpura as early as 1734.[14] Manasse provided one of the earliest experimental demonstrations of disseminated intravascular coagulation as a consequence of microbial pathogens in 1892.[15] Disseminated microthrombi were found in experimental animals subjected to endotoxic shock through injection of heat-killed Salmonella. Two years later, Sanarelli noted a generalized, preterminal purpura in monkeys subjected to a similar insult, a phenomena he labeled "epithalaxis".[16] In 1926, Zdrodowsky and Bren provided the first detailed pathological description of disseminated microthrombi in association with a bleeding diathesis in endotoxic shock.[17] Early in this century, the role of infection as a source of coagulopathy was well recognized in recommendations that source control could lead to resolution of "thrombocytopenic purpura hemorrhagica."[14] Many other overlapping terms were used to describe what is now recognized as disseminated intravascular coagulation. The first use of this term in the published literature is found in 1951, although it use did not become routine until the 1960's.[18–20]

Because patients with purpura fulminans had evidence of micro-and macrovascular clotting at the time of autopsy, and activation of the coagulation system secondary to the infection was postulated as the cause of this, treatment with anticoagulants during infection was proposed to potentially have therapeutic benefit. In one of the earliest efforts to treat infection with anticoagulant therapy, Friedman and colleagues treated a patient with aortic valve endocarditis with an infusion of heparin for 10 days in 1938.[21] The infusion had to be stopped "early" as the patient deteriorated and suffered a fatal intracranial hemorrhage (likely from pre-existing cerebral embolus). Antibiotic therapy was not given to this patient. Ironically, the next article in the journal was on the antibacterial activity of sulfanilamide. Several other reports over the ensuing years described the combination therapy of heparin and antibiotics with mixed results.

Based on this early work, other clinicians began to use anticoagulant therapy on patients with infections. In a report from 1959, Little reported the successful treatment of infection-associated purpura fulminans with heparin and antibiotic therapy.[22] The patient recovered from her infection and did not require amputation of her limbs, presumably because of the improved blood flow to her limbs because of the heparin. Little and other investigators of the period also showed that coagulation was altered and fibrinogen decreased in some patients with sepsis and septic shock.

The extreme example of the coagulation defects in sepsis is in fulminant meningococcemia. This disease results in a widespread activation of the coagulation cascade with a simultaneous suppression of fibrinolytic pathways. Although this phenomenon was reported as early as the late 1950s, there was no mechanistic explanation as to how infection could activate the coagulation cascade. It wasn't until the discovery of cytokines (see below) that the complex interactions between the coagulation system and the inflammatory system began to be appreciated.

During the 1960s and 1970s, significant and parallel discoveries regarding the coagulation and inflammatory cascades were being made. In one of the earliest reports linking pro-inflammatory mediators to a pro-coagulant state, Nawrooth and colleagues demonstrated that interleukin-1 (IL-1) induced an endothelial procoagulant that eventually became known as tissue factor.[23] Other investigators then showed that other substances related to the inflammatory cascade, namely endotoxin, complement and viruses were able to activate the coagulation cascade.

Even before the mechanistic explanations of the interaction between these two systems was elucidated, clinicians were using newly discovered and purified natural anticoagulants in severe disseminated intravascular coagulation (DIC) to attempt to prevent organ system dysfunction. In one of the earliest reports, Schipper and colleagues infused antithrombin III ([ATIII], a serine protease that affects the intrinsic, extrinsic and common coagulation pathways) into patients with DIC to try and reduce the organ damage from a dysfunctional coagulation system.[24] This approach seemed to have some beneficial effects. It wasn't until 20 years later that it was discovered that low levels of this natural anticoagulant portended a higher rate of death in human septic shock.

Eventually, several novel anticoagulant therapies were tested in humans in several large randomized controlled trials.[25-27] These included antithrombin III, tissue factor pathway inhibitor, and activated protein C. Unfortunately, only the Recombinant Human Activated Protein C Worldwide Evaluation in Severe Sepsis (PROWESS) study examining activated protein C yielded positive results with a 6.1% reduction in absolute mortality.[26] Despite this positive trial, there were some controversies with the results of the trial, due to changes in the study protocol during the study.[28,29] A subsequent trial in patients at a low risk of death of sepsis did not show a benefit of the drug.[30] As a result, the study is being repeated in patients with a high risk of death from sepsis.

CYTOKINES

It could be argued that the earliest work on cytokines dates back to the time when fever, swelling and pain were noted to be associated with wounds containing pus. The origin of modern cytokine research probably is found in the observations of Rich and Lewis in 1932; they observed antigen-mediated inhibition of neutrophil and macrophage migration in tuberculin-sensitized tissue.[31] By the 1940s, "soluble factors" derived from the white blood cells from the pus of patients with infection were found to have effects on the body.[32]

Menkin, in 1944, was the first to attempt to purify the factors possessing the ability to induce a febrile response in animals from inflammatory exudates.[33] Menkin called these factors "pyrogens" from the Greek word "pyros" meaning "fire." These factors were subsequently shown to be contaminated by endotoxin (see above). The difficulty in studying these factors prior to the 1970s was that the technology to elucidate the structure of these novel molecules was in its infancy. For the most part, scientists were left with only phenomenological observations of their purified factors.

Subsequently, a series of studies suggested the possibility of biologically active soluble factors released from a variety of cell types. One of the earliest descriptions of the effect of a purified cytokine was by Isaacs and Lindenmann who described and named "interferon" as a factor; it was produced by virus-infected fibroblasts in 1957. The substance was so named because it interfered with the production of new viruses and made uninfected cells resistant to infection.[34,35] David and colleagues, as well as Bloom and Bennett, independently described the first lymphokine, a macrophage migration inhibitory factor that inhibited migration of macrophages in response to microbial antigens in 1966.[36,37] In the 1970s and 1980s, the field of cytokine biology went through rapid expansion and several new factors were discovered. As it became apparent that a wide variety of cell types could generate soluble factors with a wide variety of biological activities related to immune function, Cohen proposed the inclusive term "cytokine" for these factors.[38,39]

In 1971, Gery and colleagues described a monocyte/macrophage-derived thymocyte mitogenic factor derived from human peripheral blood, which they termed "lymphocyte activation factor."[40] This factor, the first known monokine, is now known as interleukin-1(IL-1). The earliest studies of what would later be recognized as IL-1 probably occurred in the work of Menkin and Beeson (circa 1943–1948) when they demonstrated the pyrogenic activity of the protein component produced by cells in rabbit peritoneal exudate.[33] Despite potential contamination with endotoxin, it is likely that a significant portion of the pyrogenic activity of the exudate was related to IL-1. Interleukin-1 is now widely recognized as having a central role in the pathogenesis of sepsis, based on a large body of research spearheaded by Dinarello, Wolff, and colleagues.[41,42]

Along with IL-1, tumor necrosis factor was among the earliest monokines found to have a central role in sepsis and septic shock. The term "tumor necrosis factor" derives from its earliest known biological activity as described by Carswell in 1975.[43] His research described it as a cytotoxic protein found in the blood of endotoxic-shocked animals that could mediate hemorrhagic necrosis of mouse sarcoma tumors. Initially, this compound was also referred to as "cachectin" in recognition of its ability to modulate adipocyte function by suppressing lipoprotein lipase (producing hyptertriglyceridemia), which resulted in rapid weight loss in experimental animals.[44] Eventually, Beutler and colleagues were able to demonstrate that cachectin and tumor necrosis factor were the same compound. A group of investigators including Tracey, Beutler, Lowry, Cerami and others elucidated a central role for tumor necrosis factor in septic shock and other systemic inflammatory states.[45,46]

The discovery of the role that cytokines played in the activation of the immune system led clinicians to investigate these substances as therapeutic targets for the treatment of sepsis and septic shock. Both cytokines and anti-cytokines have been studied as potential therapies to modulate the immune response to sepsis. The pleiotropic effects of these molecules account, in part, for the failures of cytokine and anti-cytokine clinical trials in human sepsis. There has been more success in utilizing these molecules anti-inflammatory effects for conditions such as rheumatoid arthritis.

NITRIC OXIDE

Shortly after the discovery of the role of pro-inflammatory cytokines in sepsis, a central mediator of their effects on the vascular system was found. This factor dilates blood vessels and so plays a key role in the pathogenesis of sepsis. This factor was initially called endothelial-derived relaxing factor (EDRF) and eventually discovered to be nitric oxide (NO). A discussion of the history of sepsis research would not be complete without a discussion of this unique substance.

The history of the discovery of NO dates back to 1948 when Folkow and colleagues described the vasodilatory effects of cholinergic stimulation of arterial vessels in the hind limb of a cat.[47] This vasodilation was abolished by atropine and the inference was made that acetylcholine released from sympathetic nerve endings resulted in the dilation of smooth muscle. When the vessels were studied in vitro, however, acetylcholine consistently caused the vessels to contract.[48]

The discrepancy between the behavior of arteries in vivo and in vitro was explained in a serendipitous discovery by Furchgott in 1980. Arteries that were studied in vitro typically had their adventitia and endothelium removed to obtain a pure smooth muscle preparation. Furchgott's technician had inadvertently neglected to remove the endothelium for one of the experiments and the vasodilating properties of acetylcholine were again realized. This led Furchgott to hypothesize that there was an endothelial-derived factor that caused the smooth muscle to relax. He thus named it "EDRF."[49]

It was not until the 1980s that the nature of EDRF was elucidated. At the time, the vasodilatory effects of nitroglycerine (NTG) and sodium nitroprusside (SNP) were known to be mediated through the sequential generation of nitric oxide and cyclic guanosine monophosphate (cGMP).[50] In addition, acetylcholine was known to depress the contractile function of isolated cardiac myocytes through a cGMP-dependent mechanism. Nonetheless, for many years the potential link between acetylcholine mediated vascular relaxation and NO/cGMP was unrecognized. Eventually, it was shown that EDRF exerted its vasodilatory effects by working through the cGMP system.[51] The similarities between EDRF and NO were well described by 1986; in 1987, two independent laboratories published conclusive proof that NO was EDRF.[52,53] Furchgott, Ignarro and Murad were awarded the Nobel Prize in Medicine in 1998 for their part in the discovery of NO and its impact on the vasculature.

NO is now recognized to play a pivotal role in the pathophysiology of cardiovascular collapse in sepsis. In the normal state, endothelially produced NO regulates microvascular tone and is responsible for local leukocyte adhesion and platelet aggregation. When sepsis develops, NO is produced in substantial excess by endothelium and adjacent vascular smooth muscle.[54] This excess NO production results in the intense venodilation and vascular collapse of septic shock. In addition, nitric oxide also appears to be substantially responsible for sepsis-associated myocardial depression.[55]

Other investigators have found that NO also binds to cytochromes in the respiratory chain of mitochondria resulting in the termination of cellular respiration and the onset on anaerobic metabolism.[56] Thus, one of the theories about the mechanism of organ dysfunction in sepsis is that of NO-mediated mitochondrial dysfunction. Like so many other targeted therapies for sepsis, the inhibition of NO synthase in clinical trials showed no benefit, and had to be stopped early because of an increase in mortality in the treatment arm.[57]

CLASSIFICATION AND CLINICAL THEORIES OF SEPTIC SHOCK

Although work originating from the battlefields of World War I clearly linked traumatic shock associated with substantial, obvious bleeding to a loss of circulating blood volume, the origin of traumatic shock in the absence of defined hemorrhage was unclear.[58] The accepted explanation for this phenomenon remained a variation of the vasomotor paralysis theory of shock. It was postulated that nonhemorrhagic, post-traumatic shock ("wound shock") was caused by the liberation of "wound toxins" (histamine and/or other substances) that resulted in "neurogenic" vasodilation and peripheral blood pooling. However, after the war, Blalock and others demonstrated in animal models that nonhemorrhagic traumatic shock was caused by the loss of blood and fluids into injured tissue rather than circulating toxins resulting in stasis of blood within the circulation.[59] Nonetheless, this concept was one of earlier enunciations of the currently accepted pathophysiologic paradigm of sepsis and septic shock.

Although hypovolemic shock associated with trauma was the first form of shock to be recognized and studied, by the early 1900s it was broadly recognized that other clinical conditions could result in a similar constellation of signs and symptoms. Sepsis as a distinct cause of shock was initially proposed by Laennec (1831) and subsequently supported by Boise (1897).[60,61]

In 1934, Blalock developed the precursor of the most commonly used shock classification systems of the present. He subdivided shock into four etiologic categories: hematogenic or oligemic (hypovolemic), cardiogenic, neurogenic (eg, shock after spinal injury), and vasogenic (primarily septic shock). Shubin and Weil, in 1967, proposed the additional etiologic categories of hypersensitivity (ie, anaphylactic), bacteremic (ie, septic), obstructive, and endocrinologic shock.[62] However, as the hemodynamic profiles of the different forms of shock were uncovered, a classification based on cardiovascular characteristics (initially proposed in 1972 by Hinshaw and Cox) came to be accepted by most clinicians.[63] In this categorization, septic shock was considered a form of distributive shock caused by loss of vasomotor control resulting in arteriolar and venular dilation and—after resuscitation with fluids—characterized by increased cardiac output with decreased systemic vascular resistance.

HEMODYNAMICS

Since the 1960s, the understanding of the cardiovascular manifestations of septic shock has progressed through three phases. This progression in the understanding of the hemodynamic characteristics of the syndrome has been related to the application of increasingly sophisticated monitoring and investigative techniques to critically ill patients.[64,65]

The first phase, which predated the development of the flow directed pulmonary catheter by Swan and Ganz, described two progressive forms of septic shock: warm and cold. Warm skin and bounding pulses despite hypotension characterized warm shock. The other form of septic shock was characterized by cold clammy skin, a thready pulse, and hypotension. This was called cold shock. A few patients who were monitored invasively demonstrated that warm shock was associated with a high cardiac output (CO) and cold shock was associated with low CO. Based on these measurements, it was concluded that septic shock survivors went through an initial hyperdynamic phase of septic shock and then improved. Those patients who eventually succumbed to their disease went into a shock state that resulted in myocardial depression and low CO. Several clinical human studies and some experimental (endotoxin model) animal experiments seemed to confirm this observational finding.[66,67]

Further work showed that survival correlated with an increase in CO. Part of the initial confusion as to the now well-accepted hyperdynamic (high cardiac output/low systemic vascular resistance) profile of septic shock related to the lack of a simple method of measuring CO and true preload at the bedside. Initial clinicians were utilizing the central venous pressure as a surrogate of left ventricular end diastolic volume (LVEDV). Subsequently, many studies demonstrated that central venous pressure poorly correlated with measures of LVEDV in critically ill patients, especially those with sepsis.

Wilson challenged this widespread belief of the nature of the hemodynamic profile of septic shock as being a low CO state in 1965.[68] He and his colleagues were the first to describe the high CO low systemic vascular resistance (SVR) state of sepsis and distinguish it from the low CO/high SVR state of cardiogenic or hemorrhagic shock. Despite his findings, the hyperdynamic hemodynamic profile of septic shock that he noted did not become entrenched in medicine until the development of the flow directed pulmonary artery catheter.

Werner Forssmann, a German physician, was the first person to place a catheter into the heart. He performed the procedure on himself in the operating room and then climbed a stairwell to a radiographic machine to confirm the position of the catheter with a radiograph. For his efforts, he was summarily dismissed from his position and went into training in urology. Further advances in right heart catheterization were not made until 1964 when R.D. Bradley described the use of a pulmonary artery catheter (PAC) in critically ill patients.[69]

Harold Swan, a cardiologist from the University of California at Los Angeles, working with William Ganz developed the idea of a flotation-directed pulmonary artery device with a balloon on the end of the catheter. Although likely apocryphal in nature, some written accounts suggest that Swan came up with the idea of the balloon tipped catheter while watching boats in the Santa Monica Harbor. Swan and Ganz were performing studies in canines evaluating methods to place catheters into the pulmonary circulation. One afternoon they received a catheter with a balloon on its tip, and they placed the catheter in the right atrium of a dog, blew up the balloon, and the catheter "disappeared." This occurred repeatedly, until the investigators realized that the catheter was being rapidly transported to the pulmonary artery where (because of the narrow scope of the fluoroscopy machine), it was off the screen. That afternoon, Swan and Ganz immediately used the same catheter (following sterilization) in a myocardial infarction patient in the coronary care unit recording bedside pulmonary artery pressures and allowing evaluation of cardiac performance using these hemodynamic values. A description of their landmark invention was published in 1970, and the catheter is more commonly and eponymously referred to as the Swan-Ganz catheter.[8,70]

The use of the PAC resulted in the second phase in the understanding of the hemodynamics of septic shock. The widespread use of the PAC resulted in the broad acceptance of the current hyperdynamic, high cardiac output nature of resuscitated septic shock. It became clear that many patients with septic shock had low initial filling pressures, as measured by the pulmonary artery wedge (occlusion) pressure. This indicated that septic patients were often hypovolemic upon presentation, and with adequate fluid resuscitation, patients consistently demonstrated a hyperdynamic state with high CO and low SVR.

Despite the mounting evidence of a hyperdynamic state of sepsis, the belief that septic shock was associated with myocardial depression and a low cardiac output persisted. The application of portable radionuclide cineangiography led to the third phase in the understanding of the hemodynamic nature of septic shock.[64] This technique was used to prove the hypothesis that the myocardium was depressed in sepsis, despite the hyperdynamic state demonstrated with PACs. In the first described study, Calvin and colleagues in 1981 demonstrated a subgroup of septic patients with an increase in left ventricular end diastolic volume and a decrease in ejection fraction.[71] In a subsequent study of serial hemodynamics and nuclear scans by Parker and Parrillo, 15 of 20 patients with septic shock demonstrated a reduced ejection fraction during the first 2 days after septic shock onset.[72] This decrease in ejection fraction and increase in LVEDV improved within the time course of the resolution of sepsis (7–10 days) (ie, the myocardial dysfunction was reversible). Interestingly, nonsurvivors of septic shock did not demonstrate the dilated, hypokinetic ventricle that survivors developed.

It is now known that many patients with septic shock develop a reversible depression in their ejection fraction that lasts for 7–10 days. Despite this reduction in ejection fraction, CO is maintained at higher than normal levels, secondary to an increase in LVEDV that causes a higher CO. Further research has demonstrated that sepsis also causes a reversible decrease in the lusiotropic function of the heart (ie, diastolic dysfunction).[73]

Early work by Parrillo and colleagues showed that circulating myocardial depressant substances were present during sepsis. Parrillo showed that serum from patients with early sepsis decreased both the amplitude and velocity of cardiomyocyte contraction in healthy rats.[74] The substances in the serum were identified to be TNF-α and IL-1. Further work indicated that TNF-α and IL-1 cause myocardial depression through the production of intracellular mediators, particularly NO and cyclic GMP.

Other possible mediators include: sphingosine, eicosanoids, platelet activating factor, and leukocyte lysozyme.

The description of the hemodynamics of septic shock is a burgeoning field of research. The ongoing research in this area includes using the hemodynamics of sepsis to potentially predict outcome.[75]

SUMMARY

The early descriptions of sepsis date back to antiquity. The initial theories of infectious disease espoused by Hippocrates and Galen remained largely unchallenged until Lister, Koch and Pasteur rapidly advanced the field and resulted in a paradigm shift in the way we view sepsis. Building on their work, twentieth century scientists have begun to unravel the molecular mysteries of sepsis, which has allowed for an improved understanding of the pathophysiology of the disease. With the sequencing of the human genome, single nucleotide polymorphisms have started to become a new tool in the armamentarium that allows scientists to predict who will suffer adverse consequences of infectious disease. The continued research into sepsis has already resulted in a decrease in mortality when compared to historical controls, and results will no doubt continue to improve.

REFERENCES

1. Geroulanos S, Douka ET. Historical perspective of the word "sepsis." Intensive Care Med 2006;32:2077.
2. Thurston AJ. Of blood, inflammation and gunshot wounds: the history of the control of sepsis. Aust N Z J Surg 2000;70:855–61.
3. Hurlbert R. Chapter 1: a brief history of microbiology. Microbiology 101/102 internet text [online]. 1999; Available at: http://www.slic2.wsu.edu:82/hurlbert/micro101/pages/Chap1.html. Accessed December 10, 2008.
4. Majno G. The ancient riddle of sigma eta psi iota sigma (sepsis). J Infect Dis 1991;163:937–45.
5. De Costa CM. "The contagiousness of childbed fever:" a short history of puerperal sepsis and its treatment. Med J Aust 2002;177:668–71.
6. Baron RM, Baron MJ, Perrella MA. Pathobiology of sepsis: are we still asking the same questions? Am J Respir Cell Mol Biol 2006;34:129–34.
7. Francoeur JR. Joseph Lister: surgeon scientist (1827–1912). J Invest Surg 2000; 13:129–32.
8. Rosengart MR. Critical care medicine: landmarks and legends. Surg Clin North Am 2006;86:1305–21.
9. Domagk TNFG. The Nobel Foundation: Gerhard Domagk. Available at: http://nobelprizeorg/nobel_prizes/medicine/laureates/1939/domagk-biohtml. Accessed June 12, 2008.
10. The Nobel Foundation. Sir Alexander Fleming Available at: http://nobelprize.org/nobel_prizes/medicine/laureates/1945/fleming-bio.html. Accessed May 15, 2008.
11. Beutler B, Rietschel ET. Innate immune sensing and its roots: the story of endotoxin. Nat Rev Immunol 2003;3:169–76.
12. Rosenberg RD, Aird WC. Vascular-bed–specific hemostasis and hypercoagulable states. N Engl J Med 1999;340:1555–64.
13. Bernard GR. Drotrecogin alfa (activated) (recombinant human activated protein C) for the treatment of severe sepsis. Crit Care Med 2003;31:S85–93.
14. Jones H, Tocantis L. The history of purpura hemorrhagica. Ann Med Hist 1933;5: 349–58.

15. Manasse P. Virchows Arch Pathol Anatomie 1892;20:217–9.
16. Sanarelli G. Presse Med 1894;24:505–7.
17. Zdrodowsky P, Brenn E. Zentralbl Bakteriol 1926;99:159–63.
18. Hardaway RM. Pathological evidence of disseminated intravascular coagulation in human shock. Thromb Diath Haemorrh 1966;20:249–54.
19. Schneider CL. Fibrin embolism (disseminated intravascular coagulation) with defibrination as one of the end results during placenta abruptio. Surg Gynecol Obstet 1951;92:27–34.
20. Selye H. The thrombohemorrhagic phenomenon as a pluricausal disease. Perspect Biol Med 1966;9:226–43.
21. Friedman M, Hamburger WW, Katz LN. Use of Heparin in subacute bacterial endocarditis. JAMA 1939;113:1702–4.
22. Little JR. Purpura Fulminans treated successfully with anticoagulation. JAMA 1959;169:36–8.
23. Nawroth PP, Handley DA, Esmon CT, et al. Interleukin 1 induces endothelial cell procoagulant while suppressing cell-surface anticoagulant activity. Proc Natl Acad Sci USA 1986;83:3460–4.
24. Schipper HG, Jenkins CS, Kahle LH, et al. Antithrombin-III transfusion in disseminated intravascular coagulation. Lancet 1978;1:854–6.
25. Abraham E, Reinhart K, Opal S, et al. Efficacy and safety of tifacogin (recombinant tissue factor pathway inhibitor) in severe sepsis: a randomized controlled trial. JAMA 2003;290:238–47.
26. Bernard GR, Vincent JL, Laterre PF, et al. Efficacy and safety of recombinant human activated protein C for severe sepsis. N Engl J Med 2001;344:699–709.
27. Warren BL, Eid A, Singer P, et al. Caring for the critically ill patient. High-dose antithrombin III in severe sepsis: a randomized controlled trial. JAMA 2001;286:1869–78.
28. Siegel JP. Assessing the use of activated protein C in the treatment of severe sepsis. N Engl J Med 2002;347:1030–4.
29. Warren HS, Suffredini AF, Eichacker PQ, et al. Risks and benefits of activated protein C treatment for severe sepsis. N Engl J Med 2002;347:1027–30.
30. Abraham E, Laterre PF, Garg R, et al. Drotrecogin alfa (activated) for adults with severe sepsis and a low risk of death. N Engl J Med 2005;353:1332–41.
31. Oppenheim J. Foreword to the 4th Edition. In: Thomson A, Lotze M, editors. The cytokine handbook. Burlington (MA): Academic Press; 2003. p. xxiii–vii.
32. Dinarello CA. Historical insights into cytokines. Eur J Immunol 2007;37(Suppl 1):S34–45.
33. Menkin V. Chemical basis of fever. Science [New York, NY] 1944;100:337–8.
34. Isaacs A, Lindenmann J. Virus interference. I. The interferon. Proceedings of the Royal Society of London Series B, [Containing papers of a Biological character] 1957;147:258–67.
35. Isaacs A, Lindenmann J, Valentine RC. Virus interference. II. Some properties of interferon. Proceedings of the Royal Society of London Series B, [Containing papers of a Biological character] 1957;147:268–73.
36. Bloom BR, Bennett B. Mechanism of a reaction in vitro associated with delayed-type hypersensitivity. Science [New York, NY] 1966;153:80–2.
37. David JR. Delayed hypersensitivity in vitro: its mediation by cell-free substances formed by lymphoid cell-antigen interaction. Proc Natl Acad Sci USA 1966;56:72–7.
38. Cohen S. Cytokine: more than a new word, a new concept proposed by Stanley Cohen thirty years ago. Cytokines 2004;28:242–7.

39. Cohen S, Bigazzi PE, Yoshida T. Commentary. Similarities of T cell function in cell-mediated immunity and antibody production. Cell Immunol 1974;12:150–9.
40. Gery I, Gershon RK, Waksman BH. Potentiation of cultured mouse thymocyte responses by factors released by peripheral leucocytes. J Immunol 1971;107:1778–80.
41. Dinarello CA. Interleukin-1 and interleukin-1 antagonism. Blood 1991;77:1627–52.
42. Dinarello CA, Wolff SM. Pathogenesis of fever in man. N Engl J Med 1978;298:607–12.
43. Carswell EA, Old LJ, Kassel RL, et al. An endotoxin-induced serum factor that causes necrosis of tumors. Proc Natl Acad Sci USA 1975;72:3666–70.
44. Beutler B, Greenwald D, Hulmes JD, et al. Identity of tumour necrosis factor and the macrophage-secreted factor cachectin. Nature 1985;316:552–4.
45. Tracey KJ, Beutler B, Lowry SF, et al. Shock and tissue injury induced by recombinant human cachectin. Science [New York, NY] 1986;234:470–4.
46. Tracey KJ, Fong Y, Hesse DG, et al. Anti-cachectin/TNF monoclonal antibodies prevent septic shock during lethal bacteraemia. Nature 1987;330:662–4.
47. Folkow B, Haeger K, Unvas B. Cholinergic vasodilator nerves in the sympathetic outflow to the muscles of the hindlimb of the cat. Acta Physiol Scand 1948;15:401–11.
48. Sakanashi M, Furukawa T, Horio Y. Inhibition of constrictor responses of dog coronary artery by atropine. A possible effectiveness of atropine on variant form of angina pectoris. Jpn Heart J 1979;20:75–82.
49. Furchgott RF, Zawadzki JV. The obligatory role of endothelial cells in the relaxation of arterial smooth muscle by acetylcholine. Nature 1980;288:373–6.
50. Gruetter CA, Gruetter DY, Lyon JE, et al. Relationship between cyclic guanosine 3':5'-monophosphate formation and relaxation of coronary arterial smooth muscle by glyceryl trinitrate, nitroprusside, nitrite and nitric oxide: effects of methylene blue and methemoglobin. J Pharmacol Exp Ther 1981;219:181–6.
51. Rapoport RM, Draznin MB, Murad F. Endothelium-dependent vasodilator-and nitrovasodilator-induced relaxation may be mediated through cyclic GMP formation and cyclic GMP-dependent protein phosphorylation. Trans Assoc Am Physicians 1983;96:19–30.
52. Ignarro LJ, Harbison RG, Wood KS, et al. Activation of purified soluble guanylate cyclase by endothelium-derived relaxing factor from intrapulmonary artery and vein: stimulation by acetylcholine, bradykinin and arachidonic acid. J Pharmacol Exp Ther 1986;237:893–900.
53. Palmer RM, Ferrige AG, Moncada S. Nitric oxide release accounts for the biological activity of endothelium-derived relaxing factor. Nature 1987;327:524–6.
54. Kumar A, Krieger A, Symeoneides S, et al. Myocardial dysfunction in septic shock: part II. Role of cytokines and nitric oxide. J Cardiothorac Vasc Anesth 2001;15:485–511.
55. Kumar A, Brar R, Wang P, et al. Role of nitric oxide and cGMP in human septic serum-induced depression of cardiac myocyte contractility. Am J Phys 1999;276:R265–76.
56. Fink MP. Bench-to-bedside review: cytopathic hypoxia. Crit Care 2002;6:491–9.
57. Lopez A, Lorente JA, Steingrub J, et al. Multiple-center, randomized, placebo-controlled, double-blind study of the nitric oxide synthase inhibitor 546C88: effect on survival in patients with septic shock. Crit Care Med 2004;32:21–30.
58. Hunter AR. Old unhappy far off things. Some reflections on the significance of the early work on shock. Ann R Coll Surg Engl 1967;40:289–305.
59. Blalock A. Experimental shock: cause of low blood pressure produced by muscle injury. Arch Surg 1930;20:959–96.

60. Boise E. The differential diagnosis of shock, hemorrhage, and sepsis. Trans Am Assoc Obstet 1897;9:433–8.
61. Laennec R. Traite de L'uscultation Mediate et des Maladies des Poumons et du Coeur. Paris: JS Chaude; 1831.
62. Weil M. Bacterial shock. In: Weil MH, Shubin H, editors. Diagnosis and treatment of shock. Philadelphia: Williams and Wilkins Co; 1967.
63. Hinshaw L, Cox B. The fundamental mechanisms of shock. New York: Plenum Press; 1972.
64. Kumar A, Haery C, Parrillo JE. Myocardial dysfunction in septic shock: Part I. Clinical manifestation of cardiovascular dysfunction. J Cardiothorac Vasc Anesth 2001;15:364–76.
65. Rabuel C, Mebazaa A. Septic shock: a heart story since the 1960s. Intensive Care Med 2006;32:799–807.
66. Clowes GH Jr, Vucinic M, Weidner MG. Circulatory and metabolic alterations associated with survival or death in peritonitis: clinical analysis of 25 cases. Ann Surg 1966;163:866–85.
67. MacLean LD, Mulligan WG, McLean AP, et al. Patterns of septic shock in man– a detailed study of 56 patients. Ann Surg 1967;166:543–62.
68. Wilson R, Thal A, Kindling P. Hemodynamic measurements in septic shock. Arch Surg 1965;91:121–9.
69. Bradley RD. Diagnostic right-heart catheterisation with miniature catheters in severely ill patients. Lancet 1964;2:941–2.
70. Swan HJ, Ganz W, Forrester J, et al. Catheterization of the heart in man with use of a flow-directed balloon-tipped catheter. N Engl J Med 1970;283:447–51.
71. Calvin JE, Driedger AA, Sibbald WJ. An assessment of myocardial function in human sepsis utilizing ECG gated cardiac scintigraphy. Chest 1981;80:579–86.
72. Parker MM, Shelhamer JH, Bacharach SL, et al. Profound but reversible myocardial depression in patients with septic shock. Ann Intern Med 1984;100:483–90.
73. Bouhemad B, Nicolas-Robin A, Arbelot C, et al. Isolated and reversible impairment of ventricular relaxation in patients with septic shock. Crit Care Med 2008;36:766–74.
74. Parrillo JE, Burch C, Shelhamer JH, et al. A circulating myocardial depressant substance in humans with septic shock. Septic shock patients with a reduced ejection fraction have a circulating factor that depresses in vitro myocardial cell performance. J Clin Invest 1985;76:1539–53.
75. Kumar A, Schupp E, Bunnell E, et al. Cardiovascular response to dobutamine stress predicts outcome in severe sepsis and septic shock. Crit Care 2008;12:R35–46.

Cardiogenic Shock: A Historical Perspective

Fredric Ginsberg, MD[a,b,*], Joseph E. Parrillo, MD[a,c]

KEYWORDS

- Definition of cardiogenic shock
- Acute coronary thrombosis
- Hemodynamic monitoring
- Intra-aortic balloon counterpulsation
- Revascularization strategies

The description of cardiogenic shock (CS) in medical literature is a relatively recent occurrence. The term "shock" was first used in 1743 to describe a moribund condition after severe trauma. Harrison in 1935, and Blalock in 1940, were the first to classify shock according to cause: cardiogenic, oligemic, vasogenic, and neurogenic.[1] CS was applied to failure of the circulation attributable to primary diseases of the heart. In the medical literature at that time, many cardiovascular conditions were recognized that could produce CS. These included cardiac tamponade, terminal stages of chronic heart failure, beriberi heart disease, myocarditis, severe infections with septicemia, endocarditis with valve rupture, aortic dissection, massive pulmonary embolism, and supraventricular and ventricular arrhythmias. The most common cause was recognized to be acute myocardial infarction (AMI).

The first description of chest pain due to coronary artery disease (CAD) is attributed to William Heberden, who described "a disorder of the breast" before the Royal College of Physicians in 1768.[2] For more than a century, the commonly held belief was that this condition always caused death suddenly. In 1880, Carl Wiegert's description of the pathology of CAD linked atherosclerosis, coronary thrombosis, and myocardial infarction. In 1896, George Dock described four patients who had CAD, one of whom survived for 1 week after the onset of myocardial infarction. In 1910, Obrastzow and Straschesko presented two cases of AMI diagnosed clinically before death. James Herrick (**Fig. 1**) presented a classic paper in 1912 that linked clinical observations of patients ill with AMI with autopsy findings. His contention, which was not immediately accepted by the medical community, was that coronary artery thrombosis and AMI were not always immediately fatal, and that efforts needed to be made to make this diagnosis while the patient was still alive.[3] Abnormal findings

a Robert Wood Johnson Medical School at Camden, University of Medicine and Dentistry of New Jersey, Camden, NJ, USA
b Cooper University Hospital, One Cooper Plaza, Camden, NJ 08103, USA
c Department of Medicine, Cooper University Hospital, Camden, NJ 08103, USA
* Corresponding author. Cooper University Hospital, One Cooper Plaza, Camden, NJ 08103.
E-mail address: ginsberg-fredric@cooperhealth.edu (F. Ginsberg).

Crit Care Clin 25 (2009) 103–114
doi:10.1016/j.ccc.2008.12.005
0749-0704/08/$ – see front matter © 2009 Elsevier Inc. All rights reserved.
criticalcare.theclinics.com

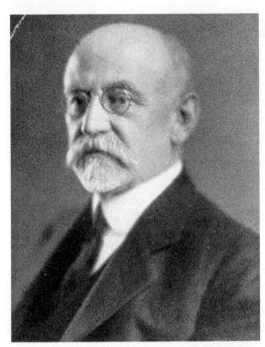

Fig. 1. James Herrick, who urged that the diagnosis of acute myocardial infarction be made prior to death.

on the ECG in patients who had AMI were described by Pardee in 1920, providing objective evidence to diagnose this condition.[2] Continuous monitoring of the ECG rhythm during AMI led to the realization that the most common cause of sudden demise was ventricular fibrillation.

Throughout the late nineteenth and early twentieth century, atherosclerosis of the coronary arteries was found at autopsy in patients dying from CAD. There was great debate as to how often coronary thrombosis was responsible for AMI, however. Various autopsy series reported widely differing frequencies of coronary thrombosis in AMI, varying from 36% to 95%.[2] Sones[4] introduced selective coronary arteriography in humans in 1962. A landmark study by DeWood and others[5] reported in 1980 described the findings of coronary angiography performed early in the course of AMI in 322 patients. When patients were studied within 4 hours of the onset of symptoms of AMI, 85% demonstrated coronary occlusion due to thrombosis. This frequency was lower, at 65%, if patients were studied 4 to 12 hours after symptom onset. This study convincingly showed that coronary thrombosis was the pathogenetic mechanism in the vast majority of patients who had AMI, and that spontaneous lysis of thrombus could occur early in the course of the illness, accounting for the inconsistent finding of thrombosis at autopsy. These results provided the rationale for applying emergency revascularization strategies with thrombolysis and emergency angioplasty for the modern treatment of acute MI.

For many decades after CS was described, there was debate as to whether the pathophysiology involved solely reduced cardiac output or whether there was associated peripheral circulatory collapse. In 1941, Grishman and Master measured cardiac output in patients after AMI and found it to be reduced. Research into the pathophysiology and treatment of CS following AMI occurred more widely in the 1950s and

1960s. In 1952, Fries and colleagues[1] were the first to measure cardiac output in patients who had shock following AMI. They also found cardiac output to be reduced but could not discern a consistent relationship between the severity of the reduction in cardiac output and the occurrence of shock. Agress and Binder attempted to produce an animal model of CS in the 1950s by producing closed chest coronary artery embolism in dogs. They found no correlation between the occurrence of shock and the size of myocardial infarction, and noted a failure of total peripheral resistance to increase in animals that had the most severe shock.

In the 1950s, CS following AMI was known to be associated with a high mortality. In a series of patients who had AMI studied in 1949 to 1951, 19.7% developed shock with a mortality of 80%.[6] Mortality rates in other series from the time varied widely, however, from 50% to 90%. This variation was due to a nonstandard definition of CS. Initially, CS was characterized as "marked hypotension for over 1 hour associated with peripheral circulatory collapse."[6] Included in series that reported lower mortality were previously hypertensive patients who had systolic blood pressures as high as 100 mm Hg during "shock," and patients who likely had transient hypotension.

A standard definition of CS attributable to AMI was proposed by Binder and colleagues in 1955.[7] They proposed a definition that included a systolic blood pressure less than 80 mm Hg, associated with a heart rate greater than 110 beats per minute with signs of peripheral circulatory collapse, such as clouded sensorium, cyanosis, cold clammy skin, and oliguria. In addition, severe hypotension needed to persist for more than 30 minutes despite administration of morphine and oxygen. Patients who had complicating conditions, such as severe arrhythmia, diabetic acidosis, hemorrhage, infection, recent stroke, or pulmonary embolism, were also excluded from their definition.

Standard therapies in the 1950s included supplemental oxygen, phlebotomy, and morphine administration. Patients who had shock and pulmonary congestion also received ethyl alcohol vapor, digitalis, and quinidine. Cortisone and intra-arterial infusions of blood or plasma were also used.[6,7]

Griffith and colleagues[6] evaluated the use of norepinephrine, methoxamine, and isoproterenol in CS. They concluded that the promptness of institution of therapy was a key factor in treating shock associated with AMI. They found isoproterenol to be useful in patients who had heart block. Binder and colleagues[7] reported no reversal of the shock state with cortisone or the use of intravenous or intra-arterial infusions. They noted an 82% mortality in patients supported with morphine and oxygen and a 92% mortality with the use of methoxamine or ephedrine. Mortality was lowered to 68% when norepinephrine was used. They also reported beneficial effects of isoproterenol in patients who had heart block accompanying shock. They concurred that early therapy for shock was important and concluded that norepinephrine was the "vasopressor drug of choice" because of its "prompt pressor response." Agress and Binder[1] also recommended routine measurement of urinary flow, the use of atropine or the Zoll external pacemaker for bradycardia, and intravenous ouabain for patients who had heart failure. A later report describing 25 patients who had CS following AMI, in whom CS was defined as systolic blood pressure less than 70 mm Hg, noted shock in 9.4% of AMIs. A wide variation in the time from onset of AMI to the onset of shock was described; shock occurred anywhere from the time of admission to hospital to more than 1 week later.[8] Norepinephrine relieved shock in 7 of 17 patients, but mortality was 100%.

Coronary care units (CCUs) were introduced in the early 1960s as a specialized area in the hospital to care for patients who had AMI. Staffed by specially trained nurses and physicians, CCUs were shown to improve in-hospital mortality from AMI. In patients who did not have shock, mortality in a representative series improved from

26% to 7%, mainly by successful treatment of life-threatening arrhythmias with rapid defibrillation.[9] Mortality in patients who had CS was not improved, however, and was reported at 81% to 85%.

Another study from the late 1960s showed hospital mortality of AMI without heart failure or shock of 4% to 6%, 15% to 21% in patients who had severe heart failure, and 83% in patients who had shock.[10] It was concluded that "the hemodynamic effect of the infarction has the greatest influence on prognosis." In a retrospective survey of patients who had AMI cared for in a CCU, a clear decrease in hospital mortality between 1970 and 1975 was observed in patients who did not have CS, but mortality in patients who had CS remained level at around 86%.[11] In 1970, the occurrence of CS continued to be reported in 10% to 20% of patients who had AMI. Women and older patients developed shock more commonly, as did patients who had higher levels of aspartate aminotransferase. Fifty percent of patients were observed to develop shock more than 1 day after presentation.[12]

Invasive hemodynamic monitoring in patients who had shock was used to obtain a better understanding of pathophysiology. In 1964, Cohn and Luria[13] described seven patients who had shock in whom bedside measurements of right atrial pressure, femoral artery pressure, blood volume, and cardiac output by dye dilution curves were performed. They described that auscultatory blood pressure was often an inaccurate reflection of central aortic pressure in patients who had shock, and that hypovolemia was often not recognized clinically. They concluded that bedside hemodynamic monitoring helped assess which patients would respond to volume expansion and when vasopressors should be prescribed. In 1966, Gunnar and colleagues[14] measured central venous pressure, central aortic pressure, and cardiac output in 23 patients who had AMI. In patients who did not have shock, average cardiac output was 3.8 ± 1.5 L/min, and cardiac output was on average 2.2 ± 0.9 L/min in patients who had shock. Six of 12 patients who had shock had low systemic vascular resistance (SVR). Methoxamine was tried but resulted in ineffective elevation of blood pressure and reduction in cardiac output. Norepinephrine was shown to increase cardiac output and SVR and was advocated for use in CS.[14]

In 1976, Forrester and colleagues[15] advocated the widespread use of hemodynamic monitoring in patients who have AMI. A balloon-tipped catheter, described by Swan and colleagues[16] in 1970, was advanced from a peripheral vein to the pulmonary artery at the bedside, without the use of fluoroscopy. Pulmonary artery occlusion pressure (PAOP) reflected left ventricular diastolic pressure (if pulmonary venous resistance was normal) and cardiac output was measured with the thermodilution technique. They compared clinical assessment of pulmonary congestion with measurements of PAOP and clinical assessment or organ perfusion with measurement of cardiac output. Pulmonary congestion correlated with PAOP greater than 18 mm Hg and pulmonary edema with PAOP greater than 30 mm Hg. Clinical hypoperfusion was described with cardiac index less than 2.2 $L/m/m^2$ and CS with cardiac index less than 1.8 $L/m/m^2$. Significant hemodynamic depression was often missed when only clinical assessment was used. Mortality of patients who had pulmonary congestion and systemic hypoperfusion was 51% (**Table 1**).

Throughout the 1970s, vasopressors and inotropic drugs were studied. Early use of vasopressors was shown to improve blood pressure and hemodynamics.[12] Mortality was not improved with the use of norepinephrine or isoproterenol, however, despite temporary clinical improvement. In 1970, Mueller and colleagues[17] showed that in patients who had CS, isoproterenol increased cardiac output because of an increase in heart rate, without improving mean arterial pressure or prognosis. Norepinephrine increased blood pressure by increasing SVR without a significant improvement in

Table 1				
Mortality rates in clinical and hemodynamic subsets				
Subsets	Pulmonary Congestion[a]	Peripheral Hypoperfusion[b]	Mortality (%)	
			Clinical	Hemodynamic
I	—	—	1	3
II	+	—	11	9
III	—	+	18	23
IV	+	+	60	51

Subset I: PAOP<18 mm Hg, cardiac index (CI)>2.2 L/min/m²; subset II: PAOP>18 mm Hg, CI>2.2 L/min/m²; subset III: PAOP<18 mm Hg, CI<2.2 L/min/m²; subset IV: PAOP>18 mm Hg, CI<2.2 L/min/m².
[a] Pulmonary capillary pressure >18 mm Hg.
[b] Cardiac index <2.2 L/min/m².
Data from Forrester JS, Diamond G, Chatterjee K, et al. Medical therapy of acute myocardial infarction by application of hemodynamic subsets (first of two parts). N Engl J Med 1976;295(24):1356–62.

cardiac index. Both agents increased myocardial oxygen consumption. In 1972, Mueller and colleagues[18] emphasized that the goal in treating patients who had CS should be "to improve myocardial oxygenation, especially in the peri-infarct ischemic 'marginal zone'" and recommended identifying factors that could improve the survival of ischemic but viable myocardium. In 1978, Mueller and colleagues[19] described the use of dopamine in patients who had CS and AMI. Peripheral perfusion improved at the expense of increased myocardial oxygen consumption, which was detrimental to ischemic myocardium. They recommended that dopamine should be used with caution.

Although inotropic and vasopressor therapy could improve hemodynamics temporarily, other therapeutic approaches were sought that could improve cardiac output and improve myocardial metabolism. In 1962, Moulopoulos, Topaz, and Kolff[20] described a device that was inserted into the descending aorta and pumped blood during diastole. Theoretic benefits included increased coronary and systemic blood flow, decreased end-diastolic pressure, and lessening the work of the left ventricle. The authors designed a polyethylene catheter with a 20-cm length latex tubing tied around the end. The tubing was filled with 25 mL of CO_2 during diastole, and was activated by a timing device synchronized to the ECG. When tested in dogs, hemodynamic benefits were achieved.

In 1968, Kantrowitz and colleagues[21] used intra-aortic balloon pumping (IABP) in five patients who had CS. The device was placed in the descending aorta by way of a femoral arteriotomy and helium was used to fill the balloon. In all five patients, hemodynamics improved and stabilized after 1 to 15 hours of balloon pumping.

After IABP was shown to be feasible and to improve hemodynamics, its effect on mortality was studied. In 1975, Dunkman and colleagues[22] reported that shock was reversed by IABP in 31 of 40 patients. Improvement generally occurred by 2 hours, with average cardiac output at baseline of 1.7 L/m/m² increasing to 2.5 L/m/m², with improvement in mean arterial pressure. Of 25 patients treated with IABP but without revascularization surgery, only 9 could be weaned from the pump and only four survived to hospital discharge. Scheidt and colleagues[23] reported on the use of IABP in 1973 in 87 patients who had CS. Although significant improvement in cardiac output was noted, only 40% of patients could be weaned from balloon support and only 17% survived to hospital discharge. Aortic dissection, renal emboli, leg ischemia, and thrombocytopenia were reported complications. Further improvements in the design of the device occurred, and a wire-guided catheter was developed allowing percutaneous insertion with fewer vascular complications.[24] IABP thus provided effective circulatory support in most patients who had CS, but mortality remained high in the absence of revascularization strategies.

Autopsy studies done throughout the 1950s and 1960s showed that patients dying from CS showed massive myocardial damage.[12,25] Page and colleagues[26] showed that patients dying from CS had larger areas of infarction than patients dying suddenly of AMI without shock. Patients who had CS demonstrated acute and old infarction involving 35% to 70% of LV myocardium (**Fig. 2**). Extensive three-vessel coronary atherosclerosis was often present. This observation, along with the failure of IABP support alone to improve mortality, lead to efforts to treat patients with coronary bypass surgery revascularization. In the series of Dunkman and colleagues[22] 15 of 40 patients who had CS who did not improve with IABP underwent coronary artery bypass surgery (CABG) with or without infarctectomy. Six of these patients survived, demonstrating that emergency CABG in this setting could result in a favorable outcome. Swan and colleagues[25] postulated that revascularization would improve left ventricular function by restoring contractile muscle mass and by improving diastolic compliance. Leinbach and colleagues[27] reported in 1973 that although 80% of patients who had CS responded to catecholamines and IABP, most could not be weaned from support. Urgent coronary angiography was shown to be feasible with IABP support. Nine of 24 patients who underwent early revascularization surgery survived. They postulated that IABP reduced infarct expansion. Johnson and colleagues[28] recommended revascularization within 12 hours of the onset of

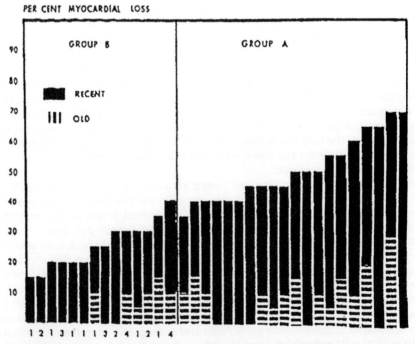

Fig. 2. Percentage of myocardium affected with acute and old infarction in groups without CS (group B) and with CS (group A). (*From* Page DL, Caulfield JB, Kastor JA, et al. Myocardial changes associated with cardiogenic shock. N Engl J Med 1971;285(3):134–7; with permission. Copyright © 1971, Massachusetts Medical Society.)

myocardial infarction for appropriate patients who had CS, with postoperative use of IABP. Mundth and colleagues[29] recommended urgent CABG with or without aneurys-mectomy if patients who had CS failed to increase cardiac index over 2 L/m/m^2 after IABP for 24 to 48 hours. DeWood and colleagues[30] reported a comparison between treatment with IABP alone and IABP combined with revascularization surgery in 1980. Although hospital mortality was similar, long-term mortality was improved in the revascularization group. In addition, those patients undergoing revascularization within 16 hours of onset of symptoms has significantly lower mortality (**Table 2**).

The mechanical complications of AMI, ventricular septal rupture, and acute severe mitral regurgitation due to papillary muscle rupture were recognized causes of CS and were associated with high mortality (**Fig. 3**). Surgical treatment of these complications was reported as early as 1957, when Cooley and colleagues[31] first reported on patch closure of ventricular septal rupture 1 day following the rupture. Surgical results for this complication were better if surgery could be delayed for 4 weeks; however, most patients died within 2 weeks of developing this complication.[28] Lajoz and colleagues[32] and Daggett and colleagues[33] reported long-term survival in patients who had ventric-ular septal rupture repaired earlier than 10 days after rupture occurred. Austen and colleagues[34] first reported successful mitral valve replacement in a patient 2.5 months after myocardial infarction complicated by papillary muscle rupture in 1964. Buckley

Table 2
Clinical and hemodynamic evaluation of patients who have acute myocardial infarction and cardiogenic shock as related to time from onset of infarction to bypass grafting and intra-aortic balloon assist

	Time from Onset of Infarction to Interventions	
	≤16 h (n = 12)	≥18 h (n = 7)
Hemodynamic measurements[a]		
CI (L/min/m^2)[b]	1.99 ± 0.42	1.77 ± 0.74
LVFP (mm Hg)	22.8 ± 1.2	25.2 ± 1.1
SBP (mm Hg)	73.9 ± 8.8	76.5 ± 9.5
Clinical description		
Age (y)[a]	51.6 ±8.4	52.0 ± 6.1
Area of MI by ECG		
Anterior	8 (66%)	5 (71.4%)
Inferior	2 (16.6%)	—
Anterior + inferior	2 (16.6%)	2 (40%)
Previous MI	6 (50%)	3 (42.8%)
No. of diseased vessels per patient		
One	2 (16.6%)	1 (14.3%)
Two	7 (58/3%)	4 (57.1%)
Three	3 (25%)	2 (28.5%)
In-hospital mortality	**3 (25%)**	**5 (71.41%)**

Abbreviations: CI, cardiac index; LVFP, left ventricular filling pressure; MI, myocardial infarction; SBP, central systolic blood pressure.
[a] Mean ± SD.
[b] $P<.05$.
Data from DeWood MA, Notske RN, Hensley GR, et al. Intraaortic balloon counterpulsation with and without reperfusion for myocardial infarction shock. Circulation 1980;61(6):1105–12.

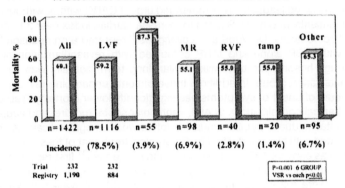

Fig. 3. Incidence of the causes of shock and associated mortality in the patients enrolled the SHOCK trial and registry. LVF, predominant LV failure; MR, acute severe mitral regurgitation; RVF, isolated RV shock; Tamp, cardiac tamponade and rupture; VSR, ventricular septal rupture. (*From* Hochman JS, Buller CE, Sleeper LA, Cardiogenic shock complicating acute myocardial infarction—etiologies, management and outcome: a report from the SHOCK Trial Registry. J Am Coll Cardiol. 2000;36:1066; with permission.)

and colleagues[35] reported two survivors of mitral valve replacement 2 to 10 days after myocardial infarction in 1971. In 1977, Bardet and colleagues[36] reported successful long-term survival in 5 of 10 patients operated on emergently for repair of ventricular septal rupture, and three of four patients who had emergency mitral valve replacement for acute severe mitral regurgitation. Current American College of Cardiology, American Heart Association guidelines for the management of patients who have ST segment elevation myocardial infarction list urgent cardiac surgical repair as a Class I recommendation for patients who have acute papillary muscle rupture, acute ventricular septal rupture, or free-wall rupture.[37]

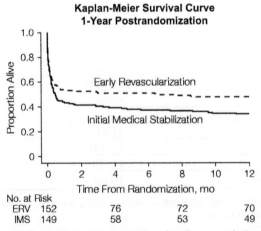

Fig. 4. Survival estimates for patients who have CS and early revascularization versus patients treated with initial medical stabilization. (*From* Hochman JS, Sleeper LA, White HG, et al. One year survival following early revascularization for cardiogenic shock. JAMA 2001;285:190–2.)

Right ventricular myocardial infarction (RVI) can accompany acute inferior wall infarction and lead to CS. The first autopsy confirmed case of a patient who had acute inferior wall MI complicated by RVI who died with heart block and probable CS was reported by Sanders in 1930.[38] The first cases of RVI diagnosed premortem and confirmed by hemodynamic study were described by Cohn and colleagues[39] in 1974. They reported six patients who had AMI (five who had inferior infarction and one who had anterolateral infarction) who had high RV filling pressure (average 20.2 mm Hg) that was equal to or greater than the simultaneously measured PAOP (average 16.3 mm Hg). Five of six patients were in shock. Three patients were treated with rapid infusion of dextran, with correction of shock in two patients. Two patients who had CS died and one had confirmation of extensive RVI at autopsy. Three patients who had CS recovered. Follow-up hemodynamic study 3 weeks after the MI showed that right-sided pressures had returned to normal. A study by Bowers and colleagues[40] showed that successful emergency percutaneous coronary intervention to an occluded right coronary artery in patients who had inferior wall MI and RVI resulted in improvement in hemodynamics within 1 hour, recovery of normal RV function in 3 to 5 days, and marked reduction in mortality.

The landmark SHOCK trial, reported in 1999, was the first prospective, randomized study in CS.[41] Emergency early revascularization with CABG or percutaneous coronary intervention was compared with a strategy of initial medical stabilization with drug therapy and IABP. Thirty-day mortality was improved in the early revascularization group, although not statistically significant (47% mortality with early revascularization versus 56% with initial medical stabilization). Mortality rates at 6 months, 1 year, and 6 years were significantly improved in the early revascularization group, however (**Fig. 4**).[42,43] The 2007 focused update of the ACC/AHA Practice Guidelines for treatment of ST segment elevation MI recommended emergency revascularization within 36 hours of onset of ST segment elevation MI complicated by CS in patients younger than 75 years of age.[37]

SUMMARY

Significant progress has been made over the past 60 years in defining and recognizing CS, and there have been tremendous advances in the care of patients who have this illness. Although there are many causes of this condition, AMI with loss of a large amount of functioning myocardium is the most frequent cause. It was recognized early in the study of CS that prompt diagnosis and rapid initiation of therapy could improve the prognosis, and this remains true today. Use of ECG for accurate diagnosis and the use of invasive hemodynamic monitoring early in the course of CS have been shown to be of benefit in diagnosis and initial pharmacologic management. Studies performed over the last 40 years demonstrated that short-term support with inotropic drugs and intra-aortic balloon counterpulsation help stabilize most patients. Pioneers in cardiac catheterization and cardiac surgery showed that these patients could be helped with aggressive interventions. Early coronary angiography with revascularization by way of percutaneous coronary intervention techniques or coronary bypass surgery are now the cornerstones of therapy. Patients who have the mechanical complications of AMI, ventricular septal rupture or acute severe mitral regurgitation due to papillary muscle rupture, should undergo emergency repair when feasible.

Although the mortality from CS remains high, especially in elderly populations, modern therapies improve the chance of survival from this critical illness. CS, once associated with near 100% mortality, is now associated with survival rates of greater than 60%.[44]

REFERENCES

1. Agress CM, Binder MJ. Cardiogenic shock. Am Heart J 1957;54(3):458–77.
2. Weisse AB. The elusive clot: the controversy over coronary thrombosis in myocardial infarction. J Hist Med Allied Sci 2006;61:66–78.
3. Ross RS, James B. Herrick Lecture. A parlous state of storm and stress. The life and times of James B. Herrick. Circulation 1983;67(5):955–9.
4. Sones FM, Shirey EK. Cine coronary angiography. Mod Concepts Cardiovasc Dis 1962;31:735–8.
5. DeWood MA, Spores J, Notske R, et al. Prevalence of total coronary occlusion during the early hours of transmural myocardial infarction. N Engl J Med 1980; 303:897–902.
6. Griffith GC, Wallace WB, Cochran B Jr, et al. The treatment of shock associated with myocardial infarction. Circulation 1954;IX:527–32.
7. Binder MJ, Ryan JA, Marcus S, et al. Evaluation of therapy in shock following acute myocardial infarction. Am J Med 1955;18:622–32.
8. Malach M, Rosenberg BA. Acute myocardial infarction in a city hospital. Am J Cardiol 1960;5:487–92.
9. Killip T III, Kimball JT. Treatment of myocardial infarction in a coronary care unit. Am J Cardiol 1967;20:457–64.
10. Killip T, Kimball JT. A survey of the coronary care unit: concept and results. Prog Cardiovasc Dis 1968;11(1):45–52.
11. Hunt D, Sloman G, Christie D, et al. Changing patterns and mortality of acute myocardial infarction in a coronary care unit. Br Med J 1977;1:795–8.
12. Scheidt S, Ascheim R, Killip T III. Shock after acute myocardial infarction. Am J Cardiol 1970;26:556–64.
13. Cohn JN, Luria MH. Studies in clinical shock and hypotension. JAMA 1964; 190(10):113–8.
14. Gunnar RM, Cruz A, Boswell J, et al. Myocardial infarction with shock. Circulation 1966;XXXXIII:753–62.
15. Forrester JS, Diamond G, Chatterjee K, et al. Medical therapy of acute myocardial infarction by application of hemodynamic subsets (first of two parts). N Engl J Med 1976;295(24):1356–62.
16. Swan HJC, Ganz W, Forrester JS, et al. Catheterization of the heart in man with the use of a flow-directed balloon tipped catheter. N Engl J Med 1970;283: 447–51.
17. Mueller H, Ayres SM, Gregory JJ, et al. Hemodynamics, coronary blood flow, and myocardial metabolism in coronary shock; response to l-norepinephrine and isoproterenol. J Clin Invest 1970;49:1885–902.
18. Mueller H, Ayres SM, Giannelli S, et al. Effect of isoproterenol, l-norepinephrine, and intraaortic counterpulsation on hemodynamics and myocardial metabolism in shock following acute myocardial infarction. Circulation 1972; XLV:335–51.
19. Mueller HS, Evans R, Ayres SM. Effects of dopamine on hemodynamics and myocardial metabolism in shock following acute myocardial infarction in man. Circulation 1978;57(2):361–5.
20. Moulopoulos SD, Topaz S, Kolff WJ. Diastolic balloon pumping (with carbon dioxide) in the aorta—a mechanical assistance to the failing circulation. Am Heart J 1962;63(3):669–75.
21. Kantrowitz A, Tjonneland S, Freed PS, et al. Initial clinical experience with intra-aortic balloon pumping in cardiogenic shock. JAMA 1968;203(2):135–40.

22. Dunkman WB, Leinbach RC, Buckley MJ, et al. Clinical and hemodynamic results in intraaortic balloon pumping and surgery for cardiogenic shock. Circulation 1972;XLVI:465–77.

23. Scheidt S, Wilner G, Mueller H, et al. Intra-aortic balloon counterpulsation in cardiogenic shock. N Engl J Med 1973;288(19):979–84.

24. Mueller HS. Cardiogenic shock. In: Parrillo JE, Ayres SM, editors. Major issues in critical care medicine. Baltimore (MD): William and Wilkins; 1984. p. 87–95.

25. Swan HJC, Forrester JS, Diamond G, et al. Hemodynamic spectrum of myocardial infarction and cardiogenic shock. Circulation 1972;XLV:1097–110.

26. Page DL, Caulfield JB, Kastor JA, et al. Myocardial changes associated with cardiogenic shock. N Engl J Med. 1971;285(3):134–7.

27. Leinbach RC, Gold HK, Dinsmore RE, et al. The role of angiography in cardiogenic shock. Circulation 1973;XLVII and XLVIIII(Suppl III):III95–8.

28. Johnson SA, Scanlon PJ, Loeb HS, et al. Treatment of cardiogenic shock in myocardial infarction by intraaortic balloon counterpulsation and surgery. Am J Med 1977;62:687–92.

29. Mundth ED, Buckley MJ, Daggert WM, et al. Surgery for complications of acute myocardial infarction. Circulation 1972;XLV:1279–91.

30. DeWood MA, Notske RN, Hensley GR, et al. Intraaortic balloon counterpulsation with and without reperfusion for myocardial infarction shock. Circulation 1980; 61(6):1105–12.

31. Cooley DA, Delmonte BA, Zeis LB, et al. Surgical repair of ruptured interventricular septum following acute myocardial infarction. Surgery 1957;41:930–7.

32. Lajos TZ, Montes M, Bunnell IL, et al. Resection of myocardial infarcts: clinical and pathologic studies. J Thorac Cardiovasc Surg 1979;60:196–206.

33. Daggett WM, Burwell LR, Lawson DW, et al. Resection of acute ventricular aneurysm and ruptured intraventricular septum after myocardial infarction. N Engl J Med 1970;283:1507–8.

34. Austen WG, Sanders CS, Averill JH, et al. Ruptured papillary muscle: report of case with successful mitral valve replacement. Circulation 1965;32:597–601.

35. Buckley MS, Mundth ED, Daggett WM, et al. Surgical therapy for early complications of myocardial infarction. Surgery 1971;70:814–20.

36. Bardet J, Masquet C, Kahn JC, et al. Clinical and hemodynamic results of intra-aortic balloon counterpulsation and surgery for cardiogenic shock. Am Heart J 1977;93(3):280–8.

37. Antman EM, Hand M, Armstrong PW, et al. 2007 focused update of the ACC/AHA 2004 guidelines for the management of patients with ST-elevation myocardial infarction. ACC/AHA Task Force on Practice Guidelines developed in collaboration with the Canadian Cardiovascular Society endorsed by the American Academy of Family Physicians 2000 Writing Group to review new evidence and update the ACC/AHA 2004 Guidelines for the management of patients with ST-elevation myocardial infarction, writing on behalf of the 2004 Writing Committee. J Am Coll Cardiol 2008;51:210–47.

38. Sanders AO. Coronary thrombosis with complete heart-block and relative ventricular tachycardia. A case report. Am Heart J 1930;6:820–3.

39. Cohn JN, Guiha NH, Broder MI, et al. Right ventricular infarction. Clinical and hemodynamic features. Am J Cardiol 1974;33:209–14.

40. Bowers TR, O'Neill WW, Grines C, et al. Effect of reperfusion on biventricular function and survival after right ventricular infarction. N Engl J Med 1998;338(14):933–40.

41. Hochman JS, Sleeper LA, Webb JG, et al. Early revascularization in acute myocardial infarction complicated by cardiogenic shock. N Engl J Med 1999;341:625–34.

42. Hochman JS, Sleeper LA, White HG, et al. One year survival following early revascularization for cardiogenic shock. JAMA 2001;285:190–2.

43. Hochman JS, Sleeper LA, Webb JG, et al. Early revascularization and long-term survival in cardiogenic shock complicating acute myocardial infarction. JAMA 2006;295:2511–5.

44. Topalian S, Ginsberg F, Parrillo JE. Cardiogenic shock. Crit Care Med 2008; 36(Suppl):S66–74.

A History of Pulmonary Embolism and Deep Venous Thrombosis

Kenneth E. Wood, DO

KEYWORDS

- Pulmonary embolism • Deep venous thrombosis
- Thrombolytic therapy • Heparin • History

Pulmonary embolism (PE) remains a common and lethal entity that continues to diagnostically and therapeutically challenge contemporary physicians. As with many aspects of medicine, insights into the historical perspective of the disease are useful in configuring contemporary advances. The purpose of this article is to review the sentinel developments related to PE and enable readers to appreciate the current status of the diagnosis and therapy of PE while providing background to facilitate the development of future strategies. A comprehensive review of the history of PE is beyond the scope of this article and interested readers are referred to works of James Dalen and his extensive historical review of PE for greater detail.[1,2]

The first written reference to thrombotic disease is probably found in the ancient Indian medical texts of the great Ayurveda physician and surgeon, Susruta (circa 600–1000 BCE), in which he describes a patient who had a "swollen and painful leg which was difficult to treat." Giovanni Batttista Morgagni recognized the presence of large blood clots in the pulmonary vessels of patients suffering sudden death in his 1761 text, "De Sedibus et Causis Morborum per Anatomen Indagatis," but was unable to provide an explanation for their presence. In the mid-1800s, Jean Cruveilhier, a prominent French pathologist of the time, proposed a central role for venous inflammation and thrombosis in all disease conditions ("phlebitis dominates all of pathology") in his texts, "Anatomie Pathologique du Corps Humain" and "Traite d'Aniatomie Pathologique Generale."

The brilliant nineteenth-century German pathologist, Rudolph Virchow (**Fig. 1**), began his research studies into thrombosis specifically to investigate Cruveilhier's proposal (at the suggestion of his anatomy professor, Robert Froriep). He since has been credited with "discovering" PE in 1846.[3,4] Virchow recognized the relationship between venous thrombosis and obstruction of the pulmonary arteries by the embolic phenomenon as depicted in his classic description: "the detachment of

Department of Medicine, Section of Pulmonary and Critical Care Medicine, University of Wisconsin Hospital and Clinics, K4/930 (9988), 600 Highland Avenue, Madison, WI 53792, USA
E-mail address: kew@medicine.wisc.edu

Crit Care Clin 25 (2009) 115–131
doi:10.1016/j.ccc.2008.12.014
0749-0704/08/$ – see front matter © 2009 Elsevier Inc. All rights reserved.

criticalcare.theclinics.com

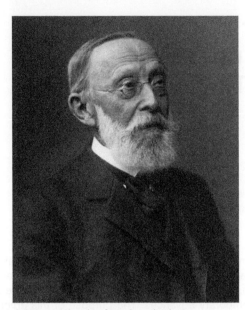

Fig. 1. Rudolf Virchow (1821–1902), who first described PE.

larger or smaller fragments from the end of the softening thrombus which are carried along the current of blood and driven into remote vessels. This gives rise to the very frequent process on which I have bestowed the name Embolia." Virchow recognized that "these stoppers originated in part of the cardiovascular system upstream of the lungs, namely the veins and right heart. They are than carried to the pulmonary artery by the blood stream." Virchow has a more dubious distinction of being among the foremost opponents of the germ theory of disease. His prominent and passionate opposition to the theory proposed by Lister and Pasteur led to prolonged delays in acceptance of this disease paradigm.[5,6] The contemporary approach regarding the genesis of venous thromboembolism (VTE) disease continues to reflect the triad, described by Virchow, consisting of intimal vessel injury, statis, and hypercoagulability.

Clinical confirmation of Virchow's discovery occurred in 1880 when Luzzatto reported a series of 160 cases that defined the clinical aspects of PE and began to recognize the role of underlying cardiopulmonary disease.[6] In 1884, Picot recognized that "venous thrombosis is always a severe disease and often fatal, because fragments of the thrombi my detach and occlude branches of the pulmonary artery....the occlusion of the main branches of pulmonary artery causes a striking rise of the blood pressure in these vessels. This rise-which the right heart must fight to insure circulation may sometimes lead to cardiac arrest."[7] The remainder of this article reviews the sentinel events related to the diagnosis and treatment of PE.

DIAGNOSIS OF PULMONARY EMBOLISM

Before the development of the objective diagnostic standards in the 1960s, the diagnosis of PE ostensibly was made on clinical grounds. The lack of sensitivity and specificity in the accuracy of the physical examination is evident in reports that reveal the majority of PEs that were defined at autopsy were not diagnosed ante mortem. Dalen and Alpert's classic report on the natural history of PE (**Fig. 2**)[8] proposed that the sensitivity of the clinical recognition of PE was approximately 29%. With a suspected incidence of 630,000 cases per year, Dalen and Alpert suggested that the diagnosis was made in only 163,000 patients, 92% of whom survived with appropriate therapy. Correspondingly, 71% of patients who survived more than 1 hour did not have the diagnosis established, with a mortality approaching 30%. The development of pulmonary angiography as an objective standard for the diagnosis of PE highlighted the lack specificity in the clinical diagnosis of PE. In one of the original angiographic reports by Dalen and colleagues in 1971, angiographic confirmation was achieved in only 89 of the 247 patients studied.[9] Subsequent work by the prospective investigation of pulmonary embolism diagnosis (PIOPED) Investigators revealed that PE was validated in only 33% of suspected patients undergoing angiography.[10] The PIOPED study was unique in that clinicians were asked to define a pretest probability of PE before obtaining a ventilation/perfusion scan. In patients who had a high clinical probability of PE, the incidence of PE at angiography was 68% compared with those who had a low probability, where the incidence was only 9%. Thus, the clinical recognition and diagnosis of PE remains nonsensitive and nonspecific. Consequently, diagnosis of PE requires objective confirmatory tests that have evolved over the past 80 years.

Electrocardiogram

The description of electrocardiographic cor pulmonale resulting from PE was reported by McGinn and White in 1935. In their landmark publication, they described a series of nine patients presenting with acute cor pulmonale accompanied, in seven patients, by electrocardiographic studies. Although the symptoms of the extensive PE were variable, the majority of the patients were reported to be in shock. Electrocardiograms taken shortly after the occurrence of PE revealed similar changes in five patients. Two others taken some time after the time of the embolic event had similar characteristics but were less definitive. The changes that seemed significant were the presence of a Q-wave and T-wave inversion in lead three and the low origin of the T wave with

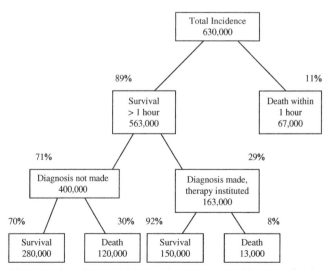

Fig. 2. Natural history of PE. (*From* Dalen JE, Alpert JS. Natural history of pulmonary embolism. Prog Cardiovasc Dis 1975;17:259–70; with permission.)

gradual staircase ascent of the ST interval in lead two with a prominent S wave with a slightly low origin of the T wave in lead one. This highly specific and classical description of the S_1-Q_3-T_3 pattern is associated with electrocardiographic cor pulmonale.[11] In 1939, Durant described two patients who had massive PE that exhibited a right bundle branch configuration. Both of these initial findings were reported by Szucs and colleagues[12] in a 1971 series of 50 consecutive patients who had angiographic documented PE. There was electrocardiographic evidence of right heart strain in only nine patients, all of whom presented with massive embolism. A similar report from the Dexter Laboratory in 1977 reviewed the electrocardiographic changes associated with syncope in massive PE. The demonstration of clot obstruction greater than 50% was associated with evidence of electrocardiographic cor pulmonale consisting of the originally described S_1-Q_3-T_3 pattern or a right bundle branch block configuration.

Arterial Blood Gases

The first report of arterial blood gas saturation with acute PE was described by Robin and coworkers in 1960. In this case series of 11 patients, the arterial saturation with patients breathing room air ranged from 34% to 90%; the investigators concluded that PE should be considered a disorder effecting gas exchange function of the lung and defined three major abnormalities: first, the development of arterial oxygen unsaturation as mechanistically defined by venoarterial shunting, decreased diffusion capacity of the lung, and relative alveolar hypoventilation; second, "an abnormality is the development of hyperventilation which serves the purpose of assisting normal arterialization of pulmonary capillary blood;" and third, "the development of significant differences between the carbon dioxide tension of arterial blood and end tidal air." The latter was proposed as produced by the dilution of alveolar air by newly formed dead space.[13] The first reported oxygen saturation in patients who had angiographically proved PE was provided by Sasahara and colleagues in 1964 in a small series of five patients, four of whom had a PaO_2 of less than 80 mm Hg.[14] The first large case report series of arterial saturation in patients who had angiographically documented PE was reported by Szucs and colleagues in 1971. PaO_2 while breathing room air was decreased to less than 80 mm Hg in all 36 patients tested. The study concluded that the PaO_2 and the lung scan were the most sensitive tests for screening; if either was normal, acute PE essentially was excluded.[12] Although a normal perfusion scan effectively may exclude PE, Stein and the PIOPED Investigators in 1995 reported that 14% of patients who had documented PE had a normal alveolar-arterial (A-a) gradient (less than or equal to 20 mm Hg). The PIOPED Investigators concluded that 20% to 23% of patients who had PE had a normal A-a gradient and that a normal A-a gradient did not exclude the diagnosis of PE.[15]

Chest Radiograph

The classic description of radiographic findings of PE was reported by Westermark in 1938. In this initial description of radiographic findings, Westermark made a clear distinction between emboli with and without infarction. In PE without infarction, Westermark noted that ischemia of the branches of the pulmonary artery was evident peripheral to the embolus. On the radiogram, he concluded that this ischemia appeared as a clarified area with diminished vascularity corresponding to the extent of the embolized artery, currently known as Westermark's sign. In contrast, when Westermark noted a wedge-shaped shadow, he concluded that is was evidence of pulmonary infarction.[16] In 1940, Hampton and Castleman published their correlation of postmortem chest radiographs with autopsy findings. **Fig. 3** illustrates the radiograph of the body suspended at autopsy. In this study, deceased patients had radiographic studies undertaken post mortem, which revealed a significant correlation between the findings at autopsy and the radiographic abnormalities. Similar to the work of Westermark, they extensively reviewed the anatomic and radiographic findings of those patients sustaining pulmonary infarction and those who did not have infarction.[17]

Pulmonary Angiograms

The development of pulmonary angiography greatly facilitated the diagnosis of PE and provided the opportunity to study the physiology of the disease process. The first report of pulmonary angiography was by Robb in 1939, who reported the visualization of the chambers of the heart, pulmonary circulation, and the great blood vessels in humans.[18] Using a large transfusion needle inserted into the basilic vein of the arm, patients were seated before a radiology cassette and a radiographic study was undertaken using a chest radiograph. Images were made at appropriate time intervals after injection and manipulation of the arm. The contrast material traveled to the superior vena cava, heart chambers, and pulmonary arteries. With this modality, the

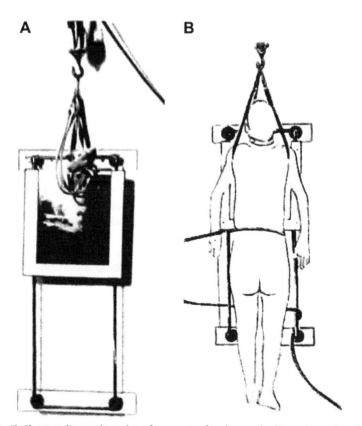

Fig. 3. (*A, B*) Chest radiograph and performance of radiograph. (*From* Hampton A, Castleman B. Correlation of postmortem chest teleroentgenograms with autopsy findings. Am J Roentgenol Radium Ther 1940;43:305–26.)

investigators were able to outline the pulmonary architecture, although they did not undertake any studies in patients who had suspected PE. The first pulmonary angiogram to define embolic obstruction was performed by Jesser in 1941;[19] the investigators injected barium into a dog and were able to find obstructions in the pulmonary artery outflow track. Similar animal studies were undertaken in 1952 by Lochhead and colleagues, who injected clots into dogs and defined the extent of anatomic obstruction.[20] The first use of pulmonary angiography in humans was reported by Aitchison and McKay in 1956 in a case report of a 47-year-old patient seen in the Royal Infirmary in Aberdeen who complained of upper gastric pain that was believed related to duodenal ulcer. The patient had no complaints referable to the respiratory system, and physical examination revealed no significant positive findings; the patient's radiograph of the chest revealed an area of translucency in the right upper lobe. The patient underwent cardiac catheterization with measurement of pulmonary artery pressures and there was no evidence of filling defect in the vessels supplying the area of radiographic abnormality. The patient was diagnosed with pneumonia.[21] The landmark study by Williams and coworkers in 1963 was the first reported series to use pulmonary angiography to diagnosis suspected PE.[22] Angiography was used in 50 patients who had suspected PE and the angiogram was reported positive in 73% of cases. Of those having positive pulmonary angiograms, 47% showed no abnormalities on the routine chest radiograph. This represented the first time that objective diagnosis of PE outside of confirmation at autopsy was achieved. Evaluation of the criteria for the angiographic diagnosis of PE was undertaken by Stein and colleagues and reported in 1967.[23] The purpose of this study was to assess the specificity of the many reported angiographic signs of acute PE in an effort to define which angiographic abnormalities could reliably indicate PE irrespective of coexistent diseases. A clinical diagnosis related to the presence or absence of PE was made in 52 patients, forming the basis of this study. The investigators divided the angiographic abnormalities into two groups: those with major or morphologic significance and those of lesser physiologic significance. Those of morphologic significance were intraluminal filling defects, cutoffs, and pruning. The investigators suggested these major signs directly indicated arterial occlusion. Physiologic significance was defined by oligemia, asymmetric filling, prolongation of arterial phase, and bilateral lower zone delay. These lesser signs were indicative of disorders of flow. The significance of underlying cardiopulmonary disease and the impact that these abnormalities can make on the pulmonary angiogram were reviewed extensively by Stein and colleagues.[23]

Lung Scans

Shortly after the first case report series of pulmonary angiograms in 1964, Wagner and coworkers[24] performed the first radioisotope perfusion scan for the diagnosis of massive PE. The investigators reported a diagnosis of avascularity consistent with PE in 14 cases in which filling defects were observed in a series of 100 consecutive patients. The diagnosis was confirmed by autopsy, pulmonary angiogram, or embolectomy. Comparison of perfusion scanning with pulmonary angiography was reported by Fred in 1966;[25] the investigators reported an excellent correlation between abnormalities seen on angiography and radioisotopes scanning. Similar results were reported by Dalen and colleagues in a 5-year period between 1964 and 1969.[9] In follow-up to the original report using perfusion scans in 1968, Wagner added radioactive xenon for ventilation assessment in the differential diagnosis of PE. Using inhaled xenon 133, the investigators described ventilation/perfusion relationships. Adding ventilation increased the specificity of the ventilation/perfusion scan. Wagner proposed that areas of absent perfusion associated with normal ventilation were consistent with the diagnosis of PE. The true value of the ventilation/perfusion scan in the diagnosis of acute PE was determined by the PIOPED Investigators.[26] In a landmark study, 1931 patients underwent scintigraphy and 755 underwent pulmonary angiography with 33% of the 755 patients who underwent angiography demonstrating PE. All the patients who had PE had abnormal scans of high, intermediate, or low probability as did most who did not have PE, leading to a sensitivity of 98% and specificity of 10%. Of the 116 patients who had high probability scans and definitively angiograms, 88% had PE although the minority who had PE had high probability scans. The overall sensitivity was 41% with specificity 97%. Of the 322 patients who had intermediate probability scans and definitive angiograms, only 33% had PE. In the group with low clinical probability, it was estimated that incidence of PE was 12%. The investigators concluded that clinical assessment in conjunction with ventilation/perfusion scans was adequate to establish the diagnosis or exclude PE for only a minority of patients. Patients who had clear and concordant clinical and ventilation/perfusion scan findings could be considered to have confirmed PE or PE excluded. The combination of high clinical probability and a high probability scan equating to the presence of PE and a low clinical probability with a low probability scan excluding PE derives from this landmark trial.[26]

Echocardiography

Echocardiography in the diagnosis of PE has its origins in a case report by Covarrubias and colleagues in 1977, in which the investigators reported a case of a 55-year-old woman who was evaluated for unresponsiveness and hypotension. Subsequent to her admission, the patient developed a significant systolic murmur with systolic clicks at the lower left sternum border that were louder in the sitting position. Echocardiography revealed multiple shaggy echoes adjacent to the tricuspid valve. Subsequently, she succumbed to her illness and at autopsy was found to have a large PE sequestered about the tricuspid valve.[27] Echocardiographic assessment of acute right ventricular overload was reported by Steckley and coworkers in 1978 when they defined echocardiographic changes that correlated with angiographic obstruction in a patient who had multiple PEs. The interval development of right ventricular dilatation and proximal septal motion coincided with the clinical event that was angiographically proved PE.[28] In 1980, Kasper and colleagues reported on 18 patients who had acute PE and were studied with right heart catheterization and M-mode echocardiography. No patients who had pre-existing cardiopulmonary disease were included and PE was documented with pulmonary angiography. This is the first case report series that correlated the extent of embolic obstruction and right heart physiology. Echocardiography revealed that right ventricular diameters were increased in 13 of the 16 patients and left ventricular diameters decreased in 10 of 15 patients. The ratio of right ventricular:left ventricular diameters correlated with extent of angiographic index of anatomic obstruction. The investigators concluded that echocardiography was valuable noninvasive tool for the assessment of acute PE and pulmonary hypertension in patients who had no prior cardiopulmonary disorder.[29] Subsequently, in 1986, Kasper and colleagues reported echocardiographic studies, in 105 patients, of acute and recurrent PE confirmed by angiography, autopsy, or lung perfusion scans. The majority demonstrated a dilated right ventricle and 42% had a reduced left ventricular cavitary diameter. Impaired septal motion was reported in 44% of the patients and right ventricular thrombi was seen in 13 patients.[30] The temporal sequence of right ventricular dysfunction in PE was first reported by Come and coworkers in 1987. This study was undertaken to assess the magnitude of the abnormalities of right heart function and their reversal when thrombolytic therapy was used to treat PE.

Coincident with clot lysis, pulmonary artery systolic blood pressure and right ventricular cavitary diameter decreased, along with an increase in left ventricular cavitary diameter. The right ventricular wall motion, initially mild, moderate, or severe in a small number of patients, normalized and improved significantly. The investigators concluded that those findings confirmed that PE results in appreciable right ventricular dysfunction and dilatation associated with tricuspid regurgitation, abnormal septal motion and that these abnormalities reversed with therapy.[31] The diagnosis and treatment of shock-related PE with transesophageal echocardiography (TEE) was reported Krivec in 1997. In 24 consecutive patients who had unexplained shock and distended jugular veins, 18 patients had right ventricular dilation with global or severe segmental hypokinesis. Central pulmonary thromboemboli in 12 patients were visualized. The sensitivity for TEE for the diagnosis of massive PE in patients who had right ventricular dilation was 92% and the specificity was 100%. Other diagnoses were achieved using the TEE assessment. The investigators concluded that bedside TEE was a valuable tool in the diagnosis of major PE as it enabled immediate therapy to be undertaken at the bedside.[32]

CT Scan of Chest

The first report using CT patterns of PE with infarction was by Sinner in 1978.[33] In this case report series of 16 patients who had clinical findings suggestive of PE, the diagnosis was corroborated by other diagnostic procedures. CT scanning revealed a variety of patterns reflecting increased attenuation. In 44% of the cases, a distinct wedge-shaped appearance was observed that was broad based against the peripheral pleural surface with the tip pointing to the perihiler area, suggestive of pulmonary infarction. In 1992, Remy-Jardin and coworkers reported the use of spiral CT scanning for central PE. Using a single breath-hold technique and comparing the results with pulmonary angiography, views were obtained with 90 mL of 30% contrast or 120 mL of 12% contrast in 98% of the examinations. Filling defects were seen in 37% of patients, complete filling defects in 46%, railroad track signs in 5%, and mural defects in 12%. In all 23 patients who had normal findings of spiral volumetric CT, normal findings were seen with pulmonary angiography. The study concluded that spiral CT had a sensitivity of 100% and specificity of 96% for a diagnosis of central PE.[34] In 1995, Goodman and colleagues reported a study of detection of PE in patients who had unresolved clinical and scintigraphic diagnosis and compared helical CT and angiography. Patients who had unresolved diagnosis and a suspicion of PE were evaluated with a contrast-enhanced helical CT and with selected pulmonary angiography. A period of 11 hours separated the two studies. The CT sensitivity was 86%, specificity 92%, and likelihood ratio 10.7. When subsegmental vessels were included, however, CT results were 63%, 89%, and 5.7, respectively. Goodman and colleagues concluded that helical CT, when inclusive of subsegmental clot, was only 63% sensitive. Discussions related to the diagnosis of PE with subsegmental clot remain unresolved and further diagnostic studies are warranted when there is a high clinical pretest probability and a negative helical CT scan, given the potential to miss subsegmental clot.[35]

Natural History

Insofar as PE is a manifestation of the continuum of VTE disease, it is helpful to review the natural history of deep venous thrombosis (DVT). In a landmark study, not likely to be repeated, Kakker and colleagues in 1969 studied 132 consecutive patients during a postoperative period using labeled ^{125}I-fibrinogen to image DVT of the legs. Thrombosis occurred in the calf veins in 40 patients (30%), which was confirmed by venography. In 14 of the 40 patients, the thrombosis lysed spontaneously within 72 hours. Thrombosis persisted for more than 72 hours in 26 patients and PE developed in four of these patients.[36] Of the many articles written about the natural history of PE, the classic manuscript defining the contemporary view of the natural history of PE was by Dalen and Alpert in 1975,[8] who defined the overall instance of PE at 630,000 cases per year and proposed that death would occur within 1 hour of presentation in approximately 11%. Of the 89% of patients who have PE who survive greater than 1 hour, they proposed that 71% of patients do not have a diagnosis made, of which 70% will survive and 30% will die. In the population that survives greater than 1 hour and in whom the diagnosis is made and appropriate therapy instituted, 92% will survive and mortality will be approximately 8%. Subsequent literature has borne out the accuracy of these approximations from 1975, which have not varied appreciably over 40 years. Similarly, this classic manuscript defined the resolution rate of acute PE based on the extent of angiographic obstruction that was reported in many case series.

TREATMENT OF PULMONARY EMBOLISM
Pulmonary Embolectomy

The first treatment for PE, thromboembolectomy, was proposed by Friedrich Trendelenburg (**Fig. 4**) (son of the famous philosopher Friedrich Adolph Trendelenburg) in his classic 1908 report,[37] which was presented at the 37th Annual Congress of the Deutsche Gesellschaft für Chirurgie (German Surgical Society). This landmark report of a failed surgery by Trendelenburg defined the surgical approach to embolectomy that he had devised on laboratory animals before 1908. **Fig. 5** demonstrates the instruments used to attempt the first thromboembolectomy.[38] Trendelenburg recorded all of the PE events at his hospital and believed that in more than half the cases, there was at least 50 minutes available for immediate operative treatment. He relied on the patient's bedside nurse for the symptoms of the embolic event and mandated that a surgeon and instruments be immediately available. The initial case reported by Trendelenburg was of a 70-year-old deaf woman who previously had sustained a fracture of the femoral neck. She collapsed with perfuse sweating and complained of severe distress. Within 3 minutes, she lost consciousness, her pupils were dilated, and there was marked parlor with jugular venous distention noted along with rapid respirations and no pulses. Trendelenburg reached the patient and undertook the operation within 18 minutes of the onset of symptoms. With a limited opening of the left side of the chest, directly over the common pulmonary artery, he divided the pulmonary artery and encircled the proximal aorta and pulmonary artery together through the pericardium. The emboli were extracted through small pulmonary artery incision. Unfortunately, this case and the subsequent two cases undertaken by Trendelenburg failed and the patients died. A subsequent trainee of Trendelenburg, Martin Kischner, performed the first successful emergency embolectomy in 1924 on a 38-year-old woman who collapsed after repair of hernia.[38] Success with surgical thromboembolectomy was reported by Crafoord[39] in 1928 when he reported two cases of successful operations using the Trendelenburg technique. Both patients survived and were discharged from the hospital. Crafoord took approximately 8 minutes from the commencement of the attack to the incision into the pulmonary artery. The first successful pulmonary embolectomy using cardiopulmonary bypass was reported by Cooley and colleagues in 1961.[40] In 1969, Greenfield and coworkers reported the first transvenous removal of PE via a vacuum cup catheter technique.[41] With local anesthesia, a cup device extracted the clot from the pulmonary artery in animals and they subsequently reported the successful of this procedure in two patients in 1971.

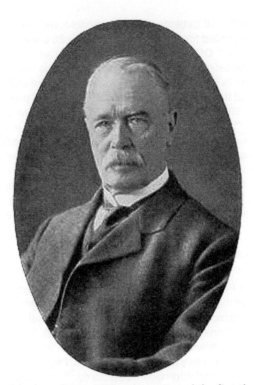

Fig. 4. Friedrich Trendelenburg (1844–1924), who proposed the first therapy for PE (thromboembolectomy). (*From* Trendelenburg F. Ueber die operatie behandlung der embolie lungenarteerie. Arch Klin Chir 1908;86:686–700 [in German].)

Using a number 12 French double-lumen balloon-tip catheter after an incision in the left common femoral vein, visualization of the secondary and tertiary branches of the pulmonary artery was undertaken with contrast for the balloon catheter device. The investigators concluded that use of this new device should prompt re-evaluation for the indications of open pulmonary embolectomy.

Venous Interruption

Although heparin was discovered in 1918, it was not part of routine clinical practice until the 1940s. In that interval, the only other therapeutic option to prevent or treat PE was venous interruption. In the classic 1934 article defining thrombosis of the veins of the lower leg causing PE,[42] Homans proposed that VTE was uncommon yet often fatal. After evaluating four patients who suffered from VTE, with two deaths from PE, Homans reported the ligation of the femoral vein for prevention PE. He reviewed four cases, including two who survived without complications. Broader application of this technique subsequently was reported by Byrne in 1955. He reported his experience with 748 patients manifesting phlebitis admitted to the hospital over 10 years. In this landmark article, Byrne segregated outcomes related to age and comorbidity. In the population that received conservative therapy, which did not include heparin, the mortality rate was 37%. In the 369 cases of surgical ligation, the mortality was 2.1%.[43] In a subsequent article published in 1944, Homans proposed that the preferred level of interruption of the venous system was at the level of inferior vena

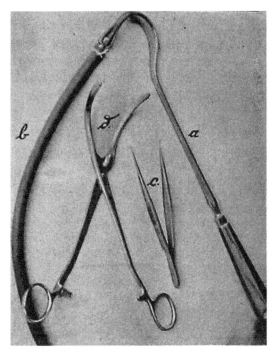

a Sonde, b Schlauch, c Sperrpincette,
d Klemmzange.

Fig. 5. Instruments used by Trendelenburg for first thromboembolectomy. (*From* Trendelenburg F. Ueber die operatie behandlung der embolie lungenarteerie. Arch Klin Chir 1908;86:686–700 [in German].)

cava (IVC). Homans suggested that interruption of the vena cava was indicated in the presence of bilateral thrombosis at the level of inguinal ligaments. This manuscript is one of the most detailed overviews of DVT and defined the process of propagation from distal to proximal rather than what had previously been proposed as proximal to distal propagation of thrombosis.[44] Subsequent to Homans' IVC ligation for DVT, Collins and colleagues[45] proposed that the IVC be ligated to prevent PE in a case report that consisted of three cases, which focused on the pelvic veins as the potential origin of thrombosis.[45] The first nonsurgical interruption of the vena cava was suggested by Mobin-Uddin and coworkers in 1969, who proposed the use of a filter to block emboli raising from the veins of the legs and pelvis. They described the long-term results of a simplified method of IVC interruption by a nonextractable prosthesis that was implanted intravenously (IV). In this case report series of 15 patients, there was no clinical evidence of PE recurrence.[46] The use of IVC filters remains controversial and contentious as there is only one randomized prospective controlled trial. Conducted by Decousus and coworkers in 1998,[47] this two-by-two study randomized 400 patients who had proximal DVT to heparin and oral anticoagulants with or without IVC filter. The incidence of PE was lower in the group that received a filter at day 12. At the 2-year follow-up, however, there was no difference in the number of deaths and major bleeding in the two groups. Although there was an insignificant decrease in the number of PE events in the group with the IVC filter, there was a higher incidence of recurrent DVT.

Heparin

Treatment

Although heparin was discovered in 1918 by Howell and Holt,[48] it was not until the 1930s that heparin was even considered in the treatment of VTE. The work of Murray and Best[49] and of Crafoord[50] established the use of heparin for the treatment of thromboembolism. Crafoord reported a case series of 21 patients who had established VTE and were treated with IV heparin and proposed that continuous heparin influenced the clinical manifestations of the thromboembolic complications.[50] This landmark article also described 135 cases of patients who were treated with heparin postoperatively for the prevention of thrombosis. In 1940, Murray summarized the state of the art of heparin therapy, reviewing the animal models and the clinical applications at that time. This classic review article and clinical case series highlighted the efficacy of heparin and the significant improvements noted with treatment.[51] Twenty years later, the first randomized controlled prospective trial of the use of heparin in treating VTE was conducted by Barritt and Jordan.[52] In this randomized controlled trial of 71 cases, PE was treated with IV heparin and concurrent oral coagulation for 14 days. The control group did not receive any anticoagulant therapy. Patients randomized to the anticoagulant group had no deaths and no nonfatal recurrences of PE. In the control group there were five deaths and five nonfatal recurrences of PE. This is the only randomized control prospective trial ever conducted related to the use of heparin in VTE and it is unlikely any further trials will be conducted. Proof of the efficacy of IV heparin in treatment of acute VTE was provided by Brandjes and colleagues,[53] who performed a randomized double-blind study comparing the efficacy and safety of continuous IV heparin plus acenocoumarol with the efficacy and safety of acenocoumarol alone in the initial treatment of outpatients who had proximal vein thrombosis. The endpoint of study was confirmed systemic extension or recurrence VTE during 6 months of follow-up. The study was terminated because of an excess number of systemic events in patients who received acenocoumarol alone— 12 of 60 patients receiving acenocoumarol (20%) compared with 4 of 60 patients (6.7%) in the combined therapy with heparin and oral anticoagulation. The extension of venous thrombosis was observed in almost 40% of the patients in oral anticoagulation group and in 8.2% of patients treated with heparin plus oral anticoagulation. This randomized controlled trial firmly established the need for IV heparin therapy in the initial phase of anticoagulation. Low molecular weight heparin was first introduced and reported in the treatment of acute PE by Thery and colleagues in 1992[54] and subsequent trials comparing low molecular weight heparin and IV unfractionated heparin were reported by Simonneau and coworkers[55] and the Columbus Investigators in 1997.[56] These studies confirmed that low molecular weight heparin seemed as effective and safe as IV unfractionated heparin in the treatment of acute PE.

Prevention

In addition to treating VTE with heparin, Crafoord and Murray and Best[49,57] used heparin for the prevention of postoperative thrombosis. Using the heparin that was available in the 1930s, both groups prophylaxed postoperative patients using clinical findings or postmortem assessment to define efficacy. Significant diminutions in the incidence of postoperative DVT, albeit via clinical diagnosis, were reported and heparin was introduced rapidly as a prophylactic measure to prevent postoperative DVT. In 1962, Sharnoff and colleagues reported the use of subcutaneous heparin to prevent postoperative VTE.[58] Kakkar and coworkers[59] similarly reported the results of a randomized controlled trial, using low-dose heparin at 5000 units 2 hours preoperatively and continued every 12 hours for 7 days, that investigated 78 high-risk patients over age 40 who underwent major surgery. The frequency of DVT, which was determined by [126]I-labelled fibrinogen testing, was 42% in the control group that did not receive prophylaxis and 8% in patients receiving heparin. It was not until the Prevention of Fatal Postperative Pulmonary Embolism by Low Doses of Heparin was reported in the International Multicentre Trial, conducted in 1975, however, that subcutaneous heparin was established as a standard for the prevention of VTE in postoperative patients.[60] In this classic landmark study, 4121 patients over age 40 undergoing elective major surgical procedures were randomized to receive heparin prophylaxis or no anticoagulation prophylaxis. The study reported that 4% of patients died during the postoperative period, 100 in the control group and 80 in the heparin group. Fifteen patients in the control group and two patients in the heparin group were found at autopsy to have died of acute massive PE. Similarly, a significant number of emboli were found at autopsy in six patients in the control group and three in the heparin group. The frequency of DVT was reduced from 24.6% in the control group to 7.2% in the heparin group. Despite overwhelming data evident in 1975, VTE prophylaxis still is significantly underused—hence, VTE prophylaxis is the number one patient safety recommendation by the Agency for Healthcare Research and Quality.

Thrombolytic Therapy

The first report of the fibrinolytic activity of hemolytic streptococci was presented by Tillett[61] in 1933, who described and demonstrated the capacity of broth cultures of hemolytic streptococci to rapidly liquefy the clotted fibrin of normal human serum. In 1964, Browse and James[62] described the use of streptokinase in PE. In a case report series of four patients, the investigators were able to define effective fibrinolysis with streptokinase. The commented that the drug was safe when used with care and occasionally precipitated hypotension but there were no apparent deleterious effects on the blood pressure of very ill patients. Steroids were used in the first 12 hours to prevent any allergic reactions, which were believed the most common complication. Some minor bleeding complications appeared and they were controlled easily with ϵ-aminocaproic acid, which specifically inhibited the fibrinolytic activity in minutes. All four patients noted striking clinical improvement, including those who were clinically near death according to the investigators' description. In 1967, the Urokinase Pulmonary Embolism Trial (UPET) was conducted to define the efficacy of thrombolytic therapy in PE.[63] In this randomized prospective controlled trial, patients were randomized to standard IV heparin therapy with and without an infusion of urokinase. Using pulmonary angiograms, lung scans, and right-sided pressure measurements, no significant differences in the recurrence rate of PE or in the 2-week mortality was observed. Bleeding, which occurred in 45% of the patients receiving urokinase, contrasted with a rate of 27% in the heparin group. The increased bleeding in the urokinase group was associated with the invasive procedures necessary to obtain angiography and hemodynamic information. The second phase of UPET[64] randomized 167 patients who had angiographically demonstrated PE to 12 hours of urokinase, 24 hours of urokinase, or 24 hours of streptokinase. Assessment of resolution by pulmonary angiogram, lung scans, and hemodynamic data revealed that clot resolution with 24 hours of urokinase was equal to that of 12 hours of urokinase therapy. Twenty-four hours of urokinase therapy resulted in greater improvement than streptokinase, which was seen in lung scans but not in angiograms. All three thrombolytic regimens were more effective in accelerating the resolution of pulmonary thromboemboli than heparin. Currently, thrombolytic therapy is approved for use in massive PE with hemodynamic deterioration and its use in hemodynamically stable patients who have right ventricular dysfunction remains a contentious discussion.

Although enormous progress has been made in understanding the physiology of PE, developing new diagnostic modalities and strategies, and constant refinement in the use of heparin therapy and thrombolytic therapy, VTE remains a common and lethal process. As the history of this disease illustrates, advances continue to be made and it is anticipated that with newer diagnostic studies and anticoagulants under development, the diagnosis and treatment of PE will continue to improve.

REFERRENCES

1. Dalen JE. Pulmonary embolism: what have we learned since Virchow? Treatment and prevention. Chest 2002;122:1801–17.
2. Dalen JE. Pulmonary embolism: what have we learned since Virchow? Natural history, pathophysiology, and diagnosis. Chest 2002;122:1440–56.
3. Morpurgo M, editor. Pulmonary embolism. New York: Marcel Dekker, Inc.; 1994.
4. von VR [Weitere untersuchungen ueber die verstopfung der lungenarterien und ihre folge]. Traube's Beitraege exp Path u Physiol 1846;2:21–31 [German].
5. Helie J. [Inflammation del'artere pulmonaire, mort subite]. Bull Soc Anat Paris 1937;8:254–7 [French].
6. Luzzatto B. Embolia dell' arteria polmonale. Milan; 1880.
7. Picot J. Lecons de clinique medicale. Paris: Masson; 1884.
8. Dalen JE, Alpert JS. Natural history of pulmonary embolism. Prog Cardiovasc Dis 1975;17:259–70.
9. Dalen JE, Brooks HL, Johnson LW, et al. Pulmonary angiography in acute pulmonary embolism: indications, techniques, and results in 367 patients. America 1971;81:175–85.
10. Levine M, Hirsh J, Weitz J, et al. A randomized trial of a single bolus dosage regimen of recombinant tissue plasminogen activator in patients with acute pulmonary embolism. Chest 1990;98:1473–9.
11. McGinn S, White PD. Acute cor pulmonale resulting from pulmonary embolism. JAMA 1935;104:1473–80.
12. Szucs MM Jr, Brooks HL, Grossman W, et al. Diagnostic senstivity of laboratory findings in acute pulmonary embolism. Ann Intern Med 1971;74:161–6.
13. Robin ED, Forkner CE Jr, Bromberg PA, et al. Alveolar gas exchange in clinical pulmonary embolism. N Engl J Med 1960;262:283–7.
14. Sasahara AA, Stein M, Simon M, et al. Pulmonary angiography in the diagnosis of thromboembolic disease. N Engl J Med 1964;270:1075–81.
15. Stein PD, Goldhaber SZ, Henry JW. Alveolar-arterial oxygen gradient in the assessment of acute pulmonary embolism. Chest 1995;107:139–43.
16. Westermark N. On the roentgen diagnosis of lung embolism: brief review of the incidence, pathology and clinical symptoms of lung embolism. Acta Radiol 1938;357–72.
17. Hampton A, Castleman B. Correlation of postmortem chest teleroentgenograms with autopsy findings. Am J Roentgenol Radium Ther 1940;43:305–26.
18. Robb GaS, Steinberg I. Visualization of the chambers of the heart, the pulmonary circulation, and the great blood vessels in man. Am J Roentgenol Radium Ther 1939;41:1–17.
19. Jesser JadT, de Takats G. Visualization of the pulmonary artery during its embolic obstruction. Arch Surg 1941;42:1034–41.

20. Lochhead RP, Roberts DJ Jr, Dotter CT. Pulmonary embolism; experimental angiocardiographic study. Am J Roentgenol Radium Ther Nucl Med 1952;68:627–33.
21. Aitchison JD, McKay JM. Pulmonary artery occlusion demonstrated by angiography. Br J Radiol 1956;29:398–9.
22. Williams JR, Wilcox C, Andrews GJ, et al. Angiography in pulmonary embolism. JAMA 1963;184:473–6.
23. Stein PD, O'Connor JF, Dalen JE, et al. The angiographic diagnosis of acute pulmonary embolism: evaluation of criteria. America 1967;73:730–41.
24. Wagner HN Jr, Sabiston DC Jr, McAfee JG, et al. Diagnosis of massive pulmonary embolism in man by radioisotope scanning. N Engl J Med 1964;271:377–84.
25. Fred HL, Burdine JA Jr, Gonzalez DA, et al. Arteriographic assessment of lung scanning in the diagnosis of pulmonary thromboembolism. N Engl J Med 1966; 275:1025–32.
26. The PIOPED Investigators. Value of the ventilation/perfusion scan in acute pulmonary embolism. Results of the prospective investigation of pulmonary embolism diagnosis (PIOPED). JAMA 1990;263:2753–9.
27. Covarrubias EA, Sheikh MU, Fox LM. Echocardiography and pulmonary embolism. Ann Intern Med 1977;87:720–1.
28. Steckley R, Smith CW, Robertson RM. Acute right ventricular overload: an echocardiographic clue to pulmonary thromboembolism. Johns Hopkins Med J 1978; 143:122–5.
29. Kasper W, Meinertz T, Kersting F, et al. Echocardiography in assessing acute pulmonary hypertension due to pulmonary embolism. Am J Cardiol 1980;45: 567–72.
30. Kasper W, Meinertz T, Henkel B, et al. Echocardiographic findings in patients with proved pulmonary embolism. America 1986;112:1284–90.
31. Come PC, Kim D, Parker JA, et al. Early reversal of right ventricular dysfunction in patients with acute pulmonary embolism after treatment with intravenous tissue plasminogen activator. J Am Coll Cardiol 1987;10:971–8.
32. Krivec B, Voga G, Zuran I, et al. Diagnosis and treatment of shock due to massive pulmonary embolism: approach with transesophageal echocardiography and intrapulmonary thrombolysis. Chest 1997;112:1310–6.
33. Sinner WN. Computed tomographic patterns of pulmonary thromboembolism and infarction. J Comput Assist Tomogr 1978;2:395–9.
34. Remy-Jardin M, Remy J, Wattinne L, et al. Central pulmonary thromboembolism: diagnosis with spiral volumetric ct with the single-breath-hold technique—comparison with pulmonary angiography. Radiology 1992;185:381–7.
35. Goodman LR, Curtin JJ, Mewissen MW, et al. Detection of pulmonary embolism in patients with unresolved clinical and scintigraphic diagnosis: helical ct versus angiography. AJR Am J Roentgenol 1995;164:1369–74.
36. Kakkar VV, Howe CT, Flanc C, et al. Natural history of postoperative deep-vein thrombosis. Lancet 1969;2:230–2.
37. Trendelenburg F [Ueber die operatie behandlung der embolie lungenarteerie]. Arch Klin Chir 1908;86:686–700 [German].
38. Meyer JA. Friedrich Trendelenburg and the surgical approach to massive pulmonary embolism. Arch Surg 1990;125:1202–5.
39. Crafoord C. Two cases of obstructive pulmonary embolism successfully operated upon. Acta Chir Scand 1928;114:172–86.
40. Cooley DA, Beall AC Jr, Alexander JK. Acute massive pulmonary embolism. Successful surgical treatment using temporary cardiopulmonary bypass. JAMA 1961;177:283–6.

41. Greenfield LJ, Bruce TA, Nichols NB. Transvenous pulmonary embolectomy by catheter device. Ann Surg 1971;174:881–6.
42. Homans J. Thrombosis of the deep veins of the lower leg, causing pulmonary embolism. N Engl J Med 1934;211:993–7.
43. Byrne JJ. Phlebitis; a study of 748 cases at the boston city hospital. N Engl J Med 1955;253:579–86.
44. Homans J. Deep quiet venous thrombosis in the lower limb. Surg Gynecol Obstet 1944;79:70–82.
45. Collins C, Jones JR, Nelson EW. Surgical treatment of pelvic thrombophlebitis: ligation of inferior vena cava and ovarian veins. New Orleans Med Sci J 1943;329–34.
46. Mobin-Uddin K, McLean R, Bolooki H, et al. Caval interruption for prevention of pulmonary embolism. Long-term results of a new method. Arch Surg 1969;99:711–5.
47. Decousus H, Leizorovicz A, Parent F, et al. A clinical trial of vena caval filters in the prevention of pulmonary embolism in patients with proximal deep-vein thrombosis. Prevention du risque d'embolie pulmonaire par interruption cave study group. N Engl J Med 1998;338:409–15.
48. Howell W, Holt E. Two new factors in blood coagulation-heparin and proantithrombin. Am J Phys 1918;47:328–33.
49. Murray GaB, Best CH. Heparin and thrombosis: the present situation. JAMA 1938;110:118–22.
50. Crafoord C. Heparin and post-operative thrombosis. Acta Chir Scand 1939;82:319–35.
51. Murray G. Experimental surgery: heparin in thrombosis and embolism. Br J Surg 1940;27:567–98.
52. Barritt DW, Jordan SC. Anticoagulant drugs in the treatment of pulmonary embolism. A controlled trial. Lancet 1960;1:1309–12.
53. Brandjes DP, Heijboer H, Buller HR, et al. Acenocoumarol and heparin compared with acenocoumarol alone in the initial treatment of proximal-vein thrombosis. N Engl J Med 1992;327:1485–9.
54. Thery C, Simonneau G, Meyer G, et al. Randomized trial of subcutaneous low-molecular-weight heparin cy 216 (fraxiparine) compared with intravenous unfractionated heparin in the curative treatment of submassive pulmonary embolism. A dose-ranging study. Circulation 1992;85:1380–9.
55. Simonneau G, Sors H, Charbonnier B, et al. A comparison of low-molecular-weight heparin with unfractionated heparin for acute pulmonary embolism. The thesee study group. Tinzaparine ou heparine standard: evaluations dans l'embolie pulmonaire. N Engl J Med 1997;337:663–9.
56. The Columbus Investigators. Low-molecular-weight heparin in the treatment of patients with venous thromboembolism. N Engl J Med 1997;337:657–62.
57. Crafoord C. Preliminary report on post-operative treatment with heparin as a preventive of thrombosis. Acta Chir Scand 1937;107:116–22.
58. Sharnoff JG, Kass HH, Mistica BA. A plan of heparinization of the surgical patient to prevent postoperative thromboembolism. Surg Gynecol Obstet 1962;115:75–9.
59. Kakkar VV, Corrigan T, Spindler J, et al. Efficacy of low doses of heparin in prevention of deep-vein thrombosis after major surgery. A double-blind, randomised trial. Lancet 1972;2:101–6.
60. Prevention of fatal postoperative pulmonary embolism by low doses of heparin. An international multicentre trial. Lancet 1975;2:45–51.
61. Tillett W. The fibrinolytic activity of hemolytic streptococci. J Exp Med 1933;58:485–502.

62. Browse NL, James DC. Streptokinase and pulmonary embolism. Lancet 1964;2: 1039–43.
63. The Urokinase Pulmonary Embolism Trial. A national cooperative study. Circulation 1973;47:II1–108.
64. Urokinase-streptokinase embolism trial. Phase 2 results. A cooperative study. JAMA 1974;229:1606–13.

Cardiopulmonary Resuscitation: From the Beginning to the Present Day

Giuseppe Ristagno, MD[a], Wanchun Tang, MD[a,b],
Max Harry Weil, MD, PhD[a,b,c],*

KEYWORDS

- Cardiopulmonary resuscitation • Cardiac arrest
- Ventricular fibrillation • Defibrillation
- Ventilation • Chest compression

Cardiac arrest represents a dramatic event that can occur suddenly and often without premonitory signs, characterized by sudden loss of consciousness and breathing after cardiac output ceases and both coronary and cerebral blood flows stop. Restarting of the blood flow by cardiopulmonary resuscitation (CPR) potentially re-establishes some cardiac output and organ blood flows. CPR has the potential of re-establishing spontaneous circulation, often in conjunction with electrical defibrillation, but CPR is likely to be successful only if it is instituted within 5 minutes after the heart stops beating.[1–3] To this extent, the American Heart Association's concept of the "chain of survival," introduced in 1991 by Cummins and colleagues[4] addresses the priorities very well. This chain includes four links, namely: (1) calling for emergency medical assistance; (2) (bystander-initiated) basic life support; (3) early defibrillation; and (4) advanced life support. The first three links are focused on out-of-hospital cardiac resuscitation by nonprofessional providers. The critical time intervals, in part based on the Utstein templates for documenting the sequence of interventions,[5] begin with the call for emergency assistance, documents arrival time of rescuers (including bystanders), the interventions performed by the emergency medical responders at the site of the victim, and the sequences of interventions that follow. In the instance of ventricular fibrillation (VF), automated external defibrillators (AEDs) have enfranchised

This project was funded by the Weil Institute of Critical Care Medicine, Rancho Mirage, CA.
[a] Weil Institute of Critical Care Medicine, 35100 Bob Hope Drive, Rancho Mirage, CA 92270, USA
[b] Keck School of Medicine of the University of Southern California, 1975 Zonal Avenue, KAM 500, Los Angeles, CA 90089-9034, USA
[c] Northwestern University Feinberg School of Medicine, 303 East Chicago Avenue, Chicago, IL 60611-3008, USA
* Corresponding author. Weil Institute of Critical Care Medicine, 35100 Bob Hope Drive, Rancho Mirage, CA 92270.
E-mail address: weilm@weiliccm.org (M.H. Weil).

Crit Care Clin 25 (2009) 133–151
doi:10.1016/j.ccc.2008.10.004
0749-0704/08/$ – see front matter © 2009 Published by Elsevier Inc.

nonprofessional rescuers to reverse VF. Current evidence supports the value of a well-organized program of bystander-initiated CPR and, in some settings, public access defibrillation.[6] Within the past year, the chain of survival has been amended to include an additional link, namely postresuscitation management.[7]

This article summarizes the major events that encompass the history of CPR, beginning with ancient history and evolving into the current commitment to "save hearts that are too young to die."[8]

THE HISTORY OF CPR

Early resuscitation attempts to reverse sudden death are as old as human history.[9] However, until the nineteenth century, routine resuscitation from death was not viewed as feasible.[10] Modern cardiopulmonary resuscitation emerged only during the latter half of the twentieth century, even though resuscitation by delivery of an electrical shock was demonstrated as early as the nineteenth century. In the 1900s, asphyxia was a major and even predominant cause of cardiac arrest because of drowning, aspiration, drug overdose, smoke inhalation, diphtheria, asthma, epiglottitis, and traumatic injuries to the head and chest. Accordingly, there was initial emphasis on airway devices and mechanical interventions for breathing. Electrical causes and, specifically electrocution, became significant causes of cardiac arrest in parallel with the emergence of electrical power in the late nineteenth and early twentieth century.[11] This prompted the development and use of defibrillation under the auspices of electrical power companies.[10,12] External mechanical methods for restoring blood circulation were a development of 1960s, when a sequence of interventions was established under the acronym ABCD:[13] Airway, Breathing, Chest compression, and Defibrillation. Although to some extent now modified to take into account priorities of chest compression over the airway, breathing, and defibrillation, the ABCD acronym continues to have practical utility, especially for other than primary cardiac causes of cardiac arrest, such as in newborns, children, and younger adults.

Airway

The earliest description of a method by which an airway could be secured may have been recorded in the Babylonian Talmud, edited between 200 BC and 400 AD.[14] The Talmud describes a lamb that sustained an injury to the neck, such that a large hole was created in the trachea. A hollow reed was inserted into the trachea and the lamb survived. More than a millennium later, Versalius,[15] the famous Belgian anatomist, inserted a tubular reed through a surgical tracheostomy. When the reed was connected to a fireplace bellows, the lungs were inflated. This anticipated the modern method of securing the airway followed by mechanical ventilation. In 1754, the first endotracheal tube was designed under the name of "air pipe." It consisted of a coiled wire that was covered by soft leather. As described by White,[16] Doctor Pugh used this device for resuscitation after neonatal asphyxia. Endotracheal intubation and mechanical ventilation with bellows thereafter evolved as primary interventions, especially for drowning victims. The primary intervention for opening the airway and thereby assuring patency of the upper airways unobstructed by the flaccid tongue was described in 1783. One hundred years later in 1877, Howard[17] proposed that the tongue of drowning victim be positioned by the rescuer such as to obtain a patent airway. He advised that the tip of the tongue be withdrawn and displaced to the extreme right corner of the mouth. In 1788, Kite introduced a curved metal cannula for blind insertion through the mouth into the trachea. Although the intent was to minimize trauma to the soft tissues of the airway, such was not possible without visualizing the larynx. During the following century, new designs of endotracheal tubes evolved, including a tube with a sponge collar, perhaps the predecessor of currently marketed cuffed endotracheal tubes. Largely through the efforts of Trendelenburg in 1871,[18] these tubes gained popularity. In the 1890s, the introduction of the laryngoscope by Kirstein[19] revolutionized nontraumatic endotracheal intubation. The S-shaped oropharyngeal airway, which continues to be used to the present, was used by Peter Safar (**Fig. 1**), together with the now routine positions of the forehead and mandible with which a patent airway is secured in unconscious victims. Correct patency of the airway was described by Safar and colleagues,[20] who observed in anesthetized, breathing patients, the return of inflated gas into a bag that was connected to the endotracheal tube.

Ventilation

The earliest recorded reference to artificial breathing is in Egyptian mythology, in which Isis resuscitated her dead husband by breathing into his mouth.[21] The Old Testament is another source of impressive historical documentation of mouth-to-mouth breathing. In II Kings, chapter 4, the prophet Elisha is described as restoring the life of a boy by placing his mouth on the mouth of the child.[22] Between 200 BC and 500 AD, the Hebrews used mouth-to-nose ventilation for resuscitation of newborn infants.[23] Early efforts for restoring life of unconscious victims focused on breathing. Primitive fireplace bellows were used for this purpose. Bellows-to-nostril ventilation in human beings was first described by Galen, who in 175 AD inflated the lungs of dead animals. In the 1500s, Paracelsus reproposed the use of bellows to attempt resuscitation of dead persons.[24] Early mouth-to-mouth techniques were subsequently described in several eighteenth century publications cited by Safar.[25] William Tossach,[26] a British surgeon, used mouth-to-mouth resuscitation of a coal miner in 1732. After 4 hours the miner is described as conscious and able to walk without support. In 1745, there was a return to mouth-to-mouth ventilation as a safer and more effective method of ventilation, in contrast to the use of fire bellows.[18] In 1800, a report

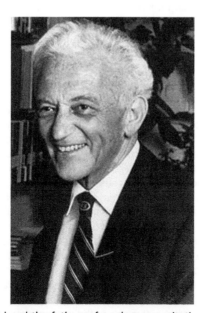

Fig. 1. Moritz Shiff, considered the fathers of modern resuscitation.

that a single, rapid inflation with bellows produced a fatal pneumothorax[27] led rescuers to discard the routine use of bellows in favor of mouth-to-mouth breathing. Yet, the use of exhaled air for resuscitation was challenged in 1770 after Scheele[28] proposed the value of oxygen in lieu of the insufflation of expired air because expired air was then perceived to be "devitalized." The combination of devitalized expired gas and the risks of lung barotrauma produced by bellows therefore prompted the search for alternative methods of mechanical ventilation.

Early revival efforts centered on drowning victims. To clear water from the trachea and lungs, the presumed causes of drowning, the unconscious patient was suspended upside down or rolled on a barrel to produce compression and decompression of the chest. Such activity produced ventilation as well as chest compression.[13,17] In 1857, Marshall Hall advanced the "chest-pressure" method, which was modified in 1861 by Silvester[29] to become the "chest-pressure arm-lift" method of artificial breathing in supine patients. The method was later modified by Howard, who placed the victim in the supine position and compressed the chest intermittently to produce expiration and recoil inspiration. Tidal volumes generated by these methods were modest, however. In the early twentieth century, Schafer[30] placed the victim into a prone position and compressed the lower back to produce expiration and recoil (passive) inspiration, a method that was widely taught, including to one of the authors (M.H.W.) when he was a Boy Scout.

The first mechanical respirator was introduced in 1838 and represented a "tank respirator." Negative pressure was generated while the chest was enclosed in an air-tight tank, thereby producing active inspiration and allowing for passive expiration when ambient pressure was restored.[31] The Drinker respirator,[32] or "iron lung" that followed, paved the way for prolonged mechanical ventilation, especially for patients afflicted with neuromuscular failure of breathing, including cervical spinal cord injury and, most of all, paralytic poliomyelitis.

Intermittent positive pressure ventilation first evolved in Europe when cuffed tracheotomy tubes became available. In 1952, Bjørn Ibsen[33] used manual positive pressure ventilation during the Danish polio epidemics, with the participation of hundreds of medical students breathing for victims who had a tracheostomy tube attached to a vented rubber bag for delivery of air or oxygen. This is incorrectly cited by some historians as the beginning of the Critical Care Medicine, yet, such that represented only protracted mechanical ventilation outside of the operating room, rather than the era of continuous hemodynamic and respiratory patient monitoring and management that ushered in care of the critical ill in modern intensive care units in the late 1950s.

In 1954, the mouth-to-mask ventilation for resuscitation was proposed by Elam, which achieved arterial oxygen saturations of more than 90%.[34] Safar,[35] instead, reproposed mouth-to-mouth ventilation as an effective ventilation method during resuscitation because it required no instrumentation. Mouth-to-mouth ventilation generated arterial oxygen saturations as high as 97%. Endotracheal positive-pressure ventilation thereafter became a standard of care for sustaining ventilation, using positive-pressure valves, both the Bennett and Bird devices.[36] These compact ventilators had advantages of patient triggering, greater accessibility, and mobility, though not yet the predictability of delivery of specified volumes of air or oxygen. Subsequently, the self-refilling bag introduced by Ruben[37] in 1958, followed by the addition of the oxygen gas-powered pneumatic demand valve resuscitator in 1964, added important advances to support breathing in emergency settings.[38] The Engstrom became the first pratical volume-controlled, patient-triggered mechanical ventilator.[39] Concurrently, the valve-mask bag became the primary manual emergency-ventilation device for resuscitation, and it continues to be in active use to the present day.[38]

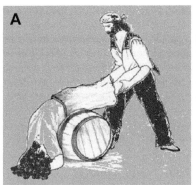
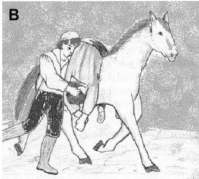

Fig. 2. The "barrel" (A) and the "trotting horse" (B) methods for chest compression (*Adapted from* Gordon AS. JAMA 1974;227(Suppl. 7)2:834–68; with permission).

Chest Compression

The importance of chest compression, also referred to in the I Kings, chapter 17, emerged again during the eighteenth century. The "barrel method" and the "horse method" (**Fig. 2**), in which victims were placed in prone position over a barrel or the back of a horse, forcefully produced chest compression during rolling or trotting.[13] Nevertheless, chest compression for restarting the circulation was still regarded as a lower priority than ventilation and, historically, even application of external pressure to the thorax was intended to produce breathing rather than circulation.[24] Indeed, it was direct cardiac compressions that Moritz Schiff[40] (**Fig. 3**) described in 1874, when he noted the carotid pulsations closely corresponding to the ejection of blood produced by directly squeezing the canine heart in a dog's open chest. This led to the term "open-chest cardiac massage." The method was effective experimentally

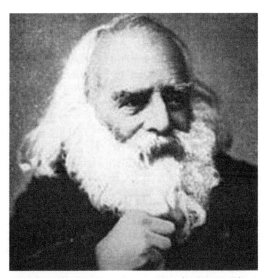

Fig. 3. Peter Safar, who first demonstrated carotid pulsations with open heart massage. (*Courtesy of* the Safar Center for Resuscitaion Research, University of Pittsburgh, Pittsburgh, PA; with permission.)

in that it returned spontaneous circulation in dogs after chloroform-induced cardiac arrest.

Soon thereafter, Rudolph Boehm[41] and Louis Mickwitz studied effects of cardiac compression in cats by pressing on the sternum and on the ribs. In 1883, Koening[42] described compressing the left precordium at the apex, which restored spontaneous circulation in a patient who had cardiac arrest accidentally induced by chloroform anesthesia. Friedrich Maass is credited with the first successful human closed-chest cardiac massage, in 1891.[10,13] However, all these initial trials remained anecdotal. A successful open-chest cardiac massage was performed in 1901 by Kristian Igelsrud, also after anesthesia-related cardiac arrest, and prompted renewed clinical interest in this resuscitation procedure.[43] Consequently, during the first half of the twentieth century, cardiac resuscitation was restricted to the operating room or in proximal in-hospital settings, which included experiences by one of the authors (M.H.W.) during his residency and fellowship training. In 1958, however, Kouwenhoven and colleagues[44] reawakened the potential value of chest cardiac massage when they observed that coincidental with the positioning of paddles on the anterior chest for delivery of an electrical shock, an arterial pulse was produced. This trio of two John Hopkins engineers and a surgeon then demonstrated that external chest compression restored spontaneous circulation in 14 of 20 victims of cardiac arrest, all of whom survived hospitalization. External compression could therefore be performed without surgical expertise or equipment, and now became widely taught and used, and open-chest cardiac massage became obsolete except for intraoperative or posttraumatic resuscitation. A combination of closed-chest compression and mechanical ventilation thereupon formed the platform after the 1960s, and remains as present-day CPR. A strong commitment to mouth-to-mouth or alternative methods of routine ventilation persisted as the co-equal of chest compression until the end of the twentieth century.

Defibrillation and External Pacing

The capability of electricity to stimulate contraction of muscle was clearly described by Galvani[45] in 1791. Ventricular fibrillation, naturally caused by lightering, was first induced experimentally by Ludwig and Hoffa in 1850, when they delivered an alternating electrical current directly to the ventricle of a dog's heart. Subsequently, John McWilliam[46] hypothesized that ventricular fibrillation rather than cardiac standstill was the predominant cause of cardiac arrest. However, the first demonstration that ventricular fibrillation could be terminated by an electrical current was in 1899, when Prevost and Battelli[47] observed that directly delivered low voltage AC currents induced ventricular fibrillation in dogs, and higher voltage currents terminated ventricular fibrillation. Hooker and colleagues[12] were specifically funded to study accidental electrocution by the Edison Electric Institute. They investigated the appropriate energy levels for effective electrical defibrillation by applying electrodes directly to dog hearts and subsequently to the intact thorax. In 1940, the famed Cleveland physiologist, Carl Wiggers,[48] confirmed both the efficacy of electrical defibrillation for reversing ventricular fibrillation and that of open-chest cardiac massage for restoring blood flow in dogs. Seven years later, the pioneer heart surgeon Claude Beck, also in Cleveland, successfully resuscitated a 14-year-old boy who developed ventricular fibrillation during a thoracoplasty for management of congenital chest deformity. Beck[49] performed cardiac massage for 45 minutes before attempted defibrillation. A supraventricular rhythm followed a second defibrillation attempt, with restoration of the pulse and therefore spontaneous circulation. Initially, alternating sinusoidal waveform currents were delivered to the myocardium with a physically large, heavy, and relatively immobile device. Dr. Paul Zoll[50] subsequently recorded the first successful closed-chest human defibrillation in 1955 in a man with recurrent syncope that terminated in ventricular fibrillation. In 1962, Dr. Bernard Lown[51] introduced direct current monophasic waveform defibrillation and demonstrated its superiority when compared with alternating currents. In 1979, the first portable external defibrillator was developed, the precursor to AEDs. A pharyngeal electrode for sensing, electrodes applied to the abdomen and tongue for delivery of a shock, and a simple algorithm to detect shockable electrocardiographic rhythms triggered automated delivery of either pacing or DC defibrillation shocks.[52] The present compact, battery-operated, portable percutaneous pacemakers and defibrillators provide for pacing in the instance of a heart block or cardioversion in the case of ventricular tachycardia or fibrillation. Such are in wide use by professional rescuers. Intelligent automated external defibrillators, which prompt the rescuer in the sequence of interventions before and during defibrillation, are now also commonplace and used by basic life support rescuers with minimal training.

MODERN CPR

The key events that provided the basis for modern CPR are summarized in **Box 1**. Clearly, the modern era of CPR emerged in 1960 with the publication by Kouwenhoven, Jude, and Knickerbocker.[44] Yet, there was little new that would soon be implemented but even more that had to be discarded. As cited above, the various prone and supine chest-pressure and arm-lift maneuvers failed to provide for either opening of the airway or effective ventilation. Mini-thoracotomy, as a routine for open-chest cardiac compressions, was discarded in favor of closed-chest compressions. Electrical defibrillation became a high priority. The now more simplified CPR interventions were extended to the larger domain of both professional and lay rescuers. In part fostered by Peter Safar, Asmund Laerdal in Stavenger, Norway created mannequins and other teaching devices and materials for CPR skill training, including devices for securing airway and for mouth-to-mouth ventilation,[53] chest compression, and defibrillation. Under the auspices of the National Academy of Science National Research Council, James Elam, Archer Gordon, James Jude, and Peter Safar formed a working committee, to which one of the authors (M.H.W.) was invited. This committee developed the first national guidelines for what to teach to whom and how, that was published in 1966.[54] Guidelines were also developed under the auspices of the World Federation of Societies of Anesthesiologists, which expanded guidelines for advanced life support, including cerebral resuscitation.[54,55] In the decade that followed the first National Conference on Standards for CPR and Emergency Cardiac Care was organized under the auspices of the American Heart Association (AHA), which thereafter assumed increasing responsibility for professional leadership of the field, both nationally and later internationally. In 1973, the second National Conference on CPR was held under the auspices of the AHA.[56] More than 3 million copies of the guidelines adopted at that conference were subsequently distributed worldwide, with the intent to promote the teaching of CPR to lay persons as well as medical professionals. Between 1973 and 1980, an estimated 12 million Americans had been trained in CPR and more than 60 million individuals worldwide.[57] Rapid-response systems evolved concurrently and emergency medical personnel, especially, were comprehensively trained in life-support interventions. In the United States, a professional group of rescuers were certified as Emergency Medical Technicians (EMTs), and subsequently, an advanced trained professional, EMT-paramedics, were in many instances organized as a part of traditional community fire rescue services.

Box 1
Key events in the emergence of modern CPR

1732— William Tossach used mouth-to-mouth ventilation for resuscitation of a coal miner.

1754—The first endotracheal tube was designed under the name of "air pipe."

1773—Scheele isolated oxygen.

1838—The first mechanical respirator was introduced, the "Tank Respirator."

1850—Ventricular fibrillation was first induced experimentally by Ludwig and Hoffa by delivering an alternating electrical current directly to the ventricle of a dog's heart.

1874—Moritz Schiff introduced the "open-chest cardiac massage."

1877—Howard proposed that the tongue of drowning victims had to be displaced cephalad such as to obtain a patent airway.

1891—Dr. Friedrich Maass performed the first documented chest compression in human beings.

1895—Kirstein introduced the laryngoscope.

1899—Prevost and Battelli observed that direct low voltage AC currents induced ventricular fibrillation in dogs and higher voltage currents terminated ventricular fibrillation.

1940—Carl Wiggers confirmed efficacy of electrical defibrillation and that of open-chest cardiac massage.

1947—Claude Beck successfully defibrillated a 14-year-old-boy who developed ventricular fibrillation during surgery.

1954—The mouth-to mask ventilation for resuscitation was proposed by Elam.

1954—James Elam proved that expired air maintained adequate oxygenation.

1955—Dr. Paul Zoll recorded the first successful closed-chest human defibrillation.

1956—Peter Safar and James Elam reproposed mouth-to-mouth ventilation for resuscitation.

1957—The United States military adopted the mouth-to-mouth resuscitation method to revive unresponsive victims.

1958—The self-refilling bag to assist ventilation was introduced by Ruben.

1958—Kouwenhoven and his colleagues, Jude and Knickerbocker, observed that compression of the anterior chest wall produced an arterial pulse.

1962—Dr. Bernard Lown introduced direct current monophasic waveform defibrillation.

1966—The first cardiopulmonary resuscitation guidelines were developed.

1979—The first portable external defibrillator was developed.

The call for resuscitation intervention is very large. Today, as many as 400,000 Americans and 700,000 Europeans sustain cardiac arrests each year.[58] Major efforts to improve outcomes from sudden cardiac death were intended to keep pace with an increasing incidence of cardiac arrest in communities with a predominance of elderly patients with ischemic heart disease.

Still, only 4% to 9% of victims of cardiac arrest survive,[59–62] and the scope of this worldwide epidemic prompted increasing international concern among industrialized nations. After the 2000 International Conference on the science of resuscitation, conferences have been scheduled on an international basis every 5 years, and the recommendations serve as the basis of national guidelines that fulfill local needs.

Yet, the emergence of well-trained rescue services have failed to continue to improve outcomes, except in unique public settings in which there is immediate access to CPR. It became apparent that CPR must be begun within less than 5 minutes of "sudden death."[63,64] It was also increasingly apparent that the promise of improved outcomes was contingent on bystander intervention. More specifically, bystander-initiated CPR by minimally trained nonprofessional rescuers became a high priority after 2000. If there was to be meaningful benefit after arrival of well-organized professional emergency medical responders in home settings, where 80% of cardiac arrest occur,[65] bystander-initiated CPR was needed. With bystander-initiated CPR, the likelihood of increased survival from out-of-hospital cardiac arrest was shown to increase as much as 10-fold.[66,67]

The latest International Conference, under the auspices of the AHA and the International Liaison Committee on Resuscitation (ILCOR)[58] in 2005, resulted in additional and major changes in CPR. The highest priority became uninterrupted precordial compression. To achieve such, interruptions for ventilations were to be minimized and lay rescuers were guided to less frequent or even abandonment of rescue breathing. The emphasis on repetitive defibrillations was moderated and only a single shock rather than three repetitive shocks was advised. The value of uninterrupted chest compression trumped the earlier procedures where chest compressions were stopped to deliver a series of up to three shocks and additional time was consumed to observe the electrocardiographic rhythm. This 2005 ILCOR/AHA conference also urged more focus on postresuscitation management, including routine use of hypothermia in the immediate postresuscitation interval.

Ventilation and Chest Compression

Although initial management of "sudden death" in the 2005 guidelines focused on chest compression rather than ventilation with which to sustain both coronary and cerebral blood flows, the airway and ventilation remain a predominant intervention for management of asphyxial cardiac arrest. These differences in priorities apply especially to the majority of neonatal, pediatric, and young adults in whom airway obstruction and loss of neural functions because of intoxications or neurotrauma are predominant.[58] Nevertheless, debate continues on airway management and the benefits of endotracheal intubation. Both optimal tidal volumes and frequencies of ventilation are still debated.[58] Out-of-hospital endotracheal intubation carries both a high failure rate[68] and as large as a 30% incidence of traumatic injury to the airway.[69] There is increasing use of the laryngeal mask airways because of the ease and predictability of placement and nontraumatic rapid insertion under the usually compromised circumstances of cardiac arrest. Assuring appropriate head and body position during nonasphyxial resuscitation is now an accepted routine. Even for asphyxial cardiac arrest, more modest rates of ventilation and, specifically 2 breaths for 30 compressions, were advised with tidal volumes of no greater than 8 mL/kg.[70] Professional rescuers have typically overventilated patients during out-of-hospital CPR, with less favorable outcomes, in part not only because of fewer interruptions of chest compression required but also because of the increases in intrathoracic pressure produced by lung inflations. The increases in intrathoracic pressure compromise venous return of blood to the heart and, therefore, the amount of cardiac output generated by chest compression.[71,72] By decreasing the frequency of ventilations, cardiac output and pulmonary blood flow are actually increased without compromise of arterial oxygen content or acid-base balance.[73] This prompted the 2005 guidelines consensus that compression/ventilation ratios of 30 to 2 be used in lieu of 15 to 2. Experts appreciated that ventilation is of little benefit unless cardiac output and, therefore, pulmonary blood flow are sufficient to allow for meaningful gas exchange. Because cardiac output during CPR is usually less than one-third of normal, correspondingly less ventilation is required to achieve optimal ventilation/perfusion ratios. Modest ventilation is generated by precordial compression alone and in amounts that are likely to be sufficient for oxygenation of the modest pulmonary blood flow.

Controversies remain regarding the value of routine oxygen breathing, either actively or passively delivered to the airway.[74–76] Spontaneous gasping itself creates pulmonary gas exchange during CPR.[77,78] However, gasping has additional and potentially favorable resuscitative benefits, not only because it produces ventilation but also because it generates compression and therefore cardiac output.[79]

In summary, ventilation has indeed become of lesser importance, except for asphyxial cardiac arrest.[58] No negative impact was observed after out-of-hospital cardiac arrest in human victims of sudden death when ventilation was omitted by the bystander CPR.[80–83] Accordingly, the American Heart Association has recently reiterated that bystanders who witness the sudden collapse of an adult should provide high-quality chest compression with minimal or no interruptions for ventilation. Exceptions include pediatric victims and victims of drowning, trauma, airway obstruction, acute respiratory diseases, and apnea of noncardiac cause.[84]

The evidence is secure that the quality of chest compressions is a major determinant of successful resuscitation.[85–89] Wik and colleagues,[85] grading bystander CPR, defined "good CPR" as generating a palpable carotid or femoral pulse. "Good CPR" improved outcomes in which 23% of victims were resuscitated, but only 1% in the absence of "good CPR." The quality of chest compressions therefore has a major effect on outcomes.[90,91] Rescuer fatigue affects the outcomes of CPR. Even well trained professional providers cannot maintain effective chest compression for intervals that exceed 2 minutes.[92–95] The challenges are even greater during evacuation and transport of victims. Pike and colleagues[96] had recorded a method of mechanical chest compression and demonstrated its use in dogs as early as 1908. Therefore, the option of using mechanical devices to perform and maintain optimal chest compression has always been attractive.[97] Mechanical chest compression potentially overcomes operator fatigue, slow rates of compression, and inadequate depth of compression. A mechanical compressor also facilitates delivery of an electrical shock without interruption of compression by a human rescuer. Several new devices have recently been introduced to facilitate mechanical chest compression, and these demonstrated equivalency and potentially greater effectiveness than manual chest compression.[98–103]

Defibrillation

More effective electrical shocks have been evolved during the last decade with greater efficacy.[51,104] The monophasic damped sinusoidal waveform for defibrillation, which replaced alternating current shocks, had remained the standard for transthoracic defibrillation for almost 30 years, together with the monophasic truncated exponential waveforms. Biphasic waveform shocks, in which initial current flows are positive for a specified duration and then reverse to negative, were introduced only a decade ago. Such biphasic low-energy waveforms have not only supplanted higher energy monophasic waveforms, but have been modified by individual manufacturers to waveform configuration with a diversity of current magnitude and duration, slopes, and total energies delivered with improved first shock efficacy.[104–110]

The relatively large impact of AEDs since 1996 has allowed for extension of defibrillation capability from emergency medical personnel to minimally trained nonprofessional providers under the AHA banner of public access defibrillation.[64,111–115] The simplicity of operation, guided by voice prompts, have the rather impressive potential of "jump starting" the heart by rapid conversion of ventricular fibrillation or ventricular tachycardia before arrival of professional providers. Survival advantage has been demonstrated in public settings, but their use in homes, in which 80% of cardiac arrests occur, has not been proven beneficial.[111-115] When the duration of untreated VF is less than 5 minutes, the immediate delivery of the electrical shock is life saving,[116-119] and that applies to public sites, including airports[64] and casinos.[120]

Another, and not as yet fully explained aspect, is the reduced incidence of ventricular fibrillation, prompting lesser value to AEDs. Ventricular fibrillation accounted for approximately 40% to 60% of initial rhythms in out-of-hospital cardiac arrest settings in the United States in the early 1990s, but is now estimated to account for only 25% of all out-of-hospital cardiac arrests.[121-124]

Postresuscitation Management

After initially successful resuscitation, more than 60% of patients fail to survive to hospital discharge.[125] Moreover, as many as 30% of survivors manifest permanent brain damage.[126] Patients who are successfully resuscitated following cardiac arrest therefore present with what is now termed "post resuscitation disease."[127] Most prominent are postresuscitation myocardial failure and ischemic brain damage. The greatest postresuscitation emphasis has been on long-term neurologically intact survival.[7] Evidence favoring correction of electrolyte and glucose abnormalities, control of postresuscitation cardiac rate, rhythm, systemic blood pressure, and intravascular volumes are cited, but objective proof of these interventions is still anecdotal. Of all interventions, the most persuasive benefits have followed the use of hypothermia.[7,128-131]

Within a short 5 years, this therapeutic intervention has proven to be neuroprotective.[132-136] The concept of hypothermia for reducing either or both ischemic and reperfusion injury of the brain represents another pioneering contribution of the late Professor Peter Safar and the persistence of his efforts through his students, and especially Professor Fritz Sterz.[132,135,137] In 1996, Professor Safar and colleagues[137] induced hypothermia by instilling Ringer's solution maintained at a temperature of 4°C into the abdominal cavity of dogs after resuscitation from cardiac arrest. Cooling was maintained for 12 hours. Functional recovery was associated with minimal histologic brain damage. Two large randomized, controlled clinical trials published in 2002[132,133] documented improved neurologic outcomes in human patients following resuscitation from cardiac arrest. This led the ILCOR, together with the AHA, to recommend routine postresuscitation hypothermia in the range of 32°C to 34°C for between 12 and 24 hours in adult victims who were comatose following out-of-hospital cardiac arrest.[7] In animal studies, hypothermia to levels of 32°C to 34°C, preferably now begun during CPR, has promise of even greater survival and functional benefits.[138-140]

SUMMARY

The attempt to restore the heart beat began with the dawn of recorded history. Yet the modern era of CPR, which began in the 1960s, followed experimental and then human trials that demonstrated that the heart beat could be effectively restarted providing that interventions were prompt. These initially included restoration of breathing, recirculation of blood, and electrical conversion of otherwise fatal ventricular fibrillation.

The early emphasis on ventilation included assuring a patent airway and externally producing gas exchange. Blood flow was initially restored by open-chest cardiac massage and superceded by closed-chest precordial compression 15 years later. Electrical defibrillation was first used simultaneously with the advent of open-chest cardiac massage and has been progressively refined for closed-chest defibrillation, with more effective currents and waveforms and lower total energies delivered.

The emergence of automated defibrillators has allowed for defibrillation by nonprofessional rescuers. Both the reduced incidence of ventricular fibrillation and the increased efficacy of defibrillation when preceded by chest compression have reordered the priorities of CPR in favor of well-executed and uninterrupted chest compressions.

Within the last decade, there has been increasing focus on bystander CPR for maintaining minimal systemic blood flow. This provides the greatest likelihood of meaningful survival after the arrival of professional rescuers.

Finally, the persistent poor yield of meaningful survival after cardiac arrest, including a large falloff of recovery after restoration of spontaneous circulation, highlights the importance of better postresuscitation management. Of all recent advances in pursuit thereof, the early start of hypothermia appears to be the best option for minimizing postresuscitation complications and especially post ischemic brain injury.

REFERENCES

1. Ristagno G, Gullo A, Tang W, et al. New cardiopulmonary resuscitation guidelines 2005: importance of uninterrupted chest compression. Crit Care Clin 2006;22(3):531–8.
2. Weil MH, Sun S. Clinical review: devices and drugs for cardiopulmonary resuscitation—opportunities and restraints. Critical Care 2005;9(3):287–90.
3. Cummins RO, Eisenberg MS. Prehospital cardiopulmonary resuscitation. Is it effective? J Am Med Assoc 1985;253(16):2408–12.
4. Cummins RO, Ornato JP, Thies WH, et al. Improving survival from sudden cardiac arrest: the "chain of survival" concept. A statement for health professionals from the Advanced Cardiac Life Support Subcommittee and the Emergency Cardiac Care Committee, American Heart Association. Circulation 1991;83(5): 1832–47.
5. Jacobs I, Nadkarni V, Bahr J, et al. Cardiac arrest and cardiopulmonary resuscitation outcome reports: update and simplification of the Utstein templates for resuscitation registries: a statement for healthcare professionals from a task force of the International Liaison Committee on Resuscitation (American Heart Association, European Resuscitation Council, Australian Resuscitation Council, New Zealand Resuscitation Council, Heart and Stroke Foundation of Canada, InterAmerican Heart Foundation, Resuscitation Councils of Southern Africa). Circulation 2004;110(21):3385–97.
6. 2005 American Heart Association guidelines for cardiopulmonary resuscitation and emergency cardiovascular care. Part 3: overview of CPR. Circulation 2005;112(Suppl I):IV-12–8.
7. 2005 American Heart Association guidelines for cardiopulmonary resuscitation and emergency cardiovascular care. Part 7.5: Postresuscitation support. Circulation 2005;112(Suppl I):IV-84–8.
8. Tjomsland N, Baskett P. Åsmund S Laerdal. Resuscitation 2002;53(2):115–9.
9. Safar P. Introduction to Wolf Creek IV Conference. New Horiz 1997;5:97–105.
10. Eisenberg MS, Baskett P, Chamberlain D. A history of cardiopulmonary resuscitation. In: Paradis NA, Halperin HR, Kern KB, et al, editors. Cardiac Arrest. The science and practice of resuscitation medicine. 2nd edition. (Cambridge): Cambridge University Press; 2007. p. 2–25.
11. d'Aubigné M, Saint-Maurice R. Cardiac fibrillation caused by electrocution. Mem Acad Chir (Paris) 1967;93(1):57–62.
12. Hooker DR, Kouwenhoven WB, Langworthy OR. The effect of alternating electrical currents on the heart. Am J Phys 1933;103:444–54.

13. Nakagawa Y, Weil MH, Tang W. The history of CPR. In: Weil MH, Tang W, editors. CPR. Resuscitation of the Arrested Heart. Philadelphia: WB Saunders; 1999. p. 1–12.
14. Rosen Z, Davidson JT. Respiratory resuscitation in ancient Hebrew sources. Anesth Analg 1972;51(4):502–5.
15. Versalius A. De humani corporis fabrica, Lib. VII Cap. XIX-De vivorum sectione nonnulla. Basle (Switzerland): Oporinus; 1543. p. 662 [Latin].
16. White GMJ. Evolution of endobronchial and endotracheal intubation. Br J Anaesth 1960;32:235–46.
17. Howard B. The direct method of artificial respiration. Lancet 1877;2:193–6.
18. Thangam S, Weil MH, Rackow EC. Cardiopulmonary resuscitation; a historical review. Acute Care 1986;12(2):63–94.
19. Kirstein A. Autoskopie des larynx und der trachea. Archiv Laryngologie Rhinologie 1895;3:156–64 [German].
20. Safar P, Escarraga LA, Chang F. Upper airway obstruction in the unconscious patient. J Appl Phys 1959;14:760–4.
21. Jayne WA. The Healing Gods of Ancient Civilization. New Hyde Park (NY): University Books Inc; 1925. p. 65.
22. Scherman N, editor. II Kings 4:32–5. Brooklyn (NY): Mesorah Publications Ltd; 2001. p. 886–7.
23. Mo'ed SederIn: The Babylonian Talmud [Shabbath]. [English translation by Rabbi I. Epstein]. vol. I. London, The Soncino Press, 1938. p. 128.
24. Cooper JA, Cooper JD, Cooper JM. Cardiopulmonary resuscitation-history, current practice, and future direction. Circulation 2006;114(25):2839–49.
25. Safar P. History of cardiopulmonary cerebral resuscitation. In: Kaye W, Bircher N, editors. Cardiopulmonary Resuscitation. (NY): Churchill Livingstone; 1989. p. 1–53.
26. Tossach WA. A man dead in appearance recovered by distending the lungs with air. Med Essays Observations 1744;5:605.
27. Le Roy J. Recherches sur l'asphyxie. J Physiol Exp Pathol 1827;7:45–65 [German].
28. C.W. Scheele Chemische abhandlung von der luft und dem feuer: Upsala und Leipzig, 1777. The Alembic Club, Edinburgh, Scotland, [translation; reprinted in Chicago, Ill: University of Chicago Press]; 1912 [German].
29. Silvester HR. A new method of resuscitating stillborn children and of restoring persons apparently dead or drowned. Br Med J 1858;2:576.
30. Schafer EA. Description of a simple and efficient method of performing artificial respiration in the human subject. Med Chir Trans 1904;87:609–23.
31. Dalziel J. On sleep and an apparatus for prompting artificial respiration. Br Assoc Adv Sci 1838;2:127–8.
32. Drinker P, McKhann CF. Landmark article May 18, 1929: the use of a new apparatus for the prolonged administration of artificial respiration. I. A fatal case of poliomyelitis. J Am Med Assoc 1986;255(11):1473–5.
33. Ibsen B. The anaesthetist's viewpoint on the treatment of respiratory complications in poliomyelitis during epidemic in Copenhagen, 1952. Proc R Soc Med 1954;47(1):72–4.
34. Elam JO, Brown ES, Elder JD. Artificial respiration by mouth to mask method; a study of the respiratory gas exchange of paralyzed patient ventilated by operator's expired air. N Engl J Med 1954;250(18):749–54.
35. Safar P. Ventilatory efficacy of mouth to mouth artificial respiration. J Am Med Assoc 1958;167(3):335–41.
36. Schorer R, Stoffregen S, Heisler N. Assisted spontaneous respiration. Comparative studies on Bird and Bennett assistors including anesthetic respiration. Anaesthetist 1966;15(4):113–6.

37. Ruben H. Combination resuscitator and aspirator. Anesthesiology 1958;19(3): 408–9.
38. Pearson JW, Redding JS. Equipment for respiratory resuscitation. 2. Anesthesiology 1964;25:858–9.
39. Sattler L. The Engström universal respirator; structural and physiological fundamentals. Dtsch Med J 1955;6(3–4):107–9.
40. Schiff M. Über direkte reizung der herzoberflaeche. Arch Ges Physiol 1882;28: 200 [German].
41. Boehm R. Über wiederbelebung nach vergiftungen und asphyxia. Arch Exp Pathol Pharm 1878;8:68 [German].
42. Koenig F. Lehrbuch der allgemeinen chirurgie. Goettingen 1883 [German].
43. Keen WW. A case of total laryngectomy (unsuccessful) and a case of abdominal hysterectomy (successful), in both of which massage of the heart for chloroform collapse was employed, with notes of 25 other cases of cardiac massage. Therap Gaz 1904;28:217.
44. Kouwenhoven WB, Jude JR, Knickerbocker GG. Closed-chest cardiac massage. J Am Med Assoc 1960;173:1064–7.
45. Galvani LA. De viribus electricitatis in motu musculari: commentarius. De Bononiensi Scientiarum et Artium Instituto atque Academia Commentarii 1791;7:363–418 [Latin].
46. McWilliam JA. Cardiac failure and sudden death. Br Med J 1889;1:6–8.
47. Prevost JL, Battelli F. La mort par les courants electriques-courants alternatifs a haute tension. J Physiol Pathol Gen 1899;1:427–42 [French].
48. Wiggers CJ. The physiologic basis for cardiac resuscitation from ventricular fibrillation-method for serial defibrillation. Am Heart J 1940;20:413–22.
49. Beck CS, Pritchard WH, Feil HS. Ventricular fibrillation of long duration abolished by electric shock. J Am Med Assoc 1947;135:985.
50. Zoll PM, Linenthal AJ, Gibson W, et al. Termination of ventricular fibrillation in man by externally applied electric countershock. N Engl J Med 1956;254(16):727–32.
51. Lown B, Neuman J, Amarasingham R, et al. Comparison of alternating current with direct current electroshock across the closed chest. Am J Cardiol 1962; 10:223–33.
52. Diack AW, Welborn WS, Rullman RG, et al. An automatic cardiac resuscitator for emergency treatment of cardiac arrest. Med Instrum 1979;13(2):78–83.
53. Tjomsland N. From Stavanger with care. Laerdal's first 50 years. Stavanger, Norway: Aase Grafiske A/S; 1991.
54. American Heart Association (AHA), National Academy of Sciences-National Research Council (NAS-NRC). Standards for cardiopulmonary resuscitation (CPR) and emergency cardiac care (ECC). J Am Med Assoc 1966;198:372–9.
55. Safar P, Bircher NG. Cardiopulmonary-cerebral resuscitation. An introduction to resuscitation medicine. World Federation of Societies of Anaesthesiologists. 3rd edition. London: WB Saunders; 1998.
56. Standards for cardiopulmonary resuscitation (CPR) and emergency cardiac care (ECC). J Am Med Assoc 1974;227(7):833–68.
57. Standards and guidelines for cardiopulmonary resuscitation (CPR) and emergency cardiac care (ECC). J Am Med Assoc 1980;244(5):453–509.
58. International Liaison Committee on Resuscitation. 2005 International consensus on cardiopulmonary resuscitation and emergency cardiovascular care science with treatment recommendations. Part 2: Adult basic life support. Resuscitation 2005;67(2–3):187–201.
59. Sanders AB, Ewy GA. Cardiopulmonary resuscitation in real world: when will the guidelines get the message? J Am Med Assoc 2005;293(3):363–5.

60. Nichol G, Stiell IG, Laupacis A, et al. A cumulative meta-analysis of the effectiveness of defibrillator-capable emergency medical services for victims of out-of-hospital cardiac arrest. Ann Emerg Med 1999;34(4 part 1):517–25.
61. Engdahl J, Bang A, Lindqvist J, et al. Time trends in long-term mortality after out-of-hospital cardiac arrest, 1980 to 1998, and predictors for death. Am Heart J 2003;145(5):749–50.
62. Eisenberg MS, Horwood BT, Cummins RO, et al. Cardiac arrest and resuscitation: a tale of 29 cities. Ann Emerg Med 1990;19(2):179–86.
63. Becker LB, Ostrander MP, Barrett J, et al. Outcome of cardiopulmonary resuscitation in a large metropolitan area: where are the survivors? Ann Emerg Med 1991;20(4):355–61.
64. Caffrey SL, Willoughby PJ, Pepe PE, et al. Public use of automated external defibrillators. N Engl J Med 2002;347(16):1242–7.
65. Bardy GH, Lee KL, Mark DB, et al. Rationale and design of the Home Automatic External Defibrillator Trial (HAT). Am Heart J 2008;155(3):445–54.
66. Larsen MP, Eisenberg MS, Cummins RO, et al. Predicting survival from out-of-hospital cardiac arrest: a graphic model. Ann Emerg Med 1993;22(11):1652–8.
67. Rea TD, Eisenberg MS, Culley LL, et al. Dispatcher-assisted cardiopulmonary resuscitation and survival in cardiac arrest. Circulation 2001;104(21):2513–6.
68. Köhler KW, Losert H, Myklebust H, et al. Detection of malintubation via defibrillator pads. Resuscitation 2008;77(3):339–44.
69. Domino KB, Posner KL, Caplan RA, et al. Airway injury during anesthesia: a closed claims analysis. Anesthesiology 1999;91(6):1703–11.
70. 2005 American Heart Association guidelines for cardiopulmonary resuscitation and emergency cardiovascular care. Part 4: Adult basic life support. Circulation 2005;112(Suppl 24):IV-19–34.
71. Aufderheide TP, Sigurdsson G, Pirrallo RG, et al. Hyperventilation-induced hypotension during cardiopulmonary resuscitation. Circulation 2004;109(16):1960–5.
72. Babbs CF, Kern KB. Optimum compression to ventilation ratios in CPR under realistic, practical conditions: a physiological and mathematical analysis. Resuscitation 2002;54(2):147–57.
73. Yannopoulos D, McKnite SH, Tang W, et al. Reducing ventilation frequency during cardiopulmonary resuscitation in a porcine model of cardiac arrest. Respir Care 2005;50(5):628–35.
74. Tang W, Weil MH, Sun S, et al. Cardiopulmonary resuscitation by precordial compression but without mechanical ventilation. Am J Respir Crit Care Med 1994;150(6 Pt 1):1709–13.
75. Noc M, Weil MH, Tang W, et al. Mechanical ventilation may not be essential for initial cardiopulmonary resuscitation. Chest 1995;108(3):821–7.
76. Hayes MM, Ewy GA, Anavy ND, et al. Continuous passive oxygen insufflation results in a similar outcome to positive pressure ventilation in a swine model of out-of-hospital ventricular fibrillation. Resuscitation 2007;74(2):357–65.
77. Noc M, Weil MH, Tang W, et al. Spontaneous gasping during cardiopulmonary resuscitation without mechanical ventilation. Am J Respir Crit Care Med 1994;150(3):861–4.
78. Fukui M, Weil MH, Tang W, et al. Airway protection during experimental CPR. Chest 1995;108(6):1663–7.
79. Xie J, Weil MH, Sun S, et al. Spontaneous gasping generates cardiac output during cardiac arrest. Crit Care Med 2004;32(1):238–40.
80. Ewy GA, Zuercher M, Hilwig RW, et al. Improved neurological outcome with continuous chest compressions compared with 30:2 compressions-to-ventilations

cardiopulmonary resuscitation in a realistic swine model of out-of-hospital cardiac arrest. Circulation 2007;116(22):2525–30.

81. Bohm K, Rosenqvist M, Herlitz J, et al. Survival is similar after standard treatment and chest compression only in out-of-hospital bystander cardiopulmonary resuscitation. Circulation 2007;116(25):2908–12.

82. SOS-KANTO study group. Cardiopulmonary resuscitation by bystanders with chest compression only (SOS-KANTO): an observational study. Lancet 2007; 369(9565):920–6.

83. Iwami T, Kawamura T, Hiraide A, et al. Effectiveness of bystander-initiated cardiac-only resuscitation for patients with out-of-hospital cardiac arrest. Circulation 2007;116(25):2900–7.

84. Sayre MR, Berg RA, Cave DM, et al. Hands-only (compression-only) cardiopulmonary resuscitation: a call to action for bystander response to adults who experience out-of-hospital sudden cardiac arrest. Circulation 2008;117(16): 2162–7.

85. Wik L, Steen PA, Bircher NG. Quality of bystander cardiopulmonary resuscitation influences outcome after prehospital cardiac arrest. Resuscitation 1994;28(3): 195–203.

86. Gallagher EJ, Lombardi G, Gennis P. Effectiveness of bystander cardiopulmonary resuscitation and survival following out-of-hospital cardiac arrest. J Am Med Assoc 1995;274(24):1922–5.

87. Van Hoeyweghen RJ, Bossaert LL, Mullie A, et al. Quality and efficiency of bystander CPR. Belgian Cerebral Resuscitation Study Group. Resuscitation 1993;26(1):47–52.

88. Abella BS, Alvarado JP, Myklebust H, et al. Quality of cardiopulmonary resuscitation during in-hospital cardiac arrest. J Am Med Assoc 2005;293(3):305–10.

89. Wik L, Kramer-Johansen J, Myklebust H, et al. Quality of cardiopulmonary resuscitation during out-of-hospital cardiac arrest. J Am Med Assoc 2005;293(3): 299–304.

90. Abella BS, Sandbo N, Vassilatos P, et al. Chest compression rates during cardiopulmonary resuscitation are suboptimal. Circulation 2005;111(4):428–34.

91. Ristagno G, Tang W, Chang YT, et al. The quality of chest compressions during cardiopulmonary resuscitation overrides importance of timing of defibrillation. Chest 2007;132(1):70–5.

92. Ashton A, McCluskey A, Gwinnutt GL, et al. Effect of rescuer fatigue on performance of continuous external chest compressions over 3 minutes. Resuscitation 2002;55(2):151–5.

93. Ochoa FJ, Ramalle-Gomara E, Lisa V, et al. The effect of rescuer fatigue on the quality of chest compressions. Resuscitation 1998;37(3):149–52.

94. Hightower D, Thomas SH, Stone CK, et al. Decay in quality of closed-chest compressions over time. Ann Emerg Med 1995;26(3):300–3.

95. Plaisance P, Adnet F, Vicaut E, et al. Benefit of active compression-decompression cardiopulmonary resuscitation as prehospital advanced cardiac life support: a randomized multicenter study. Circulation 1997;95(4):955–61.

96. Pike FH, Guthrie CC, Stewart GN. Studies in resuscitation: the general conditions affecting resuscitation, and the resuscitation of the blood and of the heart. J Exp Med 1908;10:371–418.

97. Harrison-Paul R. A history of mechanical devices for providing external chest compressions. Resuscitation 2007;73(3):330–6.

98. Steen S, Sjoberg T, Olsson P, et al. Treatment of out-of-hospital cardiac arrest with LUCAS, a new device for automatic mechanical compression and active decompression resuscitation. Resuscitation 2005;67(1):25–30.
99. Rubertsson S, Karlsten R. Increased cortical cerebral blood flow with LUCAS; a new device for mechanical chest compressions compared to standard external compressions during experimental cardiopulmonary resuscitation. Resuscitation 2005;65(3):357–63.
100. Hallstrom A, Rea TD, Sayre MR, et al. Manual chest compression vs. use of an automated chest compression device during resuscitation following out-of-hospital cardiac arrest: a randomized trial. J Am Med Assoc 2006;295(22):2620–8.
101. Ong ME, Ornato JP, Edwards DP, et al. Use of an automated, load-distributing band chest compression device for out-of-hospital cardiac arrest resuscitation. J Am Med Assoc 2006;295(22):2629–37.
102. Krep H, Mamier M, Breil M, et al. Out-of-hospital cardiopulmonary resuscitation with the AutoPulseTM system: a prospective observational study with a new load-distributing band chest compression device. Resuscitation 2007;73(1): 86–95.
103. Dickinson ET, Verdile VP, Schneider RM, et al. Effectiveness of mechanical versus manual chest compressions in out-of-hospital cardiac arrest resuscitation: a pilot study. Am J Emerg Med 1998;16(3):289–92.
104. Bardy GH, Marchlinsky FE, Sharma AD, et al. Multicenter comparison of truncated biphasic shocks and standard damped sine wave monophasic shocks for transthoracic ventricular fibrillation. Transthoracic Investigators. Circulation 1996;94(10):2507–14.
105. Bain AC, Swerdlow CD, Love JC, et al. Multicenter study of principles-based waveforms for external defibrillation. Ann Emerg Med 2001;37(1):5–12.
106. Poole JE, White RD, Kanz KG, et al. Low-energy impedance-compensating biphasic waveforms terminate ventricular fibrillation at high rates in victims of out-of-hospital cardiac arrest. LIFE investigators. J Cardiovasc Electrophysiol 1997;8(12):1373–85.
107. Greene HL, Di Marco JP, Kudenchuk PJ, et al. Comparison of monophasic and biphasic defibrillating pulse waveforms for transthoracic cardioversion. Am J Cardiol 1995;75(16):1135–9.
108. Schneider T, Martens PR, Paschen H, et al. Multicenter, randomized, controlled trial of 150-J biphasic shocks compared with 200- to 360-J monophasic shocks in the resuscitation of out-of-hospital cardiac arrest victims. Circulation 2000; 102(15):1780–7.
109. Hess EP, Atkinson EJ, White RD. Increased prevalence of sustained return of spontaneous circulation following transition to biphasic waveform defibrillation. Resuscitation 2008;77(1):39–45.
110. Didon JP, Fontaine G, White RD, et al. Clinical experience with a low-energy pulsed biphasic waveform in out-of-hospital cardiac arrest. Resuscitation 2008;76(3):350–3.
111. Weisfeldt ML, Kerber RE, McGoldrick RP, et al. Public access defibrillation. American Heart Association task force on automated external defibrillation. Circulation 1995;92(9):2763.
112. Nichol G, Hallstrom AP, Kerber R, et al. American Heart Association report on the second public access defibrillation conference, April 17–19. Circulation 1998;97(13):1309–14.

113. White RD, Bunch TJ, Hankins DG. Evolution of a community-wide early defibrillation program. Experience over 13 years using police/fire personnel and paramedics as responders. Resuscitation 2005;65(3):279–83.
114. Culley LL, Rea TD, Murray JA, et al. Public access defibrillation in out-of-hospital cardiac arrest: a community-based study. Circulation 2004;109(15):1859–63.
115. Bardy GH, Lee KL, Mark DB, et al. Home use of automated external defibrillators for sudden cardiac arrest. N Engl J Med 2008;358(17):1793–804.
116. Cobb LA, Fahrenbruch CE, Walsh TR, et al. Influence of cardiopulmonary resuscitation prior to defibrillation in patients with out-of-hospital ventricular fibrillation. J Am Med Assoc 1999;281(13):1182–8.
117. Wik L, Hansen TB, Fylling F, et al. Delaying defibrillation to give basic cardiopulmonary resuscitation to patients with out-of-hospital ventricular fibrillation. J Am Med Assoc 2003;289(11):1389–95.
118. Niemann JT, Cairns CB, Sharma J, et al. Treatment of prolonged ventricular fibrillation: immediate countershock versus high-dose epinephrine and CPR preceding countershock. Circulation 1992;85(1):281–7.
119. Berg RA, Hilwig RW, Ewy GA, et al. Precountershock cardiopulmonary resuscitation improves initial response to defibrillation from prolonged ventricular fibrillation: a randomized, controlled swine study. Crit Care Med 2004;32(6): 1352–7.
120. Valenzuela TD, Roe DJ, Nichol G, et al. Outcomes of rapid defibrillation by security officers after cardiac arrest in casinos. N Engl J Med 2000;343(17): 1206–9.
121. Bunch TJ, White RD, Friedman PA, et al. Trends in treated ventricular fibrillation out-of-hospital cardiac arrest: a 17-year population-based study. Heart Rhythm 2004;1(3):255–9.
122. Bunch TJ, White RD. Trends in treated ventricular fibrillation in out-of-hospital cardiac arrest: ischemic compared to non-ischemic heart disease. Resuscitation 2005;67(1):51–4.
123. Youngquist ST, Kaji AH, Niemann JT. Beta-blocker use and the changing epidemiology of out-of-hospital cardiac arrest rhythms. Resuscitation 2008;76(3): 376–80.
124. Polentini MS, Pirrallo RG, McGill W. The changing incidence of ventricular fibrillation in Milwaukee, Wisconsin (1992–2002). Prehosp Emerg Care 2006;10(1): 52–60.
125. Stiell IG, Wells GA, Field B, et al. Advanced cardiac life support in out-of-hospital cardiac arrest. N Engl J Med 2004;351(7):647–56.
126. Brain resuscitation clinical trial I Study Group. Randomized clinical study of thiopental loading in comatose survivors of cardiac arrest. N Engl J Med 1986; 314(7):397–403.
127. Adrie C, Laurent I, Monchi M, et al. Postresuscitation disease after cardiac arrest: a sepsis-like syndrome? Curr Opin Crit Care 2004;10(3):208–12.
128. Safar P. Resuscitation from clinical death: pathophysiologic limits and therapeutic potentials. Crit Care Med 1988;16(10):923–41.
129. Sunde K, Pytte M, Jacobsen D, et al. Implementation of a standardized treatment protocol for post resuscitation care after out-of-hospital cardiac arrest. Resuscitation 2007;73(1):29–39.
130. Knafelj R, Radsel P, Ploj T, et al. Primary percutaneous coronary intervention and mild induced hypothermia in comatose survivors of ventricular fibrillation with ST-elevation acute myocardial infarction. Resuscitation 2007;74(2):227–34.

131. Kim F, Olsufka M, Carlbom D, et al. Pilot study of rapid infusion of 2 L of 4 degrees C normal saline for induction of mild hypothermia in hospitalized, comatose survivors of out-of-hospital cardiac arrest. Circulation 2005;112(5):715–9.
132. The Hypothermia After Cardiac Arrest Study Group. Mild therapeutic hypothermia to improve the neurologic outcome after cardiac arrest. N Engl J Med 2002; 346(22):549–56.
133. Bernard SA, Gray TW, Buist MD, et al. Treatment of comatose survivors of out-of-hospital cardiac arrest with induced hypothermia. N Engl J Med 2002;346(8): 557–63.
134. Schwab S, Schwarz S, Spranger M, et al. Moderate hypothermia in the treatment of patients with severe middle cerebral artery infarction. Stroke 1998; 29(12):2461–6.
135. Fritz HG, Bauer R. Secondary injuries in brain trauma: effects of hypothermia. J Neurosurg Anesthesiol 2004;16(1):43–52.
136. Sanders AB. Therapeutic hypothermia after cardiac arrest. Curr Opin Crit Care 2006;12(3):213–7.
137. Safar P, Xiao F, Radovsky A, et al. Improved cerebral resuscitation from cardiac arrest in dogs with mild hypothermia plus blood flow promotion. Stroke 1996; 27(1):105–13.
138. Abella BS, Zhao D, Alvarado J, et al. Intra-arrest cooling improves outcomes in a murine cardiac arrest model. Circulation 2004;109(22):2786–91.
139. Maier CM, Abern K, Cheng ML, et al. Optimal depth and duration of mild hypothermia in a focal model of transient cerebral ischemia: effects on neurologic outcome, infarct size, apoptosis, and inflammation. Stroke 1998;29(10): 2171–80.
140. Tsai M, Tang W, Wang H, et al. Rapid head cooling initiated coincident with cardiopulmonary resuscitation improves success of defibrillation and post-resuscitation myocardial function in a porcine model of prolonged cardiac arrest. J Am Coll Cardiol 2008;51(20):1988–90.

Historical Aspects of Critical Care and the Nervous System

Thomas P. Bleck, MD, FCCM

KEYWORDS

- Critical care • Neurocritical care • Neurology • Neurosurgery
- Harvey Cushing • Hugh Cairns • Edwin Smith surgical papyrus
- Peter Safar

The appropriate starting point for a history of neurocritical care is a matter of debate, and the organization of facts and conjectures about it must be somewhat arbitrary. Intensive care for neurosurgical patients dates back to the work of Walter Dandy at the Johns Hopkins Hospital in the 1930s; many consider his creation of a special unit for their postoperative care to be the first real ICU. The genesis of neurocritical care begins in prehistory, however. This article gives a predominantly North American history, with some brief forays into the rest of the world community of neurointensivists.

EARLY ROOTS

Although scholars generally agree that trephination constitutes the earliest known surgical procedure, we can only speculate on the reasons for which it was performed. The archeologic record suggests that about 80% of patients subjected to this procedure survived sufficiently long for the bone to heal, suggesting a substantial degree of operative and postoperative skill (**Fig. 1**). The Edwin Smith Surgical Papyrus,[1] from approximately 3700 years ago (and believed to be a copy of a 5000-year-old manuscript dating to the Old Kingdom of Egypt), describes many conditions that now fall under the rubric of neurocritical care, including head and spinal injuries, tetanus, and status epilepticus (SE). One of the 48 cases reviewed in the text (27 of the cases are neurologic diseases or injury) describes a gaping head wound through which the surgeon can see the brain ("marrow of skull"). The papyrus also includes the earliest known descriptions of trismus ("the cord of his mandible is contracted") and nuchal rigidity in tetanus ("while he suffers with stiffness in his neck") (**Fig. 2**). Several Greek and Roman scholars also wrote about these topics, including Hippocrates and Galen. The principles elucidated by Hippocrates for the management of head injury dictated

Departments of Neurological Sciences, Neurosurgery, Medicine, and Anesthesiology, Rush Medical College, 600 S. Paulina Street, 544AF, Chicago, IL 60612, USA
E-mail address: tbleck@gmail.com

Crit Care Clin 25 (2009) 153–164
doi:10.1016/j.ccc.2008.12.004
0749-0704/08/$ – see front matter © 2009 Elsevier Inc. All rights reserved.
criticalcare.theclinics.com

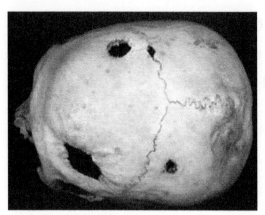

Fig. 1. Healing trephination injury in adult male. (Copyright © San Diego Museum of Man; used with permission.)

care for the next two centuries.[2] Aretaeus of Cappadocia also evinced an interest in these conditions, and noted that in tetanus, "for the most part, the patients die, for 'spasm from a wound is fatal.'"[3] One can find many subsequent descriptions of and suggestions for management of the conditions we now view as part of neurocritical care, but the unbroken intellectual string leading to the present day begins in the sixteenth century.

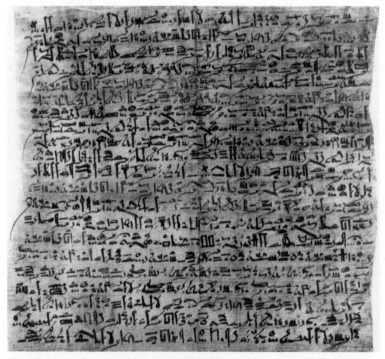

Fig. 2. The Edwin Smith surgical papyrus. This section of the papyrus displays the earliest known descriptions of trismus ("the cord of his mandible is contracted") and nuchal rigidity in tetanus ("while he suffers with stiffness in his neck").

CARDIOPULMONARY CEREBRAL RESUSCITATION

The history of cardiopulmonary resuscitation is discussed in the article by Weil and colleagues, elsewhere in this issue; however, because this is such an important thread in the development of neurocritical care a few comments here are necessary. In addition, the development of methods for mechanical ventilation is independently important in the management of neurogenic respiratory failure.[4]

The first published attempt to resuscitate a dead patient, with the implicit hope that the brain would recover, can be attributed to Paracelsus in 1530. Unfortunately, he was unsuccessful. The first technical step forward occurred 13 years later, when Vesalius described a method for the artificial ventilation of animals. In the next century, Harvey and Hooke established that respiration and cardiac contraction were independent. Another 250 years elapsed until external cardiac compression was added to resuscitation attempts, however. Throughout much of the twentieth century, the notion that the brain could tolerate only 3 minutes of cardiac arrest was firmly established. Isolated cases of recovery, often involving cold fresh water drowning of small children, led to the concept that recovery after longer periods of anoxia might be possible. Induced cardiac arrest using high-dose barbiturates and hypothermia allowed surgery on congenital heart defects. This finding prompted Peter Safar and his colleagues[5] to attempt several brain resuscitation trials using barbiturates and calcium antagonists. The failure of these trials somewhat dampened enthusiasm for this approach until the emergence of induced hypothermia for coma after cardiac arrest.

Jackson,[6] in 1746, discussed the use of a pipe in the airway for artificial respiration. He proposed the possibility that "it may be necessary to make an opening in to the wind-pipe for this purpose." Joseph Black discovered carbon dioxide in 1754, and Joseph Priestley discovered oxygen in 1774. Chaussier developed a device to deliver oxygen to humans in 1780, which closely resembles the bag-valve-mask systems we currently use (but without the valve; see later discussion). Concerns about the possible adverse consequences of positive pressure ventilation and excessive oxygen administration began shortly thereafter, and continue to this day.

Negative pressure ventilation began with the first tank respirator, invented in 1832 by Dalziel. Forty years later, Hauke reintroduced tank respirators. In 1880, Waldenburg invented the cuirass respirator, which covers only the thorax instead of the entire body below the neck.

For uncertain reasons, interest in negative pressure ventilators waned until 1918. The upsurge in poliomyelitis cases, with their attendant respiratory failure, sparked new interest in the technique. Stewart and Rogoff improved on the original tank concept in 1918, and in 1929 Drinker and McKhann described further refinements. Although seldom used today, the Drinker "iron lung" remains a technical achievement that saved uncounted lives.

Sometimes negative pressure ventilation was taken to extremes. In 1904, Sauerbruch published a description of an operating room in which everything (including the staff) was kept at varying subatmospheric pressures except the patient's head.

Long-term positive pressure ventilation required airway access, which meant a tracheostomy until the development of direct laryngoscopy by Kirstein in 1895. The subsequent use of cuffed endotracheal tubes allowed the more common use of mechanical ventilators. In the polio epidemics of the 1950s, medical students and family members using a bag system based on that used to deliver anesthetic gases in the operating room often ventilated Scandinavian patients for weeks. The valve that later converted these cumbersome systems to the Ambu-type bag-valve device was developed during World War II for use in high-altitude planes.

Bowditch invented the first automatic mechanical ventilator in 1879, although several of his contemporaries made significant contributions. The first commercial mechanical ventilator was introduced by the Bennett Corporation in 1948.

POLIOMYELITIS DEFINES NEUROCRITICAL CARE

The ability to keep patients who had polio breathing with any of these mechanical ventilatory systems was a tremendous achievement. Placing a patient in an iron lung was only the beginning of an often harrowing experience for the patient and the physician, however. The maintenance of a patent airway in nonintubated patients who cannot cough effectively and who may have lower cranial nerve dysfunction is a difficult task even in modern critical care units. Imagine the situation in the absence of fiberoptic bronchoscopy, dedicated respiratory therapists, and transcutaneous oxygen saturation monitors.

Many neurologists became the primary, if not sole, caregivers for these patients. Rigid bronchoscopy was sometimes required to clear secretions, and in several centers was a standard part of the neurologist's armamentarium. A few neurologists even operated on their patients when necessary procedures (eg, tracheostomies, appendectomies) were declined by surgeons (thankfully a rare event).

The internal medicine subspecialty of infectious disease was emerging during this same period, and the practitioners of this new area sometimes battled with neurologists regarding who should care for these patients. Some of these disagreements between giants, as between A. B. Baker and Louis Weinstein, are the stuff of legend. Although such "turf issues" seem pointless in retrospect, the territorial nature of physicians has not changed dramatically in the ensuing 40 years.

Salk's[7] development of a poliomyelitis vaccine in the early 1950s should have led to the elimination of this scourge from the face of the earth, but the disruptions in public health and medical care inherent in war and extreme poverty have thus far prevented this.

OTHER FORMS OF NEUROGENIC RESPIRATORY FAILURE

Tetanus was known as a horrible, fatal disorder since ancient times, and before modern critical care respiratory failure was a major cause of death. The earliest known authors (from about 3500 BC) advised against any treatment for patients who had tetanus. Galen noted that cutting a nerve would stop the movement of an affected limb, but that this produced paralysis. In 1829, Ceroli recommended morphine, which is still an important treatment of autonomic dysfunction in tetanus. Hutchinson and Hughlings Jackson successfully used ether at Queen Square in 1861. Claude Bernard's experimental work with curare led to its use in human cases in several countries in the mid to late nineteenth century. Melzter and Auer introduced intrathecal injection of magnesium compounds in 1906 to deal with the accentuated reflex activity of tetanus patients. This technique was still in vogue in 1925; in Tice's *Practice of Medicine*, Bartley discussed the technique of injection. He also recommended saline lavage of the subarachnoid space should respiratory paralysis ensue, and a subcutaneous injection of calcium chloride to antagonize the magnesium effect.

The development of long-term mechanical ventilation for poliomyelitis finally made effective tetanus therapy possible under conditions of neuromuscular blockade. The introduction of benzodiazepines in the 1950s, with recognition of their effect on reflex muscle contraction, promptly led to their emergence as the treatment of choice for the motor manifestations of tetanus. The mixed α/β adrenergic blocker labetalol subsequently gained acceptance as a therapy for the autonomic effects of the disease, which have become the main cause of death in tetanus.

Nicolaier[8] isolated tetanus toxin from cultures derived from soil in 1884, and Behring and Kitasato[9] proved the value of tetanus toxoid in preventing the disease in 1890. Tetanus should thus have been eliminated from the pantheon of human suffering long ago.

Scholars have not unearthed clear descriptions of the other clostridial toxin disease, botulism, in classical or medieval writings; the first report dates from 1793. The term botulism derives from the Latin word *botulus*, or sausage; blood sausage was implicated in the initial report. Outbreaks of poisoning related to sausages and other prepared foods occurred in Europe in the nineteenth century. The German physician Kerner recognized the connection between sausage and the paralytic illnesses of 230 patients in 1820, and made sausage poisoning a reportable disease. Concurrently, Russian physicians recognized a disease with similar symptoms, which they labeled fish poisoning. In 1897, van Ermengen published the first description of *Clostridium botulinum*, and showed that the organism elaborated a toxin that could induce weakness in animals. This toxin was subsequently shown to be type A toxin; type B was discovered in 1904. Wound botulism was described in 1943, and infant botulism in 1976. The occurrence of sporadic cases without an apparent cause, many related to gastrointestinal colonization, was first reported in 1986. Type A toxin was isolated and purified in 1946.

During World War I, Guillain, Barré, and Strohl[10] described the condition formally known as acute inflammatory demyelinating polyneuropathy that still bears their name. Subsequently, neurologists realized that Landry[11] had described this syndrome in 1859, but because Quincke had not yet invented the lumbar puncture needle, Landry was unable to describe the spinal fluid findings that help to distinguish the Guillain-Barré syndrome from poliomyelitis. Although Guillain stated that "his" syndrome rarely led to respiratory failure, others soon realized that this was not the case. Prolonged mechanical ventilation until recovery began was the only therapy for respiratory failure due to this condition until the 1978, when Brettle and colleagues[12] reported that a patient had improved following plasma exchange. Subsequent large randomized trials confirmed this effect, and later demonstrated that intravenous immunoglobulin therapy could also shorten the duration of mechanical ventilation and disability.[13]

Sir Thomas Willis[14] appears to have published the first description of myasthenia gravis in 1672. Early therapeutic efforts to improve airway protection and ventilatory muscle strength were limited to cholinesterase inhibitors, such as prostigmin, introduced in the 1930s, and more recently pyridostigmine. Thymectomy and corticosteroid treatments were used serendipitously. The recognition that anti-acetylcholine receptor antibodies were important in the pathogenesis of myasthenia led to treatment of myasthenic crises with plasma exchange or intravenous immunoglobulins. Surprisingly, we lack comparative trials of these modalities in this condition.

CRITICAL CARE EMERGES AS A DISCIPLINE FROM THE MANAGEMENT OF POLIOMYELITIS

With the decline in polio brought about by vaccination, the role of the neurologist in the care of seriously ill patients diminished. The first general ICU in the United States was founded in 1961 at the Baltimore City Hospital by Safar. His long-standing interests in brain protection and resuscitation make clear that the early generation of intensivists viewed neurologic function as a major part of their responsibility. Safar and his early colleagues (eg, Ake Grenvik) have maintained a keen interest in the nervous system.

As ICUs developed across the country, a few neurologists remained involved with the field. The University of Colorado was one of the early centers for critical care, under the guidance of the pulmonologist Thomas Petty. At that institution, Michael P. Earnest established a neurologic ICU in 1969.

David Jackson, a neurologist, ran a general adult critical care training program at Case Western Reserve in Cleveland in the 1970s. He also ran a critical care course at the annual meeting of the American Academy of Neurology from its inception until Allan Ropper assumed this mantle. Ropper (an internist and neurologist), Sean Kennedy (an anesthesiologist), and Nicholas Zervas (a neurosurgeon)[15] were the prime movers of the combined neurologic/neurosurgical ICU at the Massachusetts General Hospital. This group trained physicians of several disciplines as fellows. They collaborated to write the first textbook of neurocritical care, published in 1983.

Subsequently, neurocritical care units with training programs opened at Johns Hopkins (Daniel F. Hanley and Cecil Borel) and Columbia (Matthew Fink). All three of them are internists; Hanley and Fink are also neurologists, and Borel is an anesthesiologist. E. Clarke Haley and I started the unit at the University of Virginia in 1989; both of us are trained in internal medicine and neurology. In these early years, the path to neurocritical care usually involved dual residency training, which provided the neurologists with critical care experience that was not available to neurology residents at that time. In the following decade, several other programs with fellowships, and many other neuroscience ICUs have opened. These fellowships, now required to be at least 2 years in duration, train the fellows in general critical care with added emphasis on the nervous system.

In the mid-1980s, a group of neurologists interested in this field began to organize a section within the American Academy of Neurology. As befits a subspecialty based on cooperative efforts, many individuals (too numerous to detail herein) invested time and effort in this process. These efforts came to fruition in 1988, when the Academy's executive board approved a section of critical care and emergency neurology. Hanley was elected the inaugural chair of this section in 1989. The initial members of the section benefitted greatly from the experience of colleagues in Germany, especially Werner Hacke, chairman of neurology of the University of Heidelberg, and Karl Einhäupl, at that time in Munich and later the chairman of neurology at the Charité in Berlin.

During this same period, the disciplines of medical, surgical, and pediatric critical care grew tremendously. The practitioners of these fields are frequently the physicians responsible for the patients who have the most serious neurologic and neurosurgical conditions. The number of trained neurointensivists remains much too small to care for these patients, even as consultants. Recognizing that neurocritical care should remain integrated with other areas of critical care practice, the editor-in-chief of *Critical Care Medicine* made neurocritical care a permanent section of the journal in 1993, and named two neurointensivists as associate editors. In 1996, the Society of Critical Care Medicine established a neuroscience section to recognize the growing interest in the field and the increasing numbers of neurologists and neurosurgeons who are involved in critical care. Interested anesthesiologists have also been involved from the beginning, including Andrew Kofke and Donald Prough.

In 2002, a group of neurointensivists formed the Neurocritical Care Society for the purpose of furthering the field. This group held its first meeting in Phoenix AZ in February 2003. In 2008, the Neurocritical Care Society had nearly 1000 members from around the world.

The United Council on Neurologic Subspecialties, a body created by organized neurology in the United States to accredit and certify the smaller subspecialties in the field, gave its first examination in neurocritical care in 2007.

HEAD TRAUMA

As is unfortunately too often the case, advances in medicine are often the consequence of the concentration of large numbers of sick and wounded in wartime. During

World War I, Harvey Cushing (**Fig. 3**), who would become the most famous neurosurgeon of his time and who described the eponymous "Cushing [blood pressure] response," realized that 60% of deaths due to penetrating head wounds were due to infection. He introduced the concept of rapid débridement, which lowered the head trauma mortality rate from 54% early in the war to 29% at its end. Care for British patients who had head injuries during World War II was spearheaded by one of Cushing's residents, Hugh Cairns, who established mobile head injury units for the army. Each was staffed by a neurosurgeon, a neurologist, and an anesthesiologist, presaging the medical staffing of neurocritical care units in the future. These units were among the first to receive and use the new drug penicillin.

At the start of the Korean conflict, Cushing's lessons had been forgotten, and delays in débridement of penetrating head injuries initially led to a high infection rate. This rate decreased from 41% to 1% as early management improved.

In 1958, MacIver and colleagues[16] introduced a standardized management protocol consisting of early tracheostomy, drugs to reduce spasticity, and fever control. The next major advance was the introduction of CT scanning in 1973, which "did away with amateur angiograms in the middle of the night and ended the woodpecker surgery of exploratory burr holes for patients suspected of harboring a life-threatening hematoma."[17]

INTRACRANIAL PRESSURE MANAGEMENT

Intracranial shifts were recognized in the nineteenth century by Hutchinson and MacEwen, who believed that they were responsible for third cranial nerve palsies. Cushing[18] attempted to relieve these shifts by decompressing the temporal lobe, which he reported in 1908. Through clinical observation and experimental work, he realized that the tentorium formed a baffle against which the cranial contents could be compressed. In 1918 he attempted to relieve this problem with a tentorial incision, but this was not successful. Temple Fay[19] and others in Philadelphia introduced hypertonic saline to reduce intracranial volume in 1921, and reported on its use in

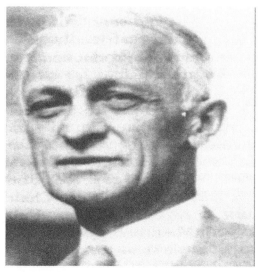

Fig. 3. Photographic portrait of Harvey Cushing (1869–1939).

head trauma in 1935.[20] Sedzimir and colleagues[21] reported on hypothermia beginning in 1955. Furness[22] reported on hyperventilation in 1957.

Until 1960, intracranial pressure could only be inferred from the pressure in the thecal sac. In that year, Lundberg[23] published his first article on intraventricular pressure measurement by a catheter, which also allowed the withdrawal of cerebrospinal fluid to manage elevated pressure. The treatment of metastatic brain tumors with steroids began in 1957.[24] Galicich, French, and Melby[25] studied the effect of dexamethasone on primary brain tumors beginning in 1961.

Decompressive craniectomy for acute head trauma was reported separately by Ransohoff and colleagues (lateral approach)[26] and Kjellberg and Prieto (bifrontal approach)[27] in 1971. Shapiro and colleagues[28] described the use of high-dose barbiturates in 1973.

Unfortunately, there have been no conceptual advances in intracranial pressure control since then. The management of cerebral perfusion pressure and brain oxygen tension has moved to the forefront.

COMA AND DEATH BY NEUROLOGIC CRITERIA

The analysis of the comatose patient, as promulgated in the classic texts of Plum and Posner,[29] is the pathway through which many neurology students are introduced to the notion of neurocritical care. Currently in its fourth edition,[30] this 400-page text is an encyclopedic approach to the analysis of acutely altered states of consciousness. Although there are many other seminal publications, this one has truly become the bible in this area. In classic neurologic style, the text presents many qualitative descriptors that may be used to summarize the examination of the comatose patient. Plum was also interested in more quantitative measures, and consulted with Teasdale and Jennett[31] on the development of the Glasgow coma scale score.

Many investigators before the 1960s concerned themselves with attempts to determine whether a comatose patient might recover, or progress to death as it was understood at the time, based on absence of spontaneous respiration, heart tones, and palpable pulses. As cardiopulmonary resuscitation techniques improved and became widespread, a small number of patients were left in an apparently permanent state of unconsciousness, without respiratory drive but with intact cardiovascular function. This state had been described in 1959 by Mollaret and Goulon[32] in the French journal *Revue Neurologique*, but was not well known in English-speaking countries. Although this was at first a predominantly academic exercise, the growth of cadaveric organ transplantation made necessary explicit criteria for determining that brain function was permanently lost.

Unfortunately, this state became known as "brain death."[33] More recently, there have been attempts to recast this notion as one in which death is defined as irreversible loss of brain (including brainstem) function, regardless of whether its cause was primarily intracranial or was a consequence of loss of cerebral perfusion on a cardiac basis. In this concept, all death is brain death, and the adjective becomes meaningless. Others have argued that death of the brain is too difficult to define or prove, and prefer the term "irreversible apneic coma." The procedures used to prove either of these terms are the same.

In 1968, a group at Harvard tried to establish criteria for the definition of brain death.[34] This report set the stage for all future work in this field. Although many of their criteria are similar to those in use today, they included some items that are no longer accepted (eg, the loss of all reflexes, including those of spinal origin). They also proposed an inadequate challenge of respiratory drive (3 minutes without mechanical ventilatory support if starting from a normal $Paco_2$). Many subsequent studies and committees have wrestled with the issues of definition, culminating in a large United States collaborative trial published in 1977.[35,36] In this study, 503 patients who were comatose and whose bodies survived 15 minutes of apnea were followed until death. The investigators reached the conclusion that the bodies of patients who reached their criteria for cerebral death would undergo death by cardiopulmonary criteria within 72 hours even if maximal supportive measures were continued. It is now clear that a small number of patients' bodies supported with mechanical ventilation and enteral feeding have been maintained for years.[37]

The current standards in the United States are those of the American Academy of Neurology's quality standards subcommittee.[38] Compliance with these guidelines is variable, however.[39]

ACUTE STROKE MANAGEMENT

Neurointensivists are closely associated with their colleagues in vascular neurology, vascular neurosurgery, and neuroradiology in the care of patients who have acute cerebrovascular disorders. In many neurocritical care units, most patients have subarachnoid hemorrhage, intracerebral hemorrhage, large ischemic strokes either requiring mechanical ventilation or management of intracranial hypertension, or a vascular disorder threatening to cause one of these. As with the rest of neurocritical care practice, an excellent collaborative relationship among these specialties is vital.

STATUS EPILEPTICUS

SE was noted in ancient times, with the earliest known description appearing on a cuneiform tablet (**Fig. 4**).[40] Until relatively recently in medical history, seizure activity

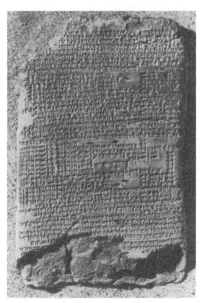

Fig. 4. First description of SE. The 25th and 26th tablets of the Sakikku cuneiform (pre-Babylonian Akkadian text) dating from 718–612 BC. (*Courtesy of* E.H. Reynolds, MD, FRCP, FRCPsych, London, UK; and J.K. Wilson, Cambridge, UK.)

was believed to be supernatural in origin (demonic possession, lunar influences, and so forth). Over the last several hundred years, various medical theories regarding its origins have been proposed. As described by Eadie,[41] hypotheses concerning the pathogenesis of epilepsy and seizures "have ranged from excess phlegm in the ventricles of the brain, through boiling up of the 'vital spirits' in the brain (Paracelsus), explosion of 'animal spirits' in the center of the brain (Willis), heightened reflex activity at a spinal (Marshall Hall) or medullary level (brown-Sequard), to Hughlings Jackson's (1870) notion of 'an occasional, an excessive, and a disorderly discharge' in part of the cerebral cortex."

Seizures are a common complication in all areas of critical care, but SE constitutes an emergency in its own right. Attempts at treating SE in the nineteenth century included bromide,[42] morphine,[43] and ice applications. Barbiturates were introduced in 1912, followed by the identification and use of phenytoin in the 1937;[44] these were the first rational treatments for SE. Paraldehyde gained brief prominence in the next decades.[45] The most recent major improvement is the use of benzodiazepines, pioneered by the French in the 1960s.[46] The Veterans Affairs Cooperative Trial constitutes the landmark clinical study in this area, and confirms the value of lorazepam as the first agent for the treatment of status.[47] Once the initial treatment with a conventional anticonvulsant has failed, SE should be considered refractory and a high-dose midazolam or another general anesthetic regimen used.[48]

ACKNOWLEDGMENTS

In many ways, I have been collecting background material for this presentation throughout my career, and have incorporated the reminiscences and ideas of so many individuals that I cannot thank them all here. A few stand out in terms of their insight, however, and I must mention some of them. Joseph Foley shared many observations and anecdotes during my visit to Case years ago; this conversation convinced me to begin recording this (still fragmentary) history. Several other individuals contributed their observations about neurology during the polio years, including Maynard Cohen and the late Frank Morrell. Ake Grenvik has an encyclopedic memory of everything about critical care, and kindly reflected on some of these issues for my benefit. Stephen Streat is a valued friend and debating adversary. Many of the contemporary neurologists mentioned in the text have also shared their stories.

REFERENCES

1. Breasted JH. The Edwin Smith surgical papyrus, published in facsimile and hieroglyphic transliteration with translation and commentary. Chicago: The University of Chicago Press, 1930.
2. Liu CY, Apuzzo ML. The genesis of neurosurgery and the evolution of the neurosurgical operative environment: part I—prehistory to 2003. Neurosurgery 2003; 52:3–19.
3. Adams F. The extant works of Aretaeus, the Cappadocian. London: Publications of the Sydenham Society; 1856.
4. Colice FL. Historical perspective on the development of mechanical ventilation. In: Tobin MJ, editor. Principles and practice of mechanical ventilation. New York: McGraw-Hill; 1994. p. 1–35.
5. Smith TL, Bleck TP. Hypothermia and neurologic outcome in patients following cardiac arrest: should we be hot to cool off our patients? Crit Care 2002;6: 377–80.
6. Baker AB. Artificial respiration, the history of an idea. Med Hist 1971;15:336–51.

7. Salk JE. Studies in human subjects on active immunization against poliomyelitis. I. A preliminary report of experiments in progress. JAMA 1953;151:1081–9.
8. Nicolaier A. Üeber infectiösen tetanus. Dtsch Med Wochenschr 1884;10:842–4 [German].
9. Behring E, Kitasato S. Üeber das zustandekommen der diphtherie-immunität und der tetanus-immunität bei thieren. Dtsch Med Wochenschr 1890;16:1113–4 [German].
10. Guillain G, Barre JA, Strohl A. Sur un syndrome de radiculo-névrite avec hyper-albuminose du liquide céphalorachidien sans reaction cellulaire. Remarques sur les caractères cliniques et graphiques des reflexes tenineux. Bull Mem Soc Med Hop Paris 1916;40:1462–70 [French].
11. Landry O. Note sur la paralysie ascendante aigue. Gazette Hebdomadaire de Médicin 1859;6:472–4 486–8 [French].
12. Brettle RP, Gross M, Legs NJ, et al. Treatment of acute polyneuropathy by plasma exchange. Lancet 1978;ii:1100.
13. Plasma Exchange/Sandoglobulin Guillain-Barré Syndrome Trial Group. Randomised trial of plasma exchange, intravenous immunoglobulin, and combined treatments in Guillain-Barré syndrome. Lancet 1997;349:225–30.
14. Willis T. De anima brutorum quae hominis vitalis ac sensitiva est, exercitationes duae. Amstelodami: Apud Joannem Blaeu; 1672 [Latin].
15. Ropper AH, Kennedy SF, Zervas NT. Neurological and neurosurgical intensive care. Baltimore (MD): University Park Press; 1983.
16. MacIver IN, Frew IJ, Matheson JG. The role of respiratory insufficiency in the mortality of severe head injuries. Lancet 1958;i:390–3.
17. Jennett B, Galbraith S, Teasdale GM, et al. EMI scan and head injuries. Lancet 1976;i:1026.
18. Cushing H. Subtemporal decompressive operations for the intracranial complications associated with bursting fractures of the skull. Ann Surg 1909;50: 1002–17.
19. Fay T. Administration of hypertonic salt solution for relief of intracranial pressure. JAMA 1923;80:1445–8.
20. Fay T. The treatment of acute and chronic cases of cerebral trauma, by means of dehydration. Ann Surg 1935;101:76–132.
21. Sedzimir CB, Jacobs D, Dundee JW. Induced hypothermia as a therapeutic measure in neurology; a clinical study of a hopeless case. Br J Anaesth 1955; 27:93–100.
22. Furness DN. Controlled respiration in neurosurgery. Br J Anaesth 1957;29:415–8.
23. Lundberg N. Continuous recording and control of ventricular fluid pressure in neurosurgical practice. Acta Psychiatr Scand Suppl 1960;36:1–193.
24. Kofman S, Garvin JS, Taylor SG 3rd. Treatment of cerebral metastases from breast carcinoma with presdnisolone. JAMA 1957;163:1473–6.
25. Galicich JH, French LA. Use of dexamethasone in the treatment of cerebral edema resulting from brain tumors and brain surgery. Am Pract Dig Treat 1961; 12:169–74.
26. Ransohoff J, Benjamin MV, Gage EL Jr, et al. Hemicraniectomy in the management of acute subdural hematoma. J Neurosurg 1971;34:70–6.
27. Kjellberg RN, Prieto A Jr. Bifrontal decompressive craniotomy for massive cerebral edema. J Neurosurg 1971;34:488–93.
28. Shapiro HM, Galindo A, Wyte SR, et al. Rapid intraoperative reduction of intracranial pressure with thiopentone. Br J Anaesth 1973;45:1057–62.
29. Plum F, Posner JB. The diagnosis of stupor and coma. Philadelphia: F.A. Davis Company; 1966.

30. Posner JB, Saper CB, Schiff N, et al. Plum and Posner's diagnosis of stupor and coma. Oxford: Oxford University Press; 2007.
31. Teasdale G, Jennett B. Assessment of coma and impaired consciousness. A practical scale. Lancet 1974;ii:81–4.
32. Mollaret P, Goulon M. Le coma dépassé (mémoire préliminaire). Revue Neurol (Paris) 1959;101:3–15 [French].
33. Wijdicks EF. Brain death worldwide: accepted fact but no global consensus in diagnostic criteria. Neurology 2002;58:20–5.
34. A definition of irreversible coma. Report of the Ad Hoc Committee of the Harvard Medical School to Examine the Definition of Brain Death. JAMA 1968;205:337–40.
35. An appraisal of the criteria of cerebral death. A summary statement. A collaborative study. JAMA 1977;237:982–6.
36. Bennett DR, Hughes JR, Korein J, et al. Atlas of electroencephalography in coma and cerebral death. New York: Raven Press; 1976.
37. Shewmon DA. Chronic "brain death": meta-analysis and conceptual consequences. Neurology 1998;51:1538–45.
38. Practice parameters for determining brain death in adults (summary statement). The Quality Standards Subcommittee of the American Academy of Neurology. Neurology 1995;45:1012–4.
39. Greer DM, Varelas PN, Haque S, et al. Variability of brain death determination guidelines in leading US neurologic institutions. Neurology 2008;70:284–9.
40. Shorvon SD. Status epilepticus: its clinical features and treatment in children and adults. Cambridge (UK): Cambridge University Press; 1994.
41. Eadie MJ. Epilepsy—from the Sakikku to Hughlings Jackson. J Clin Neurosci 1995;2:156–62.
42. Wilks S. Bromide and iodide of potassium in epilepsy. Med Times and Gaz (Lond) 1861;2:635–6.
43. Gowers WR. Epilepsy and other chronic convulsive diseases: their causes, symptoms, and treatment. London: J and A Chirchill; 1881.
44. Bleck TP, Klawans HL. Mechanisms of epilepsy and anticonvulsant action. In: Klawans HL, Goetz CG, Tanner CM, editors. Textbook of clinical neuropharmacology. New York: Raven Press; 1992. p. 23–30.
45. Weschler IS. Intravenous injection of paraldehyde for control of convulsions. JAMA 1940;114:2198.
46. Gastaut H, Naquet R, Poiré R, et al. Treatment of status epilepticus with diazepam (Valium). Epilepsia 1965;6:167–82.
47. Treiman DM, Meyers PD, Walton NY, et al. A comparison of four treatments for generalized convulsive status epilepticus. Veterans Affairs Status Epilepticus Cooperative Study Group. N Engl J Med 1998;339:792–8.
48. Bleck TP. Critical care of the patient in status epilepticus. In: Wasterlain C, Treiman D, editors. Status epilepticus. Boston: MIT Press; 2006. p. 607–13.

History of Solid Organ Transplantation and Organ Donation

Peter K. Linden, MD

KEYWORDS

- Organ transplantation • Kidney transplantation
- Lung transplantation • Liver transplantation
- Heart transplantation • Cyclosporine • Tacrolimus
- Immunosuppression • Organ donation • Organ allocation

Solid organ transplantation is one of the most remarkable and dramatic therapeutic advances in medicine during the past 60 years. This field has progressed initially from what can accurately be termed a "clinical experiment" to routine and reliable practice, which has proven to be clinically effective, life-saving and cost-effective when compared with nontransplantation management strategies of both chronic and acute end stage organ failures.[1–3] This remarkable evolution stems from a serial confluence of: cultural acceptance; legal and political evolution to facilitate organ donation, procurement and allocation; technical and cognitive advances in organ preservation, surgery, immunology, immunosuppression; and management of infectious diseases. The history of organ transplantation has also been laced with pure serendipitous discovery, tragic accidents, unfulfilled promise, abandoned paths, and incidents or practices that have produced legal or ethical quandaries; these features all combine to make the field a dynamic work-in-progress. Some of the major milestones of this multidisciplinary clinical science are reviewed in this chapter.

ANCIENT HISTORY OF ORGAN TRANSPLANTATION

Humankind has always shown an interest in the removal of tissue from one site and placement to another site in the same person or different person as cosmetic, restorative or therapeutic procedures. Although not connected to the premodern or modern era of organ transplantation, intriguing descriptions exist in mythologic, religious, and historical literature including archaeological records that allude to the concept of tissue transplantation as far back as several millennia ago.[4] Hindu text from 2500–3000 BC provide detailed descriptions of using skin grafts crudely cut and molded from a patient's own buttock or chin for reconstruction of noses mutilated

University of Pittsburgh Medical Center, Department of Critical Care Medicine, Scaife Hall Room 602A, 3550 Terrace Street, PA 15261, USA
E-mail address: lindenpk@ccm.upmc.edu

Crit Care Clin 25 (2009) 165–184
doi:10.1016/j.ccc.2008.12.001
0749-0704/08/$ – see front matter © 2009 Elsevier Inc. All rights reserved.

by punishment for crimes committed.[5] Greek mythology alludes to gods, heroes and heraldic beasts with chimeric anatomy and abilities such as Chimera beasts. The Chinese physician, Pien Chiao, reportedly exchanged hearts between a man of strong spirit but weak will and a man of weak spirit but strong will to achieve a balance in each man. The New Testament of the Bible describes several instances that, in principal, would be defined as autotransplantation today. Jesus of Nazareth restored a servant's ear that had been severed in battle by Simon Peter's sword; Saint Peter reimplanted the breasts of Saint Agatha who was injured by torture; and Saint Mark reimplanted a battle-amputated hand of a soldier. In Jacopoda Varagine's *Leggenda Aura* (348 AD), the "miracle of the black leg" describes the replacement of the gangrenous leg of the Roman deacon Justinian with the leg of a dead Ethiopian man.[6]

Evidence for autotransplantation or allotransplantation of nonvisceral tissues, such as bone, teeth and skin, have been described as far back as the prehistoric Bronze Age. Temporarily removing bone segments from the skull to relieve brain swelling, a process called "trephination", is revealed in archaeological records from that period.[7]

Transplantation of teeth from one person to another is described over a broad range of history including ancient Egypt, Greece and Rome, during the Ottoman empire, and during the sixteenth to eighteenth centuries in France, Scotland and other western European sites. For example, the Dutchman Job van Meeneren successfully grafted bone from the skull of a dog to repair a skull defect in a human patient in 1668.

Such descriptions, although providing evidence of human inquisitiveness and resourcefulness toward improving the contemporary human condition, bear no literal relationship to the yet-to-emerge modern sciences that formed the actual knowledge and technical frameworks from which modern organ transplantation evolved.

PREMODERN ERA: 1900–1959

By the early twentieth century, successful transplantation of nonvisceral tissues such as human skin and cornea had already been reported.[8,9] The most important developments in this period include: experimentation with organ transplantation in animal models; attempted but failed kidney transplantation in humans; and observational but seminal discoveries pertaining to the timing, clinical manifestations, and immunologic mechanisms of allograft rejection in immunosuppressive-naïve recipients. Rapid advances in experimental and clinical surgical skills, including vascular anastomotic methods from the late nineteenth century into the early twentieth century, forged a knowledge and technical skill base upon which experimental visceral organ transplantation, principally kidney, could be performed in animals. The french surgeon Alexis Carrel perfected vascular anastomotic suturing methods, vessel reconstruction, and cold preservation. He also successfully performed kidney reimplantation in the neck of the same dog and a few years later between dogs; he won the Nobel Laureate Prize in 1912 while at the Rockefeller Institute for Medical Research.[10,11]

Despite technical surgical success, Carrel's consistent and sobering observation was that a hostile host response to the foreign allograft was the major residual impediment to successful animal and human organ transplantation:[4]

"Should an organ, extirpated from an animal and replanted into its owner by a certain technique, continue to functionate normally, and should it cease to functionate normally when transplanted into another animal by the same technique, the physiologic disturbance could not be considered as brought about by the organ but would be due to the influence of the host, that is, the biological factors."

This did not prevent several disastrous attempts at xenotransplantation (rabbit, pig, and macaque kidney) by French (M. Princeteau and Mathieu Jaboulay) and German (Ernst Unger) surgeons between 1905 and 1909.

Advances in transplantation knowledge and experimentation were initially slowed by World War I and the Great Depression. The field was re-invigorated with the increased need for skin allografting for severe burns and other battle injuries. Success, though, continued to be limited by rejection. Peter Medawar, a British surgeon who was assigned to investigate the mechanisms of skin allograft rejection, showed that serial full-thickness skin allografts in cattle were rejected more vigorously. He also found that skin grafts between monozygotic twins (fraternal) promptly thrived and were tolerated; this finding supported the concept that allograft rejection was an immunologic phenomenon with the classic immune properties of sensitization, memory and tolerance, all concepts which have stood to the present day.[12,13] These findings, coupled with subsequent experiments in rabbits that demonstrated that allograft rejection was modified with the administration of corticosteroids harnessed from the adrenal glands, formed the rationale for ultimately targeting the host immune system of allograft recipients.[14]

While discoveries in immunologic mechanisms of allograft rejection and innovations in technical aspects of surgery were being made, there were several precocious attempts at human kidney transplantation. In 1936, Voronoy, a Russian surgeon, performed a kidney transplantation from a blood type B cadaveric donor who had expired 6 hours previously to a uremic O blood type recipient.[15] The patient survived only 2 days and the kidney failed to produce any urine. Sixteen years later Kuss and Dubost, in Paris, harvested kidneys from convicts executed by guillotine.[16,17] The subsequent transplantations were technical surgical successes but still culminated in immunologic-mediated allograft failure and recipient deaths. A living, related mother-to-son kidney transplantation also performed in France with extraperitoneal placement of the donor kidney functioned for 3 weeks before the patient succumbed to rejection.[18]

From 1951–1952, Hume and colleagues conducted a series of nine kidney transplantations at Peter Bent Brigham Hospital in Boston, Massachusetts.[19]

In the first case, the graft was implanted in the recipient renal fossa, and in the next eight, the graft was implanted in the anterior thigh with urine draining via a constructed uretero-cutaneous drain. Although several patients received cortisone, all allografts were rapidly rejected. An earlier temporary transplantation effort in a young woman with renal failure following obstetric complications by the same surgeons was reported by Joseph Murray to have occurred as early as 1945.

In 1954, a seminal report by Dr. Joseph Murray and Dr. John Merrill at The Peter Bent Brigham Hospital, documented the successful transplantation of a kidney between living identical twin brothers (Ronald and Richard Herrick). The recipient, Richard, had been supported on an artificial kidney machine invented in Holland and modified at the Peter Bent Brigham Hospital (ie, Kolff-Brigham machine).[20,21] The procedure was both a surgical and immunologic success as the recipient survived 8 years with intact renal allograft function and no evidence of rejection before succumbing to cardiovascular disease. For his work, Joseph Murray won the 1990 Nobel Prize in Medicine (shared with E. Donnell Thomas for the first successful bone marrow transplantation). The same surgical team performed a similar operation between a female twin pair in 1956 with the recipient (Edith Helm) surviving into the 1990s.

The unprecedented allograft survival achieved in these particular cases compared with the dismal failures in the prior nonmatched pairs was no doubt secondary to the opportunistic genetic matching of the donor and recipient without the aid of iatrogenic immunosuppression. Clearly, for the field to advance to a modern era and serve the genetically diverse general population needing organ transplantation, the development and refinement of immunosuppression, tissue typing and matching, and cadaveric organ harvesting and preservation would be needed.

EARLY IMMUNOSUPPRESSIVE ERA OF TRANSPLANTATION: 1960–1979
Application and Advances in Immunosuppression

Iatrogenic suppression of the recipient's immune system was the keystone to breaking the genetic compatibility barrier. At the Boston program in the late 1950s, conditioning recipients with sublethal total body irradiation was used in a series of ten kidney transplantations with nonidentical genetic lines.[22,23] Nine of ten patients expired within a month; however, the cause of death was not due to allograft failure but rather to the effects of radiation. However, one dizygotic (fraternal) twin recipient survived 20 years with intact renal function and this experience was also duplicated in Paris in another fraternal twin pair by Hamburger during the same year.[24,25]

It was becoming progressively apparent that cytoablative radiation was too blunt an immunosuppressive instrument, but it served as a "proof-of-concept" to the scientific transplantation community that a more refined and titratable modality, such as pharmacologic immunosuppression, posed an alternative possible pathway to success and safety. Fortuitously, collateral development of several antileukemia agents, including cyclophosphamide, methotrexate, 6-mercaptopurine and its analog azathioprine, was occurring during this time. Gertrude B. Elion and George H. Hitchings would share the 1988 Nobel Prize in Medicine for their contribution to the development of azothioprine in 1962. 6-mercaptopurine had already proved to delay skin graft rejection in rabbits and kidney graft rejection in dogs.[26,27] In 1960, the first renal transplantation managed with only pharmacologic immunosuppression (cyclophosphamide and methotrexate) was a female recipient of her mother's kidney.[28] Recovery of the recipient's bone marrow was accompanied by intermittent rejection managed with prednisone; however, the recipient expired after 143 days. In a series of ten kidney transplantations in the early 1960s that were immunosuppressed with either 6-mercaptopurine or azathioprine, there was only one 6-month survivor.[23,29] The resulting skepticism and pessimism about the efficacy of drug-induced myelosuppressive immunosuppression was short-lived. Landmark studies performed by Dr. Thomas Starzl in the early 1960s, while he was at the University of Colorado, showed that very high doses of prednisone (200 mg/d) added to azathioprine was able to reverse renal allograft rejection and induce host tolerance whereby the subsequent required immunosuppressive burden was diminished over time.[30]

The work of Thomas Starzl demonstrating the efficacy of a combination or "cocktail" immunosuppressive drug approach produced a frame-shift in organ transplantation on several fronts; it transformed kidney transplantation from a clinical experiment to an incipient clinical service using both cadaveric and live donors, led to a steady proliferation of transplantation centers of excellence in the United States and Europe, and opened the door for the first time to nonrenal organ transplantation including the liver, pancreas, heart and lungs, given the likely commonality of allograft rejection mechanisms across all organs. The development of rationed hemodialysis technology and vascular access led by Scribner during the 1960s also increased the potential pool of kidney transplant recipients by becoming the first "artificial bridge" to transplantation and, in the event of a failed allograft, as an alternative to death[31] Invariably, several sobering realities appeared during this immune barrier-breaking time period appeared. These focused on the secondary complications of immunosuppression, such as infection and malignancy, although paradoxically these issues only became apparent due to the longer patient survivals.[32–34]

In 1967, in a remarkable paper titled "Death After Transplantation", Starzl summarized the outcome of the first 125 organ recipients at the University of Colorado.[32] This patient group were immunosuppressed with a variable combination of irradiation, splenectomy, thymectomy, high-dose corticosteroids, and azathioprine. The first 60 deaths reported demonstrated a remarkably high rate of opportunistic bacterial, fungal, viral and protozoal infections, often multiple, and many of which were undetected and untreated ante-mortem. The dominant pathogen was cytomegalovirus as invasive disease was present in 30/60 (50%) of autopsies.

Because these findings were well before the development of many anti-infectives, preemptive and prophylaxis strategies, and sensitive monitoring methods, which were used in future decades, this report essentially portrayed the natural history of protracted corticosteroid-based immunosuppression in surgically complex patients. Opinion leaders in the more orthodox stream of medicine and surgery questioned the practicality and ethical grounds for organ transplantation.[35] This time period, as recalled by Starzl, reflected some of this opposing opinion: "As a consequence, transplantation acquired a renegade image, a burden soon compounded by difficulties in extending its reach to the replacement of vital organs other than the kidney."[1]

Nevertheless, further advances in immunosuppressive pharmacology, customized to solid organ transplantation needs, were taking place. In 1966, the development of polyclonal antilymphocyte globulin (ALG) was synthesized from the serum of horses inoculated with human leukocytes.[36] ALG supplanted the limited practice of thoracic duct drainage to achieve lymphocyte depletion and was used only in a minority of kidney and liver recipients as part of a "triple regimen" with steroids and azathioprine.

It was the class precursor of future soluble anti-lymphocyte and anti-thymocyte polyclonal and monoclonal preparations, which became valuable adjuncts for the management of refractory rejection and, at some centers, as immunosuppressive induction.

Liver Transplantation

Liver transplantation was developed only a few years after kidney transplantation. The first liver transplantation was attempted by Starzl at the University of Colorado in 1963, but it culminated in perioperative death of the patient because of overwhelming technical and hemorrhagic complications aggravated by severe portal hypertension and coagulopathy.[37] Between 1963 and 1967, liver transplantation was unsuccessfully attempted again in Colorado; Boston, Massachusetts; and Paris, France, resulting in intra- or early postoperative deaths and leading to a voluntary moratorium on further attempts. After resumption of efforts, the first one-year survivor of liver transplantation did not occur until 1967.[38] Initial attempts were unsuccessful because of a combination of technical difficulties and the unavailability of an effective means to prevent rejection. As increased experience was achieved, and with improvements in immunosuppression, prolonged liver recipient survivals were achieved. From 1963 to 1979, 170 patients underwent liver transplantation at the University of Colorado; 56 patients survived for one year, 25 for 13–22 years, and several remained alive with follow-ups of 17–31 years.[39] As with renal grafts, the long-term survival rate after liver transplantation remained poor (18%–30% one-year patient survival) until the advent of cyclosporine. Thomas Starzl also revived research efforts into xenotransplantation with a series of unsuccessful chimpanzee to human liver transplants between 1969 and 1973.

Other First Organ Transplantations

Other organ transplantation "firsts" during this era included: the first heart transplantation by Dr. Christian Barnard in Capetown, South Africa in a cardiomyopathic recipient who survived 18 days; a pancreas transplantation in 1968 at the University of Minnesota; an unsuccessful lung transplantation in 1963 by James B. Hardy in a prison inmate with chronic lung infection who survived 18 days; and a heart-lung transplantation in 1968 by Dr. Denton Cooley at Stanford, California in a 2-month-old infant with congenital heart disease who survived only 14 hours.[40–43] The first successful heart-lung transplantation in a patient with primary pulmonary hypertension is credited to Bruce Reitz of Stanford University, in California, in 1981. The patient, Mary Gohlke, lived 5 years and co-authored a book, "I'll Take Tomorrow" about her experience.[44] Despite the advances in drug-based immunosuppression and such pioneering first time transplantations, one-year graft survivals exceeding 50% were still not realized. However, an immunosuppressive agent that more accurately and effectively targeted the lymphocyte-based host response to the allogaft was just on the horizon.

THE CALCINEURIN ERA: CYCLOSPORINE AND FK-506 (1983–PRESENT)

The discovery of the immunomodulatory properties of cyclosporine by Swiss physician Jean Borel in 1977, its clinical investigational introduction in 1978, and its approval by the Food and Drug Administration as "Sandimmune" in 1983 were the most important immunosuppressive developments in organ transplantation.[45–47] This compound is a natural peptide product of the fungi *Cylindrocarpon lucidum* and *Trichderma polysporum*.[48] Its potent immunologic effects are directed toward both cell-mediated T-helper lymphocyte and lymphocyte-derived antibody synthesis but without the bone marrow suppressive effect of azathioprine or the broad immune nonlymphocyte collateral effects of steroids.[49]

The increases in graft and patient survival when cyclosporine was part of a multidrug immunosuppressive regimen across all categories of existing solid organ transplantation was nothing short of stunning in the 1980s when 1-year graft survival rates exceeded 89% in kidney transplantation recipients and 70% in heart and liver transplantation recipients (**Fig. 1**).[50–53] In 1983, Joel Cooper of the Toronto General Hospital performed the first successful single lung transplantation on Tom Hall who was suffering from pulmonary fibrosis.[54] The patient lived for 6 years before succumbing to renal failure. Dr. Cooper extended his success to the first double lung transplantation in 1986.[55]

Significant adverse events were still common, particularly during the early part of the cyclosporine-related learning curve; they included: neurotoxicity, nephrotoxicity, opportunistic infection, de novo diabetes, and B-cell lymphoma. These complications were only partially responsive to dose-reduction strategies.

A major technical advance in liver transplantation during this period was the implementation of venovenous bypass circuitry that rerouted blood after venous clamping of the cava and portal vein in extracorporeal circuit back to the axillary vein to decompress venous congestion created by the cross-clamp of the portal vein and inferior vena cava at the time of native liver hepatectomy.[56]

In the early 1990s, FK-506 (tacrolimus) was clinically investigated in human liver recipients with cyclosporine-refractory rejection.[57] Approximately 75% of such allografts were rescued with the conversion to FK-506.[58] The sequential increment in both graft and patient survival in liver transplantation with the introduction of the calcinreurin-inhibitors compared with the precalcineurin immunosuppressive era was impressive (see **Fig. 1**). Although many centers maintained some allegiance to

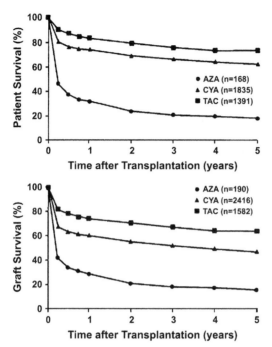

Fig. 1. Patient and liver allograft survival in the azathiporine, cyclosporine, and tacrolimus eras.

cyclosporine, the greater potency and equivalent safety of FK-506 compared to that of cyclosporine resulted in significant conversion to FK-506 based immunosuppression for liver, kidney, pancreas and thoracic organ transplantation.[59–62]

Intestinal transplantation, an endeavor that was abandoned in the 1970s, remained hampered by poor graft survival with cyclosporine. Many experts in the field at the time considered the bowel nontransplantable because of the high immunosuppressive burden required to suppress the host-response because of the bowel's high antigenic load and the converse problem of graft-versus-host disease. FK-506 provided a major boost to overcome the immunologic hurdle of intestinal and multivisceral transplantation in patients with short gut syndrome who were otherwise relegated to lifelong parenteral nutrition.[63–65] The first bowel transplantation occurred in conjunction with a liver transplantation at the London Health Sciences Center in 1988.

Novel immunosuppressive agents that also became available during this time, such as antilymphocyte drugs (OKT3 eg, Orthoclone, anti-thymocyte globulin eg, thymoglobulin), a new antiproliferative agent (mycophenolate mofetil), interleukin-2 receptor antagonists, and sirolimus, have increased the degrees of freedom for clinicians who may tailor a combination immunosuppressive regimen based upon the recipient's toxicity risks and degree of allograft tolerance.

Tissue Typing and Immunologic Methods

Transplantation across the major blood antigen groups had long been known to result in rapid humoral-mediated rejection and failure of the kidney or heart allograft caused by the presence of preformed isoagglutinins that attacked the vascular endothelial resulting in vasculopathic necrosis.[66,67] However, successful liver transplantation using a type O organ donor in a type A, B, or AB recipient can be performed—albeit with lower graft survival and hemolysis in the recipient. Successful liver transplantation had also been reported in the converse and more hostile antigen mismatch of an O recipient of a nonblood type O liver.[68,69]

Discoveries of the major histocompatibility complex (MHC) and the existence of human leukocyte antigens (HLA) occurred in the late 1950s. French physician Jean Dausset shared the 1980 Nobel Prize in Medicine for the description of the first known leukocyte antigen (now called HLA-A2) in 1958.[70] These key discoveries regarding immune function and graft rejection were not put into clinical use until the 1970s when a sensitive and rapid assay, the "HLA-crossmatch," that could detect the presence of preformed lymphocytotoxic HLA antibodies in the recipient that were destructive to the renal and nonrenal allograft was developed.[71,72] Such sensitized patients might be prospectively managed with a more aggressive immunosuppressive regimen or other antibody depleting interventions, such as plasmapheresis.

What unexpectedly became clear over time, however, was that—unlike bone marrow transplantation where perfect HLA compatibility was required for marrow engraftment—a single or multiple antigen disparity in HLA matching did not create an insurmountable hurdle for graft survival amongst all the major organ categories. Thus, HLA-matching would not become a significant prospective eliminating factor for allocating donor organs to the prospective organ recipient.[73]

ORGAN DONATION

A system for procuring large numbers of cadaveric donor organs was not a concern during the early years of clinical transplantation. As summarized above, a significant number of the earliest kidney donors were living donors because of the lack of refined immunosuppression and reliable preservation methods for the donated organ. Thus, the timing and process of procuring a suitable donor organ for transplantation was highly individualized in the earliest days of experimental organ transplantation. There is remarkably little information on the dynamics of identifying, consenting, and retrieval of the early cadaveric organs in the early clinical transplantation era in the 1960s.[1]

Important historical aspects within this realm include: earlier conceptions of death, modern and legal definitions of brain death and cardiac death, timing and techniques of organ procurement or harvesting, and organ preservation methods. The legislative landmarks that influenced the cadaveric organ donation process landscape are summarized in **Box 1**.

Death and brain death: "a person is dead when a physician says so"
—(Kenneth V. Iserson).[74]

During its relatively brief modern history, human organ transplantation has been intimately tied to the legal definitions of brain death in the prospective organ donor. Prior to the early period of organ transplantation, a cardiorespiratory definition of death (defined as the cessation of detectable heartbeat and breathing) prevailed. Lazarus phenomena and even cases of premature burials were reported from the eighteenth to mid-twentieth centuries and amply highlighted the imperfection of such a concept.[75,76] With the increasing sophistication of mechanical, pharmacologic and other intensive care life support technology beginning in the mid-twentieth century, such an exclusive definition became more untenable. The technology to maintain organ perfusion and oxygenation created the patient–donor substrate from which cadaveric organ procurement could yield donor organs with recoverable ischemic injury and ultimately viable function for the recipient. This situation also

---

Box 1
Major legislative and regulatory landmarks relevant to organ donation and transplantation in the United States

1968 Harvard Commission defines "brain death"

1968 Uniform Anatomic Gift Act legalizes organ/tissue donation for transplantation

1971 Uniform Anatomic Gift Act mandates legality of donor card

1981 Uniform Determination of Death Act

1984 National Organ Transplant Act (NOTA) prohibits organ and tissue selling and establishes Organ Procurement and Transplantation Network (OPTN)

1986 Required Request Legislation

1986 United Network for Organ Sharing (UNOS) receives federal contract to ensure equitable access and organ allocation and oversight of procurement programs and transplant centers

1987 Uniform Anatomic Gift Act prioritized descendant's wishes for donation over family wishes, requires hospitals to inquire about organ donation

1988 Joint Commission on Accreditation of Health Care Organizations (JCAHO) establishes requirement for hospitals to have identification and notification procedures to identify potential organ donors and referral for procurement

1991 Patient Self Determination Act

1996 Organ Donation Insert Card Act, authorizing mailing information about organ and tissue donation with income tax refunds

1998 National Conditions of Participation

1999 The Department of Health and Human Services issues "Final Rule" for Organ Procurement and Transplantation. Requests broader sharing of organs and more consistent medical criteria to be used for allocation. The goal is to make the allocation system fairer and to assure that patients with the most urgent medical conditions receive transplants.

2002 United Network Organ Sharing employs MELD scoring for liver allocation

2003 United Network Organ Sharing issues guidelines for extended donor criteria for kidney transplantation

---

produced both medical and ethical uncertainties for both potential organ procurement and/or continued life support.

Medicolegal efforts to standardize an alternate definition of death based on the absence of brain function began, in part, during the same time period that organ transplantation programs required clarity or a "dead-donor rule" to initiate an organ procurement process.[77,78]

The concept of brain death was introduced in 1968 by the Ad Hoc Committee of the Harvard Medical School to Examine the Definition of Brain Death whose requirement included unreceptivity and unresponsivity, no movements or spontaneous breathing, and no reflexes.[79] A flat electroencephalogram and ruling out reversible causes of loss of brain function, such as hypothermia or drug intoxication, were also recommended. The legislative complement to this working definition as it related to organ transplantation was the congressional passage of the Uniform Anatomic Gift Act, which made it legal to donate a deceased person's organs and tissues for transplantation and reduced variations in legal guidelines the different states—although notably this failed to produce an increase in organ donation. Organ procurement for transplantation programs functioned through the 1970s with this first definition.

Further consensus and refinement was achieved with the President's Commission in 1981 that defined brain death as "whole brain" and explicitly excluded nonbrain and higher (cortical) brain criteria.[80] Quoted from this piece: "This view give the brain primacy not merely as the sponsor of consciousness but also as the complex organizer and the regulator of bodily functions...only the brain can direct the entire organism."

The legal consequence of the Commission's report was the Uniform Determination of Death Act requiring " irreversible cessation of all functions of the brain, including the brainstem". Critics would argue that preserved neurohumoral function (antidiuretic hormone secretion from the posterior pituitary evidenced by the absence of diabetes insipidus) as well as rare cases of detectable electroencephalogram and evoked potential activity in patients meeting brain death criteria by clinical examinations made a whole-brain concept of brain death untenable.[81] Medical consultants to the same commission stipulated coma with responsiveness to any stimuli, standard bedside cranial nerve function tests, and an apnea test plus a specified time period after which such tests are repeated. Although this definition of brain death was generally accepted uniformly among physicians and became a legal definition throughout the United States, there remain significant cultural and religious variations in acceptance and understanding of the definition that hampered organ donation, despite the burgeoning success of transplantation in future years.[82]

Organ Donation After Cardiac Death

The rising demand for cadaveric organs relative to a static cadaveric organ supply in the 1990s gave impetus to programs that deployed rapid procurement techniques after cessation of the heartbeat after elective withdrawal of life support in a patient with irreversible conditions and no contraindications for organ donation (controlled donation after cardiac death [DCD]) or rarely patients receiving cardiopulmonary resuscitation who may or may not be stabilized with cardiopulmonary bypass.[83–86] The transformation from a brain-death-only definition to a DCD-definition was and remains a major bioethical controversy. However, before the introduction of the brain death definition in 1968, this practice was how cadaveric organs were retrieved in the earliest days of clinical transplantation.

This practice has diversified the source of cadaveric organ donation, although brain death donation remains the dominant source of donor organs (**Fig. 2**).

In 2006, a special commission on DCD donation advocated the practice as "an ethically acceptable practice of end-of-life care, capable of increasing the number of deceased donor organs available for transplantation".[87]

The DCD protocols varied across centers; however, a recent guideline from United Network of Organ Sharing formalized the serial components of donor identification, next-of-kin consent and approval, withdrawal of life-sustaining measures, pronouncement of death, and organ recovery are required.[88]

Kidney and liver organs have been the most frequent organs harvested from DCD donors, although rare reports of successful lung and heart retrieval and transplantation have been reported. Although renal transplant graft and patient survivals appear equivalent to patients receiving kidneys from brain-death donors, outcomes in DCD liver recipients have been consistently inferior across the same comparison with one-year graft survival rates of 72% between 2002–2007 compared with 84% one-year graft survival in brain death donors.[89] This result has dampened the enthusiasm for DCD liver donation in the last several years and increased the level of caution about which recipients should receive a DCD donor liver.[89]

Donor selection practices changed as a consequence of organ shortage. The timeless adage "necessity is the mother of invention" has always been the ethic in the field of solid organ transplantation, particularly as it pertains to organ supply. As of

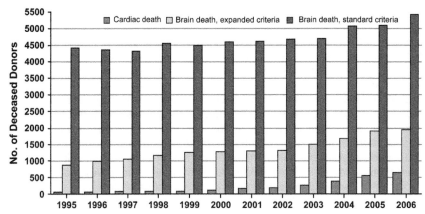

Fig. 2. Distribution of organ donation from brain death and cardiac death in the United States, 1995–2006.

November 21, 2008 there were 100,745 UNOS waiting-list candidates for organ transplantation in the United States; 8659 transplants were performed from 9490 donors during the first 8 months of 2008.[90] The increasing annual trend in the organ supply deficit for all organ transportation categories in the United States is shown (**Fig. 3**).

Cadaveric organ donation increased annually during the 1980s and 1990s because of increasing public education and awareness, the organization of hospital-based or free standing local organ procurement programs, and the sheer proliferation of transplantation centers. However, the list of patients who became transplantation-eligible rose at a much greater rate during the same time period. The margin of listed but

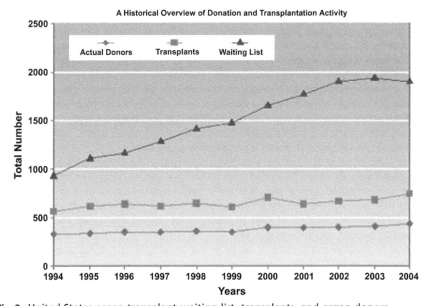

Fig. 3. United States organ transplant waiting list, transplants, and organ donors.

nontransplanted patients grew substantially and has become an area of public, political and medical concern and controversy.

In addition to DCD donation, several innovative practices emerged during this period to expand the finite and inadequate organ supply. Extended donor criteria for cadaveric organ donors were employed in high-volume kidney and liver transplantation centers.

In 2003, UNOS formalized extended donor criteria for kidney transplantation to include: donor age > 60 years and donors age 50–59 years with a history of stroke, hypertension, or a creatinine of greater than 1.5 mg/dL.[91] Prospective recipients of extended criteria kidneys needed to be informed at the time of consent that receiving an extended-donor kidney might increase the risk of poor graft function and other complications. Extended-donor criteria for liver transplantation evolved on a "by-transplantation center" basis with some variances across centers as to what defined an extended-criteria liver donor. A partial list includes: patient age, gender, race, weight, cause of brain death, length of hospital stay, prolonged warm or cold ischemia, donor hypernatremia, higher degrees of macrosteatosis, and the use of pressors.[92,93] Significant risks of primary nonfunction or delayed graft function has come with the use of such donors; this change is particularly critical because such organs are often paired with a recipient who is less severely ill.

Utilization of donors with positive serology for hepatitis C in hepatitis C positive recipients and hepatitis B core antibody donors in hepatitis B naïve and positive recipients, when coupled with post-transplantation hepatitis B antiviral treatment, have shown comparable graft and patient survival to seronegative liver donors.

Liberalization of donors with antemortem bloodstream infection and lung donors with infiltrates, when coupled with appropriate antimicrobial treatment of the recipient, have enhanced organ supply as well.

Live organ donation has its longest historical connection with kidney transplantation. Because of the increasing organ shortage and lengthening waiting times, living related kidney donation rose dramatically during the 1980s and 1990s to comprise about 50% of all performed kidney transplantation since 2000.[90] Advances in laproscopic-guided donor nephrectomy has no doubt also accelerated such practice.[94] Living donation has more recently expanded to liver, and partial pancreas, lung and small bowel donation that—due to the nature of the partial organ dissection and compromised residual organ reserve—have higher complication rates for the organ donor.[95–97]

Careful donor and recipient selection, technically perfect organ extraction, and meticulous postoperative care are obligatory to minimize donor jeopardy. A recent multidisciplinary consensus conference on the live organ donor was convened to provide guidelines to promote the well being of the living organ donor; donor complication rates are closely monitored by regulatory agencies.[98]

Other innovative strategies have evolved to expand the donor pool and shorten waiting list times. Directed living donation of kidneys across otherwise incompatibles related or nonrelated donor–recipient pairs has appeared in large transplantation centers that can accommodate a high operative work load in a short interval.[99] In situ or ex vivo cadaveric split liver transplantation allows transplantation of a left segment to a child and the remaining liver to a larger child or adult; this procedure has been successful but is risky because of the small split liver donor size and associated liver trauma.[100–102] Uncommonly, "domino" transplants are performed thta use an organ from one recipient for subsequent transplantation to a second recipient in recipient disease states that permit such a strategy (ie, end stage liver disease due to a metabolic defect or amyloidosis).[103,104]

Organ Procurement and Preservation

Removal of an organ from the body creates an obligatory ischemic insult whose sequelae may be subclinical organ dysfunction including delayed or permanent non-function. The role of temperature in its relation to organ ischemia was already known based on animal experimental transplantation that showed ischemia-sparing effects with the use of external iced saline or local graft arterial instillation of cooled fluids; hypothermic methods began to be applied in human kidney and liver transplantation.[105] Total body hypothermia of the living kidney donor during the donor nephrectomy was achieved with both external and internal cooling in the early 1960s. Core cooling was also employed before machine infusing into the distal aorta, an approach that was simplified later in the decade to aortic infusion of cooled crystalloid solution, a technique that persists to the present day.[106–108] Organ sharing across multiple centers and the rising success of all categories of organ transplantation after the introduction of cyclosporine prompted combined organ procurement of multiple organs en bloc or in sequence after in situ vascular cooling followed by ex vivo or back table dissection of the procured organs.[109]

Initial enthusiasm for ex vivo sanguinous or asanguinous artificial pulsatile perfusion for a period of up to 24–48 hours failed to produce significant improvements in allograft function, although interest and practice with modern devices have been rekindled in recent years for both cadaveric kidney and other organs.[110,111]

Organ immersion or the "slush" technique became the dominant standard of postprocurement storage from the 1980s to the present day.[1] A variety of flush solutions have been formulated; however, all have constituents to prevent cellular swelling, provide adequate osmolality, and acid buffering, inhibit auto-degradation of cell constituents, and promotion of metabolic recovery after reperfusion. The development of Collins solution, Euro-Collins solution, and University of Wisconsin solution were the major historical landmark advances in graft flush solutions. The latter, developed by James Southard and transplantation surgeon Folkert Belzer of the Unversity of Wisconsin, Madison, has emerged as the preferred solution since the 1980s.[112] Upper limits of preservation time were extended to 48–72 hours for kidneys, 24 hours for livers, and 12 hours for hearts.

Pitfalls and Perils

It should come as no surprise that with the accelerated volume of organ transplantation and the proliferation of many more transplantation centers and programs to serve the medical need, some unintended and unforeseen consequences have occurred, often with spectacular exposure in the lay media.

During the period of HIV-1 penetration into the general population and before the to the availability of HIV-1 antibody screening tests in 1985, a cluster of catastrophic case reports of HIV-1 transmission with rapid progression to AIDS caused by the high viral inoculum transferred to the recipient were documented.[113,114] Since the advent of HIV-screening, there have only been a few isolated cases of organ transplantation-related transmission.

Fatal transmission of rabies to four recipients from a donor dying of an enigmatic encephalitis after an undocumented bat-bite was proved only at the time of brain biopsy or postmortem in the recipients,[115] as was a similar transmission of West Nile Virus to four recipients who received organs from a polytransfused trauma victim.[116]

Accidental organ blood type mismatches caused by human error, although extremely rare, have resulted in rapid allograft failure and death in some cases. The last high profile case occurred at Duke University and involved the accidental transplantation of a mismatched heart with consequential death of the recipient due to heart failure.[117]

Xenotransplantation to humans has been performed only a handful of times in the twentieth century with poor outcomes,[118–121] mostly using primate organs.

Although it is a fascinating and efficient way to expand organ supply, the unknown risks of xenozoonosis (particularly due to animal virus transmission), animal rights opposition, and the very high immunosuppressive burden needed to cross the inter-species immune barrier have made this field an appropriately slow and cautious work in progress.[122]

Many ethical questions continue to arise particularly related to promoting both cadaveric and living organ supply given the current limits of altruistic donation. Financial incentivization for both living and cadaveric organ donation has been a common practice in third world countries with emerging transplantation programs but no developed organ allocation system. Recently, a modified approach of indirect or direct compensation has been proffered by some in the United States, although concerns about exploitation, allocation fairness principles, and other potentials for misuse persist.[123,124]

The practice of obtaining organs from executed convicted prisoners in China has been long known and condemned by the global transplantation community.[125]

Because of organ shortages, refusal to transplantation caused by medical reasons, or the lack of local organ transplantation programs, individuals from other parts of the world have traveled to China for transplantation at their own expense. This practice has been termed "transplant tourism."[126] Subsequent post-transplantation care has been met with resistance in the receipients' native countries.

The battle amongst transplantation centers with competing interests for fewer organs has partially driven organ allocation policies in the United States. Basic to this dispute is whether to transplant the sickest patients or the less sick patients who inherently are more likely to survive the transplantation procedure and post-transplantation period.

This dynamic set large volume centers and geographic regions with a low organ supply against smaller transplantation centers and geographic regions with a higher organ supply.

In 2002, UNOS adopted the Model of Endstage Liver Disease (MELD), a scoring system using three objective parameters (bilirubin, serum creatinine, and international normalized ratio) that best predict short-term mortality. Subsequent analysis has shown indications that such a system results in better allocation by prioritizing patients at greatest need for a liver transplantation within organ procurement regions, although geographic disparities in organ availability and waiting times still remain unresolved.[127,128]

SUMMARY

The history and advancement of organ transplantation to its current status is a remarkable collaboration of surgical, medical, legal, political and bioethical inputs over multiple generations and the foresight and diligence of pioneers in the field. The current stresses created by the increasing gap between organ supply and demand are in fact because of transplantation's remarkable success rather than its failure. Existing and new challenges toward further improving outcome and access to organ transplantation will no doubt persist; however, there is little reason not to expect the same level of adaptive innovation to meet and overcome these realities.

REFERENCES

1. Starzl TE. History of clinical transplantation. World J Surg 2000;24(7):759–82.
2. Suthanthiran M, Strom TB. Renal transplantation. N Engl J Med 1994;331(6): 365–76.
3. Sayegh MH, Carpenter CB. Transplantation 50 years later – progress, challenges and promises. N Engl J Med 2004;351(26):2761–6.
4. Hossein S. Organ transplantation: from myth to reality. J Invest Surg 2001;14:135–8.
5. Bergan A. Ancient myth, modern reality. A brief history of transplantation. J Biocommun 1997;24(4):2–9.
6. Gutkind L. Many sleepness nights. New York: WW Norton; 1998.
7. Sabiston DC Jr. Textbook of surgery: the biological basis of surgical practice. 12th edition. Philadelphia: WB Saunders; 1981.
8. Chick LR. Brief history and biology of skin grafting. Ann Plast Surg 1988;21(4): 358–65.
9. Zirm ME. Eduard Konrad Zirm and the 'wondrously beautiful little window'. Refract Corneal Surg 1989;5(4):256–7.
10. Carel A. The operative technique for vascular anastomoses and transplantation of viscera. Lyon Med 1902;98:859.
11. Carrel A, Guthrie CC. Functions of a transplanted kidney. Science 1905;22:473.
12. Ono SJ. The birth of transplantation immunology: the Billingham-Medawar experiments at Birmingham University of University College London. 1951. J Exp Biol 2004;207(Pt 230):4013–4.
13. Billingham RE, Brent L, Medawar PB. Activity acquired tolerance of foreign cells. Nature 1953;172:603–6.
14. Billingham RE, Krohn PL, Medawar PB. Effect of cortisone on survival of skin homografts in rabbits. Br Med J 1951;4716:1157–63.
15. Hamilton DNH, Reid WA. Yu Yu Vjronoy and the first human kidney allograft. Surg Gynecol Obstet 1984;159:289–94.
16. Kuss R, Teinturier J, Millieez P. Quelques essais de greffe rein chex l'homme. Mem Acad Chir 1951;77:755–64.
17. Dubost C, Oeconomos N, Nenna A, et al. Resulstats d'une tentative de greffe renale. Bull Mem Soc Med Hop Paris 1951;67:105–6.
18. Michon L, Hamburger J, Oeconomos N, et al. Une tentative de transplantation renale chez l'homme aspects medicaux et biologiques. Presse Med 1953;61: 1419–23.
19. Hume DM, Merrill JP, Miller BF, et al. Experiences with renal homotransplantation in the human: report of nine cases. J Clin Invest 1955;34:327–82.
20. Merrill JP, Murray JE, Harrison JH, et al. Successful homotransplantation of the human kidney between identical twins. JAMA 1956;160:277–82.
21. Merrill JP. The artificial kidney. N Engl J Med 1952;246:17–27.
22. Murray JE, Merrill JP, Dammin GJ, et al. Study of transplantation immunity after total body irradiation. Clinical and experimental investigation. Surgery 1960;48: 272–84.
23. Murray JE, Merrill JP, Dammin GJ, et al. Kidney transplantation in modified recipients. Ann Surg 1962;156:337–55.
24. Merrill JP, Murray JE, Harrison JH, et al. Successful homotransplantation of the kidney between non-identical twins. N Engl J Med 1960;262:1251–6.
25. Hamburger J, Vaysse J, Crosnier J, et al. Transplantation of a kidney between non-monozygotic twins after irradiation of the receiver: good function at the fourth month. Presse Med 1962;67:671–4.

26. Meeker W, Condie R, Weiner D, et al. Prolongation of skin homograft survival in rabbits by 6-mercaptopurine. Proc Soc Exp Biol Med 1959;192:459.

27. Calne RY. The rejection of renal homografts: inhibition in dogs by 6-mercaptopurine. Lancet 1960;1:417–8.

28. Goodwin WE, Kaufmann JJ, Mims MM, et al. Human renal transplantation. Clinical experience with six cases of renal homotransplantations. J Urol 1963;183:12–24.

29. Murray JE, Merrill JP, Harrison JH, et al. Prolonged survival of human-kidney homografts by immunosuppressive drug therapy. N Engl J Med 1973;268: 315–23.

30. Starzl TE, Manchioro TI, Waddell WR. The reversal of rejection in human renal homografts with subsequent development of homograft tolerance. Surg Gynecol Obstet 1963;117:385–95.

31. Scribner BH, Buri R, Caner JE, et al. The treatment of chronic uremia by means of intermittent hemodialysis: a preliminary report. Trans Am Soc Artif Intern Organs 1960;6:114–22.

32. Starzl TE. Death after transplantation (editorial). Am J Med 1967;42(3):327–34.

33. Hill RB, Rowlands DT, Rifkind D. Infectious pulmonary disease in patients receiving immunosuppressive therapy for organ transplantation. N Engl J Med 1964;271:1021–7.

34. Penn I, Hammond W, Brettschneider L, et al. Malignant lymphomas in transplantation patients. Transplant Proc 1969;1:106–12.

35. Elkinton JR. Moral problems in the use of borrowed organs, artificial and transplanted. Ann Intern Med 1964;60:309–10.

36. Starzl TE, Marchioro TL, Porter KA, et al. The use of heterologous antilymphoid agents in canine renal and liver homotransplantation and in human renal homotransplantations. Surg Gynecol Obstet 1967;124(2):301–8.

37. Starzl TE, Marchioro TL, Vonkaulla KN, et al. Homotransplantation of the liver in humans. Surg Gynecol Obstet 1963;117:659–76.

38. Starzl TE, Groth CG, Brettschneider L, et al. Extended survival in 3 cases of orthotopic liver homotransplantation of the human liver. Surgery 1968;63(4): 549–63.

39. Starzl TE, Koep LJ, Halgrimson CG, et al. Fifteen years of clinical liver transplantation. Gastroenterology 1979;77(2):375–88.

40. Barnard CN. The operation. A human cardiac transplant: an interim report of a successful operation performed at Groote Schuur Hospital, Cape Town. S Afr Med J 1967;41(48):1271–4.

41. Kelly WD, Lillehei RC, Merkel FK, et al. Allotransplantation of the pancreas and duodenum along with the kidney in diabetic nephropathy. Surgery 1967;61(6): 827–37.

42. Hardy JD, Webb WR, Dalton ML Jr. Lung homotransplantations in man. JAMA 1963;186:1065–72.

43. Cooley DA, Bloodwell RD, Hallman GL, et al. Organ transplantation for advanced cardiopulmonary disease. Ann Thorac Surg 1969;8(1):30–46.

44. Gohlke M, Jennings M. I'll take tomorrow. New York: M Evans Publishing; 1985, ISBN 0871314584.

45. Kahan B. Cyclosporine. N Engl J Med 1989;321(25):725–38.

46. Calne R. Cyclosporine, a milestone in immunosuppression. Transplant Proc 2004;36(Suppl 2):13S–5S.

47. Starzl TE, Iwatsuki S, Shaw BW Jr, et al. Immunosuppression and other nonsurgical factors in the improved results of liver transplantation. Semin Liver Dis 1985;5(4):334–43.

48. Dreyfuss M, Harri E, Hofmann H, et al. Cyclosporin A and C: new metabolites from Trichoderma polysporum. Eur J Appl Microbiol 1976;3:125–30.
49. Borel JF, Feurer C, Gubler HU. Biological effects of cyclosporin A: a new antilymphocytic agent. Agents Actions 1976;6:468–75.
50. Rosenthal JT, Hakala TR, Iwatsuki S, et al. Cadaveric renal transplantation under cyclosporine-steroid therapy. Surg Gynecol Obstet 1983;157(4):309B–15B.
51. Starzl TE, Klintmalm GB, Porter KA, et al. Liver transplantation with use of cyclosporine a and prednisone. N Engl J Med 1981;305(5):266–9.
52. Griffith BP, Hardesty RL, Deeb GM, et al. Cardiac transplantation with cyclosporine A and prednisone. Ann Surg 1982;196(3):324–9.
53. Reitz BA, Wallwork JL, Hunt SA, et al. Heart-lung transplantation: successful therapy for patients with pulmonary vascular disease. N Engl J Med 1982; 306(10):557–64.
54. Cooper JD, Pearson FG, Patterson GA, et al. Technique of successful lung transplantation in human. J Thorac Cardiovasc Surg 1987;93(2):173–81.
55. Cooper JD, Patterson GA, Grossman, et al. Double-lung transplant for advanced chronic obstructive lung disease. Am Rev Respir Dis 1989;139(2):303–7.
56. Griffith BP, Shaw BW Jr, Hardesty RL, et al. Veno-venous bypass without systemic anticoagulation for transplantation of the human liver. Surg Gynecol Obstet 1985;160:270–2.
57. Fung JJ, Todo S, Jain A, et al. Conversion of liver allograft recipients with cyclosporine related complications from cyclosporine to FK 506. Transplant Proc 1990;22(1):6–12.
58. Fung JJ, Todo S, Tzakis A, et al. Conversion of liver allograft recipients. from cyclosporine to FK506-based immunosuppression: benefits and pitfalls. Transplant Proc 1991;23(1 part 1):14–21.
59. Armitage JM, Kormos RL, Griffith BP, et al. The clinical trial of FK 506 as primary and rescue immunosuppression in cardiac transplantation. Transplant Proc 1991;23:1149–54.
60. Todo S, Fung JJ, Starzl TE, et al. Liver, kidney, and thoracic organ transplantation under FK 506. Ann Surg 1990;212:295–305.
61. Starzl TE, Fung J, Jordan M, et al. Kidney transplantation under FK 506. JAMA 1990;264:63–7.
62. Fung JJ, Todo S, Jain A, et al. The Pittsburgh randomized trial of tacrolimus versus cyclosporine for liver transplantation. J Am Coll Surg 1996;183: 117–25.
63. Todo S, Tzakis AG, Abu-Elmagd K, et al. Intestinal transplantation in composite visceral grafts or alone. Ann Surg 1992;216:223–33.
64. Todo S, Tzakis AG, Abu-Elmagd K, et al. Cadaveric small bowel and small bowel–liver transplantation in humans. Transplantation 1992;53:369–76.
65. Frezza EE, Tzakis A, Fung JJ, et al. Small bowel transplantation: current progress and clinical application. Hepatogastroenterololgy 1996;43(8): 363–76.
66. Starzl TE. Patterns of permissible donor-recipient tissue transfer in relation to ABO blood groups. In: Hill GJ, editor. Experience in renal transplantation. Philadelphia: Saunders; 1964. p. 37–47.
67. Starzl TE, Marchioro TL, Holmes JH, et al. Renal homografts inpatients with major donor-recipient blood group incompatibilities [addendum]. Surgery 1964;55:195–200.
68. Warner PR, Nester TA. ABO incompatible solid organ transplantatoin. Am J Clin Pathol 2006;125(Suppl):S87–92.

69. Farges O, Kalil AN, Samuel D, et al. The use of ABO-incompatible grafts in liver transplantation: a life-saving procedure in highly selected patients. Transplantation 1995;59(8):1124–33.
70. Dausset J. Iso-leuco-anticorps. Acta Haemetol 1958;20:156–66.
71. Van Rood JJ, Eernisses JG, van Leeuwen A. Leucocyte antibodies in sera from pregnant women. Nature 1958;181:1735–6.
72. Terasaki PK, McClelland JD. Microdroplet assay of human services cytotoxins. Nature 1964;204:998–1000.
73. Starzl TE, Eliasiw M, Gjertson M, et al. HLA and cross reactive antigen group matching for cadaver human kidney allocation. Transplantation 1997;64:983–91.
74. Kenneth V. Iserson. Death to dust. Tuscon: Galen Press Ltd; 1994. p. 19.
75. Whetstine LM. End of life communication in the ICU. In: Crippen D, editor. A global perspective. New York: Springer; 2008.
76. Pernick MS. Back from the grave; Recurring controversies over defining and diagnosing death in history. In: Zaner RM, editor. Death: beyond whole brain criteria. Boston: Kluwer Academic Publishers; 1988. p. 17–74.
77. Robertson JA. The dead donor rule. Hastings Cent Rep 2000;29:6–14.
78. Truog RD, Robinson WM. Role of brain death and the dead-donor rule in the ethics of organ transplantation. Crit Care Med 2003;31(9):2391–6.
79. A definition of irreversible coma. Report of the Ad Hoc Committee of the Harvard Medical School to examine the definition of brain death. JAMA 1968;205: 337–40.
80. Guidelines for the determination of death. Report of the Medical Consultants on the Diagnosis of Death to the President's Commission for the Study of Ethical Problems in Medicine and Biomedical and Behavioral Research. JAMA 1981; 246:2184–6.
81. Halevy A, Brody B. Brain death: reconciling definitions, criteria, and tests. Ann Intern Med 1993;119(6):519–25.
82. Siminoff LA, Burant C, Youngner SJ. Death and organ procurement; public beliefs and attitudes. Soc Sci Med 2004;59:2325–34.
83. Foley DP, Fernandez LA, Leverson G, et al. Donation after cardiac death. The University of Wisconsin experience with liver transplantation. Ann Surg 2005; 242(11):724–31.
84. Casavilla A, Ramirez C, Shapiro R, et al. Experience with liver and kidney allografts from non-heart beating donors. Transplantation 1995;59:197–203.
85. Alvarez J, del Barrio R, Arias J, et al. Non-heart beating donors from the street: an increasing donor supply pool source. Transplantation 2000;70:314–7.
86. D'allessandro AM, Hofmann RM, Knechle SJ, et al. Liver transplantation from controlled non-heart-beating donors. Surgery 2000;128:579–88.
87. Bernat JL, D'Alessandro AM, Port FK, et al. Report of a national conference on donation after cardiac death. Am J Transplant 2006;6:281–91.
88. Steinbrook R. Organ donation after cardiac death. N Engl J Med 2007;357(3): 209–13.
89. Selck FW, Grossman EB, Ratner LE, et al. Utilization, outcome and retransplantation of liver allografts from donation after cardiac death. Implications for further expansion of the deceased donor pool. Ann Surg 2008;248(4):599–607.
90. United Network for Organ Sharing. Available at: www.unos.org [website] Accessed November 29, 2008.
91. UNOS Policy 3,5.1. Expanded criteria donor definitions and point system. Richmond: VA United Network for Organ Sharing; 2002.

92. Cameron AW, Ghobrial M, Yersiz H, et al. Optimal utilization of donor grafts with extended criteria. A single center experience in over 1000 liver transplants. Ann Surg 2006;243(6):748–55.
93. Feng S, Goodrich NP, Bragg-Gresham JL, et al. Characteristics associated with liver graft failure: The concept of donor risk index. Am J Transplant 2006;6:783–90.
94. Handschin AE, Weber M, Demartines N, et al. Laparoscopic donor nephrectomy. Br J Surg 2003;90(11):1323–32.
95. Busuttil RW, Goss JA. Split liver transplantation. Ann Surg 1999;229:313–21.
96. Starnes VA, Woo MS, MacLaughlin EF, et al. Comparison of outcomes between living donor and cadaveric lung transplantation in children. Ann Thorac Surg 1999;68:2279–83.
97. Margreiter R. Living related pancreas and small bowel transplantation. Langenbecks Arch Surg 1999;384:544–9.
98. Authors for the Live Organ Donor Consensus Group. Consensus statement on the liver organ donor. JAMA 2000;284(22):2919–26.
99. Roth AE, Sonmez T, Unver MU, et al. Utilizing list exchange and nondirected donation through chain paired kidney donations. Am J Transplant 2006;6: 2695–705.
100. Killic M, Seu P, Stribling RJ, et al. In situ splitting of the cadaveric liver for two adult recipients. Transplantation 2001;72(11):1853–8.
101. Reyes J, Gerber D, Mazariegos GV, et al. Split-liver transplantation: a Comparison of ex vivo and in situ techniques. J Pediatr Surg 2000;35(2):283–9.
102. Rogiers X, Malago M, Gawad K, et al. In situ splitting of cadaveic livers. The ultimate expansion of a limited donor pool. Ann Surg 1996;224(3):331–9.
103. Lowell JA, Smith C, Brennan DC, et al. The domino transplant: transplant recipients as organ donors. Transplantation 2000;69(3):372–6.
104. Astor TL, Galantowicz M, Phillips A, et al. Domino heart transplantation involving infants. Am J Transplant 2007;7(11):2626–9.
105. Starzl TE, Brittain RS, Stonington OG, et al. Renal transplantation in identical twins. Arch Surg 1963;86:600–7.
106. Starzl TE. Experience in renal transplantation. Philadelphia: Saunders; 1964. p. 68–71.
107. Marchioro TL, Huntley RT, Waddell WR, et al. Extracorporeal perfusion for obtaining postmortem homografts. Surgery 1963;54:900–11.
108. Merkel FK, Jonasson G, Bergan JJ. Procurement of cadaver donor organs: evisceration techniques. Transplant Proc 1972;4:585–9.
109. Starzl TE, Miller C, Broznick B, et al. An improved technique for multiple organ harvesting. Surg Gynecol Obstet 1987;165(4):343–8.
110. Shah AP, Milgrom DP, Mangus RS, et al. Comparison of pulsatile perfusion and cold storage for paired kidney allografts. Transplantation 2008;86(7):1006–9.
111. Imber CJ, St Peter SD, Lopez de Cenarruzabeitia I, et al. Advantages of normothermic perfusion over cold storage in liver preservation. Transplantation 2002; 73(5):701–9.
112. Van der Werf WJ, D'Alessandro AM, et al. Procurement, preservation and transport of cadaver kidneys. Surg Clin North Am 1998;78(1):41–54.
113. Quarto M, Germinario C, Fontana A, et al. 1 HIV transmission through kidney transplantation from a living related donor. N Engl J Med 1989;320(26):1754.
114. Kumar P, Pearson JE, Martin DH, et al. Transmission of human immunodeficiency virus by transplantation of a renal allograft with development of the acquired immunodeficiency syndrome. Ann Intern Med 1987;106(2):244–5.

115. Srinivasan A, Burton EC, Kuehnert MJ, et al. Transmission of rabies virus from an organ donor to four transplant recipients. N Engl J Med 2005;352(11):1103–11.
116. Iwamoto M, Jernigan DB, Guasch A, et al. Transmission of West Nile virus from an organ donor to four transplant recipients. N Engl J Med 2003;348(22): 2196–203.
117. Sloane A. Grading duke; "A" for acknowledgement. J Health Law 2003;36(4): 627–45.
118. Reemtsma K. Renal heterotransplantation from nonhuman primates to man. Ann NY Acad Sci 1969;162:412–8.
119. Bailey LL, Nehlsen-Cannarella SL, Concepcion W, et al. Baboon-to-human cardiac xenotransplantation in a neonate. JAMA 1985;254:3321–9.
120. Starzl TE, Marchioro TL, Peters GN, et al. Renal heterotransplantation from baboon-to- man: experience with 6 cases. Transplantation 1964;2:752–6.
121. Starzl TE, Fung JJ, Tzakis A, et al. Baboon-to-human liver transplantation. Lancet 1993;341:65–71.
122. Soin B, Vial CM, Friend PJ. Xenotransplantation. Br J Surg 2000;87:138–48.
123. Monaco AP. Rewards for organ donation: the time has come. Kidney Int 2006; 69(6):955–7.
124. Sells R. Incentives for organ donation: some ethical concerns. Ann Transplant 2004;9(1):23–4.
125. Hillman H. Harvesting organs from recently executed prisoners. Practice must be stopped. BMJ 2001;323(7323):1254.
126. Khamash HA, Gaston RS. Transplant tourism: a modern iteration of an ancient problem. Curr Opin Organ Transplant 2008;13(4):395–9.
127. Freeman RB, Weisman RH, Harper A, et al. The New Liver Allocation System moving towards evidence based transplantation policy. Liver Transpl 2002;8: 851–8.
128. Moylan CA, Brady CW, Johnson JL, et al. Disparities in liver transplantation before and after introductioin of the MELD Score. JAMA 2008;300(20):2371–8.

History of Technology in the Intensive Care Unit

Nitin Puri, MD[a],*, Vinod Puri, MD[b], R.P. Dellinger, MD[a]

KEYWORDS

- History • Renal replacement therapy • Echocardiogram
- Pulmonary artery catheter • Pulse oximetry
- Mechanical ventilation

THE HISTORY OF INVASIVE MONITORING
Early Invasive Monitoring

Invasive monitoring in the intensive care unit owes a great deal to many forward-thinking pioneers in this field. In 1929, the German resident Forssmann, in an attempt to deliver drugs more effectively for cardiac resuscitation, inserted a nonflow directed (no balloon) catheter into his own arm and advanced it to what was calculated to be his right heart (**Fig. 1**). He walked to the radiology department to verify its placement by radiography.[1] Forssmann's successful experiment was considered a stunt by the German medical community and he was forced to change his career to urology. Ultimately, he was recognized for his contribution to the development of cardiac catheterization with a Nobel Prize in science in 1956.[1] The next two decades saw the creation of cardiac catheterization laboratories to investigate and treat congenital, rheumatic, and eventually ischemic heart disease. In the 1960s, the only physiologic tool available for bedside evaluation was the central venous pressure (CVP) measurement as first described by Wilson.[2] The limitations of CVP monitoring were becoming evident over the first decade of its use in clinical practice.[3]

During this same time Myocardial Infarction Research Units (MIRU) and Shock Research Units (SRU) demonstrated the value of hemodynamic measurements in acutely ill patients with both cardiogenic and other forms of shock.[4,5] Del Guercio and colleagues[6] applied similar techniques for surgical patients. However, for measurement of cardiac output, investigators had to rely on indocyanine green dye dilution techniques. Indocyanine green dye had to be injected into the right atrium

[a] Division of Critical Care Medicine, Department of Medicine, Cooper University Hospital, 3 Cooper Ave, Camden, NJ 08103, USA
[b] Division of Critical Care Medicine (Rtd), Providence Hospital, 1450 Covington Road, Southfield, MI 48301, USA
* Corresponding author.
E-mail address: puri-nitin@cooperhealth.edu (N. Puri).

Crit Care Clin 25 (2009) 185–200
doi:10.1016/j.ccc.2008.12.002
0749-0704/08/$ – see front matter © 2009 Elsevier Inc. All rights reserved.
criticalcare.theclinics.com

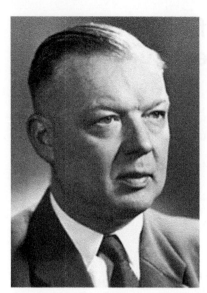

Fig. 1. Werner Forssmann. (Copyright © The Nobel Foundation.)

and a sensor detected the dye in the radial or femoral artery. The cardiac output was calculated from a curve that could be recorded on paper.[7] Cardiac dilution curves in turn were both tedious and specialized enough to be available to a select few clinicians. Bedside procedures in the early 1970s were also improved by the percutaneous cannulation of central veins and arteries using the modified Seldinger techniques in the intensive care units.[8] Along with the miniaturization and development of disposable pressure transducer systems, new intravascular catheters were becoming available. Thus the stage was set for an explosive growth in the art and science of critical care medicine.

Pulmonary Artery Catheter

Right heart catheterization at the bedside has helped enormously in our understanding of critical illness. Swan's lyrical description of his epiphany while watching sailboats in the Santa Monica Bay that led him to develop the flow directed catheters is well ingrained in critical care lore.[9] However, credit must also go to Lategola and Bradley[10,11] for the first descriptions of a flow-directed pulmonary artery catheter (PAC) placement. Swan and Ganz[12] ushered in the era of bedside hemodynamic monitoring in the critically ill patients using the flow-directed catheter to enable noncardiologists to perform bedside hemodynamic monitoring, which contributed to the popularity and usefulness of the technique. Cardiac anesthesiology flourished because of the PAC and afterload reduction became a common practice in both the operating room and ICU.[9]

However, there was ongoing controversy about the utility of monitoring pulmonary artery pressures. The classic opinion article of Eugene Robins divided the scientific community into proponents and opponents of Swan-Ganz catheter.[13] The acceptance and widespread use of the expensive and invasive monitoring technique rankled the skeptics. Proponents argued that the PAC was a diagnostic not a therapeutic device. The performance of the procedure by inexpert physicians and the lack of interpretive skills amongst physicians were cited by the enthusiasts. Connors,[14] who previously had produced an article citing the usefulness of PAC over clinical skills, now authored the widely disseminated study to understand prognosis and prefer-ences and risk of treatment (SUPPORT) study that cast doubt about the life-saving potential of the technique. His article showed a correlation between use of the PAC and mortality. Animated discussion followed in forums of scientific meetings and in the medical literature. Critics of the article noted that it was not designed as a trial of PAC and the propensity score used to create statistical equivalence in the compared groups had limitations. In an editorial response to this study, Bone and Da-len called for a moratorium on the use of the PAC.[15]

A consensus conference grading the evidence supporting the use of the PAC in different clinical situations was convened.[16] The consensus statement disagreed with a moratorium, but it did advocate for further educating physicians about how to place the catheters and the use of data that the catheters provided. One outcome of the consensus process was the creation of the American College of Chest Physi-cians online Pulmonary Artery Catheter Education Program started in 2001.[17] The consensus group further advocated prospective, randomized clinical trials using the PAC to determine its effect on morbidity and mortality in multiple conditions. Prospec-tive clinical trials about the PAC continue to be equivocal.[18,19] Even though the decline in the use of the catheters is well documented, a case can be made for invasive hemo-dynamic monitoring in persistently unstable patients.[18,20]

The PA catheter likely jump-started the field of critical care medicine by offering insight into patient hemodynamics at the bedside. The questions about its utility and safety as well as new technology have a led to a significant decline in its use. However, it remains an important tool for intensivists and standardized educational programs now exist to help ensure the proper use of the catheter. PAC-derived hemo-dynamic profiles and the required interpretation continue to be commonplace on critical care board examinations.

ECHOCARDIOGRAPHY
The Early Years

The origins of clinical echocardiography date back to the 1950s under the leadership of Edler and Hertz. Echocardiography was initially performed in the motion-mode, which provided a one-dimensional axial view of the heart displayed as monochromic dots.[21] The technology progressed in the early 1970s with primitive two-dimensional (2D) imaging obtained by recording the various levels of brightness from ultrasonic reflections of the heart. Clinicians were able to visualize cardiac structures and subse-quently Doppler was first integrated into echocardiography using Bernoulli's equation to calculate hemodynamic data as a marker of severity of valvular stenosis.[22] Linear array probes, flat probes that provided square images of superficial structures, allowed real time imaging in the 1970s. However, these probes had limited echocar-diographic utility because of rib shadows. Subsequently, the development of phased array scanners (ie, flat probes that provided images based on timing of ultrasonic reflections) moved the field forward in the mid-1970s; this advancement allowed for high quality real time imaging of the heart.[21] Color flow Doppler was developed in the 1980s and it gave clinicians knowledge about the direction of blood flow.[22] These advances allowed the use of echocardiography in critically ill patients to calculate stroke volume and cardiac output.[23–25] In 1984, echocardiography was shown to correlate with radionuclide cinematography findings of reversible myocardial depres-sion in patients with septic shock.[26,27] However, echocardiography continued to have limited clinical utility in the critically ill, being mainly used for the diagnosis of cardiac tamponade, aortic dissection, and the complications of myocardial infarctions.[25]

Advances in the technology and the controversies surrounding right heart catheterization led to a explosive growth of echocardiography in critically ill patients in the 1990s. Perhaps its greatest utility is its bedside application in a patient with shock of unknown etiology.

Expanding Indications

In 1994, Jardin and colleagues[28] published a study where he used transthoracic echocardiography (TTE) to show that right heart catheterization (RHC) does not reliably estimate left ventricular end diastolic pressure (LVEDP) in comparison to TTE in patients with septic shock. The development of flexible endoscopes, multiplane views, and the miniaturization of transducers made echocardiography a more viable option to be used in the ICU setting.[29,30] The refinement of transesophageal echocardiography (TEE), first described by Frazin and colleagues[31] in the 1970s, increased its clinical utility in the critically ill. TEE was demonstrated to directly change management decisions in 20% of critically ill patients in one study, where the imaging showed an immediate need for pericardiocentesis or a surgical procedure.[32] Viellard-Baron (a colleague of Jardin) and his colleagues[33] described his group's use of TEE in mechanically ventilated patients who were in shock and their institution's replacement of right heart catheterization by echocardiography to monitor serial hemodynamics. Echocardiography measurement of inferior vena cava diameter changes has been shown to be an indicator of volume status of patients with shock. In echocardiography-based ICU care, these measurements can guide volume resuscitation.[25] The use of the echocardiogram has helped us to further define critical care disease states. Jardin and colleagues[34,35] challenged the concept of left ventricular end-diastolic dilatation in early septic shock and showed that more than 30% of patients have hypodynamic shock. Echocardiography has been used to calculate the LVEDP in patients with mitral valve disease, a well-known condition in which the measurement with PA catheter can be inaccurate.[36] The accepted limitation of right heart catheterization pressure measurements and physical examination for estimating left heart pressures have been a stimulus for echocardiography as a better estimation tool.

Summary

Echocardiography is still evolving as a tool in the care of critically ill patients. In some institutions, intensivists have used it to replace the PA catheter as the primary modality for monitoring hemodynamics to determine management decisions. Its use in shock of unknown etiology can help narrow clinicians differential diagnosis.[37] The addition of postgraduate courses on ultrasound for intensivists at United States' critical care meetings is a recent but positive development.

RENAL REPLACEMENT THERAPY
Brief History of Dialysis

Since the eighteenth century, physicians have been aware that the peritoneum could be used as a conduit to remove excess and potentially "toxic" fluid from the peritoneal space. Peritoneal dialysis first clinical application was in Germany in 1923 by George Ganter.[38] He was concerned about the attempts of others to use extracorporeal membranes to dialyze patients that required the use of hirudin, an extract from leeches to provide anticoagulation. He instilled a sterile solution into the peritoneum of a woman with acute renal failure and let it dwell for multiple hours until her electrolytes had corrected. The patient subsequently died when she was discharged from the hospital, which caused Ganter to realize she needed continued therapy.[38]

During this same era, Georg Haas performed the first intermittent dialysis on a human being when he cannulated the radial artery and antecubital vein and cleansed approximately 150 cc of blood in 15 minutes.[39] The further progression of dialysis was buoyed by the replacement of hirudin with heparin for anticoagulation and the transition from collodion to cellophane for dialysate membrane. Hirudin was associated with significant histamine release in patients resulting in substantial morbidity. Collodian tubing was delicate and was difficult to reuse. Cellophane by comparison was not as fragile and easily sterilized, therefore reusable.[40] These advancements allowed Kolff in 1943 to dialyze a woman with malignant hypertension and treat both her renal failure and hypertension. In 1945, he was able to save a woman's life with acute renal failure, which was the first time a patient lived because of dialysis.[41,42] Both intermittent and peritoneal dialysis have made significant technological advances since their origins and are now used routinely in the critically ill patient with renal failure.

Renal Replacement Therapy in ICU

The incidence of renal failure in critically ill patients is difficult to precisely quantify because of the multitude of definitions used in the past for renal failure and the heterogeneous nature of the disease. One multinational observation study reported that 6% of critically ill patients have acute renal failure and 70% of these patients required renal replacement therapy.[43] Traditional dialysis techniques, such as intermittent hemodialysis and peritoneal dialysis, have potential limitations in critically ill patients. Intermittent hemodialysis exposes ICU patients to severe hypotension in 20%–30% of cases and peritoneal dialysis inadequately clears solutes from the blood.[44] The exposure to hypotension and concern for its deleterious effect as to worsening of renal function was a major impetus for the development of continuous renal replacement therapy (CRRT).[45] Kramer provided the first continuous dialysis option when he created continuous arteriovenous hemofiltration (CAVH) by accessing the femoral artery in 1977.[46] The method was broadly accepted in the United States after Lauer and colleagues[47,48] published their successful use of CAVH in critically ill patients in 1983. CAVH was an advancement, but its reliance on the patient's blood pressure to remove fluid and the morbidity associated with cannulating the femoral artery provided the rationale for developing other techniques. After the invention of CAVH, the next two major developments in continuous renal replacement therapy were the introduction of double lumen catheters and peristaltic pumps. The double lumen catheters avoided the need for arterial puncture and the peristaltic pumps made it easier to take off larger volumes of fluid. These developments and the use of countercurrent diasylate comprise the continuous veno-venous hemofiltration (CVVH) system that is used in today's ICU.[49]

Which Modality is Better to Treat Acute Renal Failure in the ICU?

The use of CRRT in the ICU has both anecdotal and scientific rationale. The continuous volume control usually avoids worsening of hypotension in hemodynamically unstable patients. Improved uremia control, more rapid improvement of metabolic acidosis, and control of serum phosphate have all been suggested.[44] Disadvantages of CRRT include the need for anticoagulation, its labor intensive nature, the clotting of the coil in low flow states despite anticoagulation and the clotting that occurs when anticoagulation is contraindicated.[50]

Multiple studies comparing intermittent versus continuous hemodialysis in patients who have acute kidney injury have been inconclusive as to the outcome benefit.[51] Biesin and colleagues[52] suggested that the two technologies have positively influenced each other as CRRT has gone from a low efficiency to a high efficiency treatment while intermittent dialysis can be done daily and for extended sessions. The influence of the technologies on each other has led to a relatively new modality known as slow low efficient dialysis (SLED), which is traditional dialysis done under low intensity over a longer period of time.[53,54] The adaptation of renal replacement technology to the needs of the critically ill has been likened by Ricci and colleagues[54] to the plethora of mechanical ventilation options which exist for patients with respiratory failure. Multiple modes of renal replacement therapy in critically ill patients are used interchangeably. If a CRRT coil clots in a patient, clinicians have the option of using SLED or daily intermittent hemodialysis if the critically ill patients can hemodynamically tolerate it.

Treating Sepsis with Hemofiltration

The relationship between sepsis and acute kidney injury (AKI) is well known with a large, international observational study attributing 50% of AKI in critically ill patients to sepsis.[43] The role, if any, of CRRT as a blood purification treatment in septic patients is not clear. Hemofiltration in sepsis showed beneficial results in animals in 1990 when Stein demonstrated improved hemodynamics associated with hemofiltration in pigs with endotoxemia. These results were confirmed by multiple other animal studies, but they have not been reproduced in humans.[55] In a study by Ronco and colleagues,[56] a small subset of patients with sepsis had increased survival with high-dose hemofiltration, but the results were not generalizable. Pulsed high-dose hemofiltration in humans has shown lower than expected mortality by acute physiology and chronic health evaluation (APACHE) II score prediction in patients with septic shock and decreased vasopressor requirements.[57–59] The use of renal replacement therapy to clear toxic metabolites as a treatment for septic shock requires confirmation with additional research. The literature supporting use of hemofiltration as a therapy consists of small case series, uncontrolled human trials and animal models. A recent prospective clinical trial showed increasing the dose of CRRT in septic patients with AKI did not decrease mortality or improve kidney injury.[60] More prospective clinical trials are needed to see if CRRT can be used to decrease mortality as a treatment independent of renal function in critically ill septic patients.

Summary

The morbidity and mortality from AKI remains high in critically ill patients despite new dialysis techniques. No significant mortality benefits have been noted using CRRT instead of intermittent hemodialysis, but intensivists now have a wider array of methodologies to dialyze critically ill patients. Limited studies have shown that use of hemofiltration in septic patients may have clinical benefit, but more research needs to be done.

PULSE OXIMETRY
The Early Years

Historically, the clinical lack of sensitivity to detect hypoxemia is well documented.[61] This problem perplexed investigators for over forty years. Pulse oximeters saw limited use in a few pulmonary research laboratories. The oximeters used were bulky, required recalibration after each use and were capable of causing second degree skin-burns. In 1972, the Japanese engineer Ayogi accidentally discovered the basis for modern pulse oximetry while experimenting with dye techniques to measure cardiac output.[62] He discovered that by using photoplethysmography, he could isolate the pulsatile variations in oxygenated and deoxygenated hemoglobin. Ayogi noted that the differences in the wavelengths between oxyhemoglobin and reduced hemoglobin amounted to changes in arterial saturation. His innovation allowed the pulse oximeter to transition from a research device to an important clinical tool.[63]

Introduction into Clinical Practice

The Minolta Camera Corporation introduced the modern-day pulse oximeter into the United States with little fanfare in the early 1980s. This pulse oximter was modified by Scott Wilbur for the Biox Corporation who made it less bulky and more convenient for clinical use.[64] William New, a Stanford anesthesiologist, recognized the clinical utility of the new less bulky pulse oximeter. He made an adhesive probe and introduced the pulse oximeter into the operating room for noninvasive monitoring of patient's oxygenation.[65,66] Willam New, Jack Lloyd, and Jim Corenman later started the Nellcor corporation, which became almost synonymous with pulse oximetry.

The pulse oximeter migrated relatively quickly from the operating room to the intensive care unit after New published his work in 1983.[67] The spread of the technology was supported by small studies which verified its accuracy in ventilated patients. Mihm and colleagues[68,69] affirmed the arterial saturation correlation in 18 critically ill patients and their work was later supported by Van de Louw and colleagues in a larger study in 2001. The oximeter provided real-time insight into ventilator changes when clinicians tried to wean oxygen concentration and the need for arterial blood gases was shown to be reduced.[70,71] It was subsequently dubbed the "fifth" vital sign in the critically ill patients.[72] By the late 1980s, the pulse oximeter was accepted as a standard instrument for monitoring critically ill patients, but even today no study exists showing its survival benefits.

Limitations of the Technology

Pulse oximetry has significant limitations, which have been well documented in the literature.[73,74] Skin pigmentation and dark nail polish have been shown to reduce the accuracy of readings. Anemic patients may have abnormal readings of their arterial saturation. The primary limitation in the critically ill is the inaccuracy of pulse oximetry in shock and those with hypothermia. Pulse oximetry in patients with low cardiac output may not reflect the true oxygen saturation because of peripheral vasoconstriction. Pulse oximeters are notoriously inaccurate when the patient's saturations are below 70%. A significant plunge in arterial oxygenation is needed for patients to drop their saturation below 100% at high partial pressures of oxygen (this is the flat part of the sigmoid oxygen saturation curve).[69]

Advancements of Technology

Oximeters have transitioned from reusable probes to disposable ones that can now be applied to multiple sites on patient's bodies (eg, forehead, fingers, ear lobe). A major advancement in pulse oximetry technology occurred in the mid-1980s with the ability to alter the tones of audible sound as a patient saturation varied. Nellcor modulated their second-generation oximeter pulse tone to different saturations and it was widely adopted (Jeffrey Littman, MD, Camden, NJ, personal communication, May 2008). The major advancement in the 1990s was the Masimo Corporation's signal extraction technology, which reduced motion and low perfusion artifact.[75]

Summary

No studies have attributed a specific decrease in mortality to the use of the pulse oximeter in critically ill patients. Its use is omnipresent in ICUs because of physician's inability to detect subclinical hypoxemia. The pulse oximeter has significant limitations, but technological improvements continue to increase its clinical utility.

MECHANICAL VENTILATION
The Modern Origins

The nineteenth century saw the development of negative pressure ventilation with little clinical utility until Drinker-Shaw invented the iron lung in 1929. This machine was first effectively used to manage the respiratory paralysis caused by polio. The iron lung was a cylindric tank in which patients would be enclosed with only their head protruding. This machine created negative pressure around the patient's body to create inhalation and exhalation occurred passively.[76] The Cuirass ventilator, an armored sealed vest limited to the thorax that allowed greater nursing access during negative pressure ventilation, was the other primary mode of ventilation for polio patients. The Copehagen polio epidemic of 1952 brought to the forefront the limitations of the iron lung, including its expense, size, the inability to secure a patient's airway, and pulmonary atelectasis.[77]

Ibsen, an anesthesiologist, understood these limitations when he was brought in as a consultant to help the overwhelmed Danish medical system cope with the epidemic. He suggested the use of positive pressure ventilation (PPV) outside the operating theater. Also, he learned of Bower's successful use of intermittent positive pressure breathing to supplement negative pressure ventilation for treatment of respiratory acidosis in polio patients.[78] Over a thousand medical students were required to manually ventilate patients during the Copehagen polio epidemic. However, medical centers with less manpower sought machines to ventilate patients.[79] Thus, Ibsen's advocacy of PPV was the impetus for modern mechanical ventilators and, arguably, for the development of intensive care units.[80] Before his experience, ICUs were set up for the summer polio epidemics and then disbanded.[81]

The Early Ventilators

For PPV, the machine forced air into the patient's lungs either to a preset pressure or volume. The first volume ventilator to receive widespread praise was Engstrom's, which he developed in the early 1950s.[82] It was a piston-powered, volume-cycled ventilator, which provided a constant minute ventilation. The ventilator was used successfully in Europe for both postoperative and polio patients.[83] The integration of PPV into United States respiratory practice was drawn by the insistence of cardiothoracic surgeons and anesthesiologists.[77] Morch's (an anesthesiologist's) surgical ventilator had been widely used in Europe for fifteen years before it was introduced to the United States in 1955. It represented a definitive improvement in ventilatory management during surgical procedures because it allowed measurement of tidal volume, sterilization of ventilator components in contact with airflow, and it could function in either pressure or volume cycled mode.[84]

An explosion in ventilatory technology occurred over the next sixty years with the early United States pioneers being Bennett, Bird and Emerson. The inventions of all three men were significantly influenced by their World War II experiences with the provision of oxygen for pilots during high-altitude flights.[85] Bennett invented a flow-sensitive valve, which Bower had used to augment NPV with PPV at Los Angeles County Hospital in the late-1940s. Both Bird and Bennett used a variation on this same valve and developed pressure-cycled ventilators that allowed airflow until a predetermined pressure was reached. At this pressure, a valve would close and exhalation would occur. Their ventilators were powered by compressed oxygen.[86] Emerson created a volume cycled ventilator where the tidal volume was delivered by a piston powered motor.[87] In this environment of invention, studies comparing PPV ventilators with iron lungs (which persisted in use till the early 1960's in the USA) showed the benefits of PPV.[80,88]

Volume-Controlled Ventilation

As a dramatic increase in the number of patients receiving artificial ventilation occurred in the 1960s, volume ventilation became the ventilatory method of choice. This dominance was because of its ability to deliver a preset tidal volume independently of a patient's lung mechanics—unlike pressure control ventilation.[81,89] An alternative method of breath delivery was to provide a fixed pressure through inspiration that was time cycled (pressure controlled). The increased use of PPV was due to the wider development of multidisciplinary ICUs and the ability to obtain blood gases. In Europe, the Servo 900 was the workhorse in the ICUs and it was the first ventilator with capability to display pressure and flow curves and provide the option of either volume or time cycled breaths. (Jennie Haag, Edgewick, NJ, personal communication, August 2008) In the United States, the Puritan-Bennett MA-1 followed distantly by the Ohio-560 were the most commonly used ventilators in the seventies (**Fig. 2**).[83] Both were bellow-based volume cycled ventilators that were electronically controlled as opposed to the piston-powered ventilators of the previous two decades. They both had high peak pressure capabilities and were able to deliver preset tidal volumes even if patients had decreased lung compliance.[84,90]

Positive End Expiratory Pressure for Adult Respiratory Distress Syndrome

Patients with decreased lung compliance because of acute infiltrative and edematous lungs occasionally caused physicians great consternation as the patients' lungs were difficult to oxygenate. Frumin and colleagues[91] were the first to scientifically demonstrate the value of continuous positive pressure inside the expiratory circuit to increase arterial oxygenation. They hypothesized that this positive end expiratory pressure (PEEP) recruited closed alveoli and improved oxygenation.[92] In 1967, Ashbaugh and colleagues[93,94] recognized in twelve heterogeneous patients a similar difficulty of oxygenation and named it acute respiratory distress syndrome, only to change it in 1971 to adult respiratory distress syndrome (ARDS). Petty saw the value of PEEP in increasing oxygenation and the initial work of his team provided the basis for the treatment of hypoxia (caused by ARDS) with PEEP. PEEP had significant hemodynamic

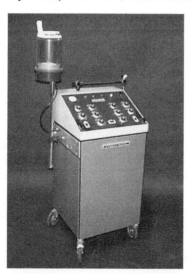

Fig. 2. Puritan-Bennett MA-1 ventilator. (*Courtesy of* W. Neal Witwer, RN, CLNC, Galveston, TX. Available at www.nealwitwer.com; used with permission.)

effects on critically ill patients, including decreasing cardiac output and arterial blood pressure, therefore it was recommended that PEEP levels greater than 10 required vigilance by intensivists.[95]

PEEP was first applied by immersing the expiratory limb of the ventilator in a small bucket of water with the depth of immersion representing the PEEP applied by the ventilator. The introduction of PEEP valves with threshold resistors allowed clinicians to avoid this encumbrance.

Evolution of Ventilatory Modes

Besides optimizing methods to oxygenate patients, more thought was given to weaning patients from ventilators. The classic mode of ventilation for volume control was controlled mandatory ventilation (CMV). The ventilator provides every breath and this result is achieved only by heavily sedating the patient. Assist-control ventilation (AC) is a preset tidal volume delivered to patients, but patients can initiate additional breaths. In 1973, Downs and colleagues introduced intermittent mandatory ventilation (IMV), which allowed patients to receive their preset ventilatory support and then initiate their own breaths receiving fresh humidified gas flow from a separate circuit. Between positive pressure ventilator breaths patients were able to inspire and generate their own spontaneous tidal volume without ventilator interference.[96] IMV was later refined to synchronized intermittent mandatory ventilation (SIMV) to prevent patients from initiating breath when the ventilator was attempting to provide a breath ("stacking"). While the merits of IMV were vigorously debated in the medical literature, IMV was widely adopted into clinical practice. The MA-1 design was limited by the need for an additional circuit to be setup for IMV. Emerson recognized the importance of the new ventilatory mode and was amongst the first to invent a commercially viable machine that incorporated IMV.[87]

Pressure Support Ventilation and Pressure Control Ventilation

In the early 1980s, Norlander proposed a method of ventilatory support to help patients with their inspiratory effort.[97] Pressure was applied in the inspiratory limb to help augment patients' tidal volume and decrease their work of breathing. This mode of ventilation, pressure support ventilation (PSV), was revolutionary as patients controlled their own respiratory rate and had partial control over their tidal volume.[80] It was primarily used to wean patients from the ventilator and, by 1998, it was reported that 45% of practitioners used PSV for weaning.[98] PSV was widely recognized as an important modality and it was incorporated into ventilators of that era including the Servo 900c and Bennett 7200.

PCV was available on most ventilators by the mid-1990s. The recognition of the significant impact of volutrauma on the lungs and a greater tolerance of permissive hypercapnia made clinicians reconsider PCV.[80] Inverse ratio ventilation (IRV) was a modification on PCV in which the patients' inspiratory time for ventilation was made longer than their exhalation time. IRV was less frequently applied using volume ventilation with an inspiratory hold. The modality was designed for patients who were difficult to oxygenate (eg, ARDS), but it had significant limitations. Because of the prolonged inspiratory phase, patients had to be heavily sedated or paralyzed, and the benefit in oxygenation was at the cost of high mean airway pressures cardiovascular compromise.[99]

Microprocessors-Based Ventilators

The advent of microprocessors in ventilators allowed for peak inspiratory pressure, mean airway pressure, and continuous positive airway pressure to be measured.

Safety was improved because of internal alarms, which sensed abnormalities when ventilating patients.[84] The mechanics of ventilators became enhanced, for example, the transition from inspiration to expiration in the machine was now electronically controlled because the ventilator sensed the end of inspiration as opposed to previously waiting for pressure to decrease.[80] The first commercially available ventilator in the United States to have a microprocessor was the Bennett 7200. Microprocessors allowed for the development of graphics to enable real-time visualization of pressure flow and volume during ventilatory cycles. A few examples of ventilators that provide advanced graphics are the Servo-I, Drager-Evita-4 and GE Care Station-Engstrom.

Airway Pressure Release Ventilation (APRV)

In 1987, Stock and Downs introduced airway pressure release ventilation (APRV) as a new mode of ventilation in anesthetized dogs.[100] They asserted that contemporary mechanical ventilation modes because of their historical design for patients with neuromuscular illness were inadequate for patients with intrinsic lung disease. APRV is the application of continuous positive airway pressure (CPAP) at alternating high and low levels in time limited cycles (T_{high} and T_{low}). APRV has a time sensitive pressure release valve in the expiratory circuit which decreases pressure in the airway to aide exhalation.[101] The mode currently allows the physiologic benefits of spontaneous breathing. The mode as currently used employs a very short T_{low} which is referred to as a "dump" period, which facilitates CO_2 removal. Literature is limited as to any advantage or superiority of APRV over other modes.[102]

Summary

The merits of PPV were recognized during the polio epidemic of 1952 and that experience helped spur generalized ICUs. A great number of innovators and investigators have developed ventilators that have contributed to the care of the critically ill and injured patients. Modern day intensivists on a daily basis must decide which mode of ventilation is compatible with the needs of an individual patient. Moreover, newer ventilators allow intensivists to combine dual breaths. In the future, new insights and design innovations in ventilators may advance beyond the current machines and modes of ventilation.

SUMMARY

The history of technology in the ICU spans five decades of pioneering work by dedicated investigators from medical, bioengineering and other fields. Technology has played a significant role in the advancement of the practice of critical care medicine. The understanding of hemodynamics, first by the PAC and subsequently by echocardiogram, has enhanced our understanding of the physiology of critical illness. The development of CRRT has allowed practitioners to dialyze ICU patients; the monitoring of oxygen saturation with pulse oximetry has provided continuous feedback for early warning systems. Mechanical ventilation and its history parallel the development of ICUs and its further development will likely lead to better care for patients. Technology will continue to play an important role in the ICU as new challenges in the care of critically ill and injured patients are faced.

ACKNOWLEDGMENTS

We would like to thank Denise McGinly for her help in preparing this article. We are also grateful to Karen Mitchell, Rosemary Schwedel and Betty Jean Swartz at Cooper University Hospital, New Jersey.

REFERENCES

1. Forssmann-Falck R. Werner Forssmann: a pioneer of cardiology. Am J Cardiol 1997;79(5):651–60.
2. Wilson JN, Grow JB, Demong CV, et al. Central venous pressure in optimal blood volume maintenance. Arch Surg 1962;85:563–78.
3. Sprung CL, Jacobs LJ. Indications for pulmonary artery catherization. In: Sprung CL, editor. The pulmonary artery catheter: methodology and clinical applications. 2nd edition. Baltimore (MD): University Park Press; 1984. p. 7–21.
4. Forrester JS, Diamond G, Chatterjee K, et al. Medical therapy of acute myocardial infarction by application of hemodynamic subsets. N Engl J Med 1976; 295(24):1356–62.
5. Weil MH, Shubin H, Rosoff L. Fluid Repletion in Circulatiory Shock: Central Venous Pressure and Other Practical Guides. JAMA 1965;192:668–74.
6. Cohen JD, Del Guercio LRM. Physiological assessment of patients who are high surgical risks. In: Weil MH, Henning RJ, editors. Handbook of critical care medicine. Chicago: Pub Yearbook Med Publishers; 1979. p. 9–30.
7. Shubin H, Weil MH, Rockwell MA Jr. Automated measurement of cardiac output in patients by use of a digital computer. Med Biol Eng 1967;5(4):353–60.
8. Jernigan WR, Gardner WC, Mohr MM, et al. Use of internal jugular vein for placement of central venous catheter. Surg Gynecol Obstet 1970;130(3):520–4.
9. Swan HJ. The pulmonary artery catheter. Dis Mon 1991;37(8):473–543.
10. Lategola M, Rhan H. A self-guiding catheter for cardiac and pulmonary arterial catheterization and occulsion. Proc Soc Exp Biol Med 1953;84(3):667–8.
11. Bradley RD. Diagnostic right-heart catheterization with miniature catheters in severely ill patients. Lancet 1964;2(7366):941–2.
12. Swan HJC, Ganz W, Forrester J, et al. Catheterization of the heart in man with use of a flow-directed balloon-tipped catheter. N Engl J Med 1970;283(9): 447–51.
13. Robin E. The cult of the Swan-Ganz catheter: overuse and abuse of pulmonary flow catheters. Ann Intern Med 1985;103(3):445–9.
14. Connor AF Jr, Speroff T, Dawson NV, et al. The effectiveness of right heart catheterization in the Initial care of critically ill patients. JAMA 1996;276(11):889–97.
15. Dalen JE, Bone RC. Is it time to pull the pulmonary artery catheter? JAMA 1996; 276(11):916–8.
16. Pulmonary Artery Catheter Consensus conference. Pulmonary Artery Catheter Consensus conference: consensus statement. Crit Care Med 1997;25(6): 910–25.
17. Watson R, Connors A, Bernard G. The Connors et al PAC Study, with expert commentary by Dr. Gordon Bernard. J Crit Care 2005;20(2):181–6.
18. Rubenfield G, McNamara-Aslin E, Rubison L. The pulmonary artery catheter 1967–2007 rest in peace? JAMA 2007;298(4):458–61.
19. Cotter G, Cotter OM, Kaluski E. Hemodynamic monitoring in acute heart failure. Crit Care Med 2008;36(1 Suppl):S40–3.
20. Wiener RS, Welch HG. Trends in the use of the pulmonary artery catheter in the United States 1993–2004. JAMA 2007;289(4):423–9.
21. Edler I, Lindstrom K. The history of echocardiography. Ultrasound Med Biol 2004;30(12):1565–644.
22. Feigenbaum H. History of echocardiography. In: Feigenbaum H, Armstrong WF, Ryan T, editors. Feingenbaum's echocardiography. 6th edition. New York: Lippincott Williams & Wilkins; 2004. p. 1–9.

23. Shors C. Cardiac function determined by echocardiogram. Crit Care Med 1975; 3(1):5–7.
24. Levy BI, Payen DM, Tedgui A, et al. Non-invasive ultrasonic cardiac output measurement in intensive care unit. Ultrasound Med Biol 1985;11(6):841–9.
25. Vieillard-Baron A, Slama M, Cholley B, et al. Echocardiography in the intensive care unit: from evolution to revolution? Intensive Care Med 2008;34(2):243–9.
26. Ozier Y, Gueret P, Jardin F, et al. Two-dimensional echocardiographic demonstration of acute myocardial depression in septic shock. Crit Care Med 1984; 12(7):596–9.
27. Parker MM, Shelhamer J, Bacharach S, et al. Profound but reversible myocardial depression in patients with septic shock. Ann Intern Med 1984;100(4):483–90.
28. Jardin F, Valtier B, Beauchet A, et al. Invasive monitoring combined with two-dimensional echocardiographic study in septic shock. Intensive Care Med 1994;20(8):550–4.
29. Krishnamoorthy VK, Sengupta PP, Gentile F, et al. History of echocardiography and its future applications in medicine. Crit Care Med 2007;35(8 Suppl): S309–13.
30. Seward JB, Khandheria BK, Freeman WK, et al. Multiplance transesophageal echocardiography: image orientation, examination technique, anatomic correlations and clinical applications. Mayo Clin Proc 1993;68(6):523–51.
31. Frazin L, Talano JV, Stephanides L, et al. Esophageal echocardiography. Circulation 1976;54(1):102–8.
32. Sohn DW, Shin GJ, Oh JL, et al. Role of transesophageal echocardiography in hemodynamically unstable patients. Mayo Clin Proc 1995;70(10):925–31.
33. Vieillard-Baron A, Prin S, Chergui K, et al. Hemodynamic instability in sepsis: bedside assessment by Doppler echocardiography. Am J Respir Crit Care Med 2003;168(11):1270–6.
34. Jardin F, Fourme T, Page B, et al. Persistent preload defect in severe sepsis despite fluid loading: a longitudinal echocardiographic study in patients with septic shock. Chest 1999;116(5):1354–9.
35. Vieillard-Baron A, Caille V, Charron C, et al. Actual incidence of global left ventricular hypokinesia in adult septic shock. Crit Care Med 2008;36(6):1701–6.
36. Diwan A, McCulloch M, Lawrie GM, et al. Doppler estimation of left ventricular filling pressures in patients with mitral valve disease. Circulation 2005;111(24):3281–9.
37. Jones AF, Tayal V, Sullivan D, et al. Randomized, controlled trial of immediate versus delayed goal-directed ultrasound to identify the cause of nontraumatic hypotension in the emergency department. Crit Care Med 2004;32(8): 1703–8.
38. Teschner M, Heidland A, Klassen A, et al. Georg Ganter a pioneer of peritoneal dialysis and his tragic academic demise at the hand of the Nazi regime. J Nephrol 2004;17(3):457–60.
39. Gottschalk CW, Fellner SK. History of the science of dialysis. Am J Nephrol 1997; 17:289–98.
40. Twardoski ZJ. History of hemodialyzers' designs. Hemodial Int 2008;12: 173–210.
41. Kolff WJ. First clinical experience with the artificial kidney. Ann Intern Med 1965; 62(3):608–19.
42. Malchesky PS. Artificial organs and vanishing boundaries. Artif Organs 2001; 30(2):75–88.
43. Uchino S, Kellum JA, Bellomo R, et al. Acute renal failure in critically ill patients. A multinational, multicenter study. JAMA 2005;294(7):813–8.

44. Bellomo R, Ronco C. Blood purification in the intensive care unit: evolving concepts. World J Surg 2001;25(5):677–83.
45. Bellamo R, Ronco C. Continuous versus intermittent renal replacement therapy in the intensive care unit. Kidney Int Suppl 1998;53(66):S125–8.
46. Kramer P, Kaufhold G, Grone HJ, et al. Management of anuric intensive-care patients with arteriovenous hemofiltration. Int J Artif Organs 1980;3(4):225–30.
47. Lauer A, Saccaggi A, Ronco C, et al. Continuous arteriovenous hemofiltration in the critically ill patient. Ann Intern Med 1983;99(4):455–60.
48. Burchardi H. History and development of continuous renal replacement techniques. Kidney Int Suppl 1998;53(66):S120–4.
49. Ricci Z, Bonello M, Salvatori G, et al. Continuous renal replacement technology: from adaptive technology and early dedicated machines towards flexible multipurpose machine platforms. Blood Purif 2004;22(3):269–76.
50. Dirkes S, Hodge K. Continuous renal replacement therapy in the adult intensive care unit: history and current trends. Crit Care Nurse 2007;27(2):61–80.
51. Bagshaw SM, Berthiaume LR, Delaney A, et al. Continuous versus intermittent renal replacement therapy for critically ill patients with acute kidney injury: a meta-analysis. Crit Care Med 2008;36(2):610–7.
52. Van Biesen W, Lameire N, Vanholder R. A tantalizing question: Ferrari or Rolls Royce? A meta-analysis on the ideal renal replacement modality for acute kidney injury at the intensive care unit. Crit Care Med 2008;36(2):649–50.
53. Kumar VA, Craig M, Depner TA, et al. Extended daily dialysis: a new approach to renal replacment for acute renal failure in the intensive care unit. Am J Kidney Dis 2000;36(2):294–300.
54. Ricci Z, Ronco C. Dose and efficiency of renal replacement therapy: continuous renal replacement therapy versus intermittent hemodialysis versus slow extended daily dialysis. Crit Care Med 2008;36(4 Suppl):S229–37.
55. Kellum JA, Bellamo R. Hemofiltration in sepsis: where do we go from here? Crit Care 2000;4(2):69–71.
56. Ronco C, Bellomo R, Homel P, et al. Effects of different doses in continuous veno-venous haemofiltration of outcomes of acute renal failure: a prospective randomized trial. Lancet 2000;356(9223):26–30.
57. Ratanarat R, Brendolan A, Ricci Z, et al. Pulse high-volume hemofiltration in critically ill patients:a new approach for patients with septic shock. Semin Dial 2006; 19(1):69–74.
58. Honore PM, Joannes-Boyau O, Gressens B. Blood and plasma treatments: high volume hemofiltration–a global view. Contrib Nephrol 2007;156:371–86.
59. Cruz D, Bellomo R, Kellum JA, et al. The future of extracorporeal support. Crit Care Med 2008;36(4 Suppl):S243–52.
60. Palvesky PM, Zhang JH, O'Connor TZ, et al. Intensity of renal support in critically ill patients with acute kidney injury. N Engl J Med 2008;359(1):7–20.
61. Severinghaus J, Kelleher J. Recent developments in pulse oximetry. Anesthesiology 1992;76(6):1018–38.
62. Ayogi T. Pulse oximetry: its invention, theory and future. J Anesth 2003;17(4): 259–66.
63. Severinghaus JW, Honda Y. History of blood gas analysis VII. Pulse oximetry. J Clin Monit 1987;3(2):135–8.
64. Tremper KK. Noninvasive monitoring of oxygenation and ventilation. 40 years in development. West J Med 1992;156(6):662–3.
65. Wukitsch MW, Petterson MT, Tobler DR, et al. Pulse oximetry: analysis of theory, technology and practice. J Clin Monit 1988;4(4):290–301.

66. Yelderman M, New W Jr. Evaluation of pulse oximetry. Anesthesiology 1983; 59(4):349–52.
67. Kelleher JF. Pulse oximetry. J Clin Monit 1989;5(1):37–62.
68. Mihm FG, Halperin BD. Noninvasive detection of profound arterial desaturations using a pulse oximetry device. Anesthesiology 1985;62(1):85–7.
69. Van de Louw A, Cracco C, Cerf C, et al. Accuracy of pulse oximetry in the intensive care unit. Intensive Care Med 2001;27(10):1606–13.
70. Jabran A, Tobin MJ. Reliability of pulse oximetry in titrating supplemental oxygen therapy in ventilator dependent patients. Chest 1990;97(6):1420–5.
71. Imman KJ, Sibbald WJ, Rutledge FS, et al. Does implementing pulse oximetry in a critical care unit result in substantial arterial blood gas savings. Chest 1993; 104(2):542–6.
72. Neff TA. Routine oximetry. A fifth vital sign? Chest 1988;94(2):227.
73. Tremper KK, Barker SJ. Pulse oximetry. Anesthesiology 1989;70:98–108.
74. Brown M, Vender JS. Noninvasive oxygen monitoring. Crit Care Clin 1988;4(3): 493–509.
75. Gehring H, Hornberger C, Matz H, et al. The effects of motion artifact and low perfusion on the performance of a new generation of pulse oximeters in volunteers undergoing hypoxemia. Respir Care 2002;47(1):48–60.
76. Petty TL. A historical perspective of mechanical ventilation. Crit Care Clin 1990; 6(3):489–504.
77. Somerson SJ, Sicilia MR. Historical perspectives of the development and use of mechanical ventilation. AANA J 1992;60(1):83–94.
78. Trubhovich RV. On the very first, successful, long-term, large scale use of IPPV. Albert Bower and V Ray Bennett: Los Angeles, 1948–1949. Crit Care Resusc 2007;9(1):91–100.
79. Zorab J. The resuscitation greats Bjorn Ibsen. Resuscitation 2003;57(1):3–9.
80. Colice G. Historical perspective on the development of mechanical ventilation. In: Tobin M, editor. Principles and practice of mechanical ventilation. 2nd edition. New York: McGraw-Hill; 2006. p. 1–36.
81. Snider GL. Historical ethical perspective on mechanical ventilation: from simple life support to dilemma. Am Rev Respir Dis 1989;140(2 Pt 2):S2–7.
82. Engstrom CG. Treatment of severe cases of respiratory paralysis by Engstrom universal respirator. Br Med J 1954;2(4889):666–9.
83. Petty TL. The modern evolution of mechanical ventilation. Clin Chest Med 1988; 9(1):1–10.
84. Morch ET. History of mechanical ventilation. In: Kirby R, Banner M, Downs J, editors. Clinical applications of ventilatory support. 2nd edition. New York: Churchill Livingstone; 1990. p. 1–62.
85. Morris MJ. Acute respiratory distress syndrome in combat casualties: military medicine and advances in mechanical ventilation. Mil Med 2006;171(11):1039–44.
86. Pontoppidan H, Wilson RS, Rie MA, et al. Respiratory intensive care. Anesthesiology 1977;47(2):96–116.
87. Banner MJ, Kirby DR. Mr. Jack Emerson–a matter of life and breath. Chest 1997; 112(2):307–8.
88. Safar P, Berman B, Daimond E, et al. Cuffed tracheotomy vs. tank respirator for prolonged artificial ventilation. Arch Phys Med Rehabil 1962;43:487–93.
89. Shapiro BA. A historical perspective on ventilator management. New Horiz 1994; 2(1):8–18.
90. McPherson SP, Spearman CB. Bellows ventilators. In: Respiratory therapy equipment. St. Louis (MO): C.V. Mosby Company; 1985. p. 398–467.

91. Frumin MJ, Berman NA, Holaday DA, et al. Alveolar-arterial O_2 differences during artificial respiration in man. J Appl Phys 1959;14:694–700.
92. Falke KJ. The introduction of positive end expiratory pressure into mechanical ventilation: a retrospective. Intensive Care Med 2003;29(8):1233–6.
93. Ashbaugh DG, Bigelow DB, Petty TL, et al. Acute respiratory distress in adults. Lancet 1967;2(7511):319–23.
94. Bernard G. Acute respiratory distress syndrome a historical perspective. Am J Respir Crit Care Med 2005;172:798–806.
95. Lozman J, Powers SR Jr, Older T, et al. Correlation of pulmonary wedge and left atrial pressures. A study in the patient receiving positive end expiratory pressure ventilation. Arch Surg 1974;109(2):270–7.
96. Downs JB, Klein EF Jr, Desautels D, et al. Intermittent mandatory ventilation: a new approach to weaning patients from mechanical ventilators. Chest 1973; 64(3):331–5.
97. Norlander O. New concepts of ventilation. Acta Anaestesiol Belg 1982;33(4): 221–34.
98. Esteban A, Anzueto A, Frutos F, et al. Characteristics and outcomes in adult patients receiving mechanical ventilation: a 28-day international study. JAMA 2002;287(3):345–55.
99. Mercat A, Titiriga M, Anguel N, et al. Inverse ratio ventilation (I/E = 2/1) in acute respiratory distress syndrome: a six-hour controlled study. Am J Respir Crit Care Med 1997;155(5):1637–42.
100. Stock MC, Downs JB, Frolicher DA. Airway pressure release ventilation. Crit Care Med 1987;15(5):462–6.
101. Rasanen J, Downs JB, Stock MC. Cardiovascular effects of conventional positive pressure release ventilation and airway pressure release ventilation. Chest 1988;93(5):911–5.
102. Habashi NM. Other approaches to open-lung ventilation: airway pressure release ventilation. Crit Care Med 2005;33(3):S228–40.

Historical Perspectives in Critical Care Medicine: Blood Transfusion, Intravenous Fluids, Inotropes/Vasopressors, and Antibiotics

Ryan Zarychanski, MD, FRCPC[a], Robert E. Ariano, PharmD[b],
Bojan Paunovic, MD, FRCPC[a], Dean D. Bell, MD, FRCPC[c],*

KEYWORDS

- Critical care • History of medicine • Blood transfusion
- Anti-bacterial agents • Vasoconstrictor agents
- Infusions • Intravenous

The field of Critical Care Medicine is now recognized as a distinct and essential medical specialty, providing care to those who are most severely ill and who need intensive monitoring. Key therapeutic advances in medicine, such as mechanical ventilation and invasive hemodynamic monitoring, have geographically defined the specialty within a hospital setting, but the needs of critically ill patients go beyond the walls of the intensive care unit (ICU). Though the need to care for seriously ill patients has been constant throughout time, the ability to fully appreciate the needs of the most critically ill and the capacity to provide meaningful care are recent advances in the history of medicine.

Significant progress in critical care medicine has been the result of tireless observation, dedicated research, and well-timed serendipity. This article provides a historical perspective for four meaningful therapies in critical care medicine: blood transfusion, fluid resuscitation, vasopressor/inotropic support, and antibiotics. For each therapy,

[a] Section of Critical Care Medicine, University of Manitoba, JJ399-700 William Avenue, Winnipeg, Manitoba, R3E 0Z3, Canada
[b] Department of Pharmacology & Therapeutics, Faculty of Medicine & Pharmacy, University of Manitoba, Department of Pharmacy, St. Boniface General Hospital, 409 Tache Avenue, Winnipeg, Manitoba R2H 2A6, Canada
[c] Section of Critical Care Medicine, Departments of Anesthesia and Medicine, University of Manitoba, JJ399-700 William Avenue, Winnipeg, Manitoba R3E 0Z3, Canada
* Corresponding author. Section of Critical Care Medicine/Health Sciences Centre, JJ399 - 700 William Avenue, Winnipeg, Manitoba R3E 0Z3, Canada.
E-mail address: dean1@mts.net (D.D. Bell).

Crit Care Clin 25 (2009) 201–220
doi:10.1016/j.ccc.2008.10.003
criticalcare.theclinics.com
0749-0704/08/$ – see front matter © 2009 Elsevier Inc. All rights reserved.

key discoveries and events that have shaped medical history and helped define current practice are discussed. Prominent medical and social pressures that have catalyzed research and innovation in each domain are also addressed, as well as current and future challenges.

HISTORY OF BLOOD TRANSFUSION IN CRITICAL ILLNESS

The transfusion of blood and blood components is a relatively recent practice in the history of medicine, but man's fascination with blood dates back to before the common era. Blood was revered by the Greeks as one of four essential humors, and was thought to contain a person's vital essence according to Romans.[1] Believed to have mercurial powers, blood was drained to expunge evil and transfused to soothe mental illness. Rooted in our understanding of physiology and perfected by war, blood transfusions are now routine practice among the critically ill and are administered to 42% to 50% of patients during the course of an ICU admission.[2,3] Expensive and not without risk, blood transfusions are nonetheless an indispensible therapy administered to millions of patients per year.

Venesection, or blood letting, was widely practiced from the time of Hippocrates into the nineteenth century; however, transfusion only gained acceptance as a necessary medical therapy in the last 100 years.[1] The transfusion of blood first required a working knowledge of anatomy and circulation, credited to the British physician William Harvey in 1628.[4] Direct transfusion between two animals was reported by Richard Lower (Oxford) in 1665 and, ironically, though Lower successfully resuscitated hypovolemic dogs, blood transfusions would not be used to treat hemorrhage for more than 150 years. In 1667, Jean-Baptiste Denis (France), published his experience with transfusion of lamb's blood to a human being (**Fig. 1**).[4] The indication in this case was mental illness, with the idea that the blood of a docile animal would impart calm when administered to the deranged.[1]

Blood transfusion in the sixteenth century was controversial and poor outcomes prompted bans on the practice. Bans were imposed by the British Royal Society (1668), the French Government, and the Vatican in 1669.[5] Significant progress did not occur until 1795, when Philip Syng Physick suggested human-to-human transfusion.[5] It was not until 1818 that James Blundell, a London obstetrician, reported the first human-to-human transfusion to treat postpartum hemorrhage. At the time, Blundell knew nothing of human blood groups or aseptic technique; successes were frequent enough to encourage the operation's continued use, while failures were attributed to clotted blood or to the hopeless state of the patient.[6]

Karl Landsteiner (Vienna) transformed the practice of transfusion with his discovery of the ABO blood antigen system in 1901—a discovery for which he would later receive the Nobel Prize for Medicine and Physiology. Landsteiner carefully observed that serum from some individuals would cause clumping of reds cells isolated from other patients. The next defining event in the evolution of transfusion occurred in 1915, when Richard Lewinsohn (Mt. Sinai Hospital, NY) showed that a 0.2% solution of sodium citrate could safely anticoagulate collected blood.[1] The following year, the addition of dextrose was shown to reduce hemolysis of blood that was stored for 2 weeks.[7] These advances meant that the physical presence of a live donor was no longer a requirement. Red cell viability and storage would be later optimized and prolonged with cold storage and the addition of phosphate. As the world prepared for World War I, the practice of blood transfusion gained in popularity throughout America. British physicians, however, were more interested in the merits of saline as a blood alternative.

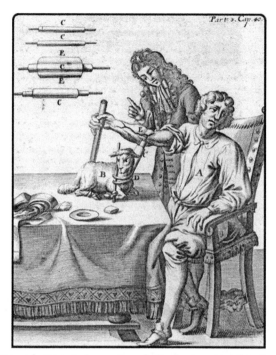

Fig. 1. Early depiction of attempted xeno-transfusion by Jean-Baptiste Denis.

Blood and War

The practice of blood transfusion has been, and continues to be, shaped by trauma and violence. At the start of World War I, American physicians were the most experienced with transfusion. However, because the United States did not enter the war for 3 years after Britain and Canada, it was Bruce Robertson, a Canadian physician with United States training, who first introduced blood transfusions to war surgery. Robertson was convinced that whole blood was superior to the saline infusions used by the British, and first described the use of transfusion to treat secondary hemorrhage (not battlefield resuscitation) in four soldiers.[8] Given the urgency of treatment, Robertson decried the value of pretransfusion compatibility testing, and regarded hemolysis as "unlikely." In his original publication, one of four transfused soldiers appeared to have died from an acute hemolytic reaction. Robertson generally used citrate as an anticoagulant and performed the procedure using a syringe and cannula.

When America entered World War I in 1917, transfusion gained wider acceptance and practice. As this was before the days of blood banks, "front-line units" were collected from soldiers willing and ready to give blood in an instant. In World War I, appreciation for the significance of time to resuscitation developed. Though transfusions were not widely performed in the setting of primary shock, the speed of resuscitation was correlated to survival; death came to those with significant treatment delays.[9]

World War II provided the stimulus for mass organized transfusion services. Convinced of the importance of whole blood resuscitation, the British moved quickly to establish blood depots in London as war approached. The British model was to collect blood centrally and to forward the product to the battlefront. America, however, initially decided that transfusion was too difficult and dangerous to disseminate on a global scale. That decision would later be regretted and revisited as a result of constant blood shortages and perceived reductions in survival of American, compared with British, casualties.[10] As the war progressed, a national blood program was established in the United States that would eventually collect and provide massive quantities of blood for use overseas. With the need to transport, store, and use blood more effectively, the concept and technique of blood fractionation was developed at Harvard Medical School by Edwin Cohn in the 1940s.[11] The following year, albumin produced with Cohn's methods would be used for the first time to treat the wounded at Pearl Harbor.[1]

Since its introduction in World War I, blood transfusion has been, and continues to be an integral component of armed conflicts involving United States military personnel. The successes seen with blood transfusions and wartime blood banking were quickly adapted for peace-time use. At the end of World War I, hospital blood banks and national blood services were established around the world. The demand for blood fractions, especially plasma-derived products, created new a global commercial market for blood.[12]

Recent Developments

Fractionation of blood has created a variety of therapeutic products for patients diagnosed with bleeding disorders or immunologic diseases. However, the arrival of human immunodeficiency virus and hepatitis altered the practice and business of transfusion forever, after it was discovered that the products administered to hemophiliacs or to patients with severe bleeding were also a source of infection. With the late 1980s and 1990s came an expensive new medical armamentarium of recombinant factors, blood substitutes, and blood-conserving therapies. Physicians increasingly pursued the unattainable goal of zero-risk transfusion strategies. While some of these products, such as recombinant factors VIII and IX, have restored health and confidence to those with hemophilia, the role of other products, such as recombinant factor VIIa, are still being evaluated in clinical trials. Leukoreduction (removal of white cells from donated blood) has been shown to decrease febrile nonhemolytic transfusion reactions[13] and to decrease postoperative infection.[14] Universal leukoreduction has been implemented in many developed countries, such as Canada, Britain, and France since the late 1990s. The United States has been slow to adopt this technology universally, but is moving toward this goal. Interest in autologous blood donations has expanded in light of concerns regarding transfusion-transmitted infections, but this modality has a limited role in combat or severe unexpected bleeding, and has not been proven to be associated with decreased risk of viral infection. The future of this transfusion option is uncertain amid the remarkable safety of the present-day blood supply.

Blood is a limited resource and, given the shrinking available donor pool and real or perceived risks associated with transfusion, substantial effort has been made to reduce patient exposure to allogeneic blood. On the battlefield, compression devices and early evacuation, combined with the use of factor VIIa and a high ratio of plasma to red cells, are employed with the intention of limiting shock and reducing transfusion requirements. In the ICU, multiple strategies can be employed to reduce blood loss and lessen anemia, including closed blood sampling, small-volume sample tubes, and point-of-care testing.[15] Furthermore, the recently demonstrated safety of a lower pretransfusion hemoglobin concentration among ICU patients has given physicians the opportunity to withhold transfusions when they previously would have administered blood.[16]

Future Challenges

While substantial progress has been made in the field of transfusion, significant challenges remain. Several artificial blood substitutes, oxygen-carrying compounds that are stable over time, do not require pretransfusion testing, and do not transmit disease, have been evaluated in clinical trials. Unfortunately, those that have been tested have been found to increase mortality.[17] Platelet substitutes may be closer to clinical fruition but are still under development. Red cell stimulating agents (eg, erythropoietin) are not associated with improvements in clinically significant outcomes and likely do not alter transfusion requirements when a restrictive transfusion practice is adopted.[18] The in vitro culture and differentiation of human stem cells to produce specific blood components is conceivable, but far from reality.

Observations and experience from current armed conflicts continue to shape our thinking of blood transfusion. Recent experiences from Iraq have demonstrated the benefit of increased transfusion of plasma relative to red cell units. Increased plasma-to red cell-ratio has been associated with decreased mortality, primarily because of less uncontrolled hemorrhage.[19] The observed benefit has prompted a call for increased up-front transfusion of coagulation factor-containing products for patients requiring massive transfusion.[20,21] Moreover, combat support hospitals and some large civilian trauma centers are now using thawed plasma, which is released 1:1 with emergency red cell units.[19] Fresh whole blood has been used in every combat operation since World War I and has been demonstrated to improve hemoglobin concentration while limiting dilutional coagulopathy. While fresh whole blood is not feasible in civilian blood banks, how we order and administer fractionated blood products represents an important consideration in our global quest to use this scare resource as effectively as possible.

HISTORY OF INTRAVENOUS FLUIDS

The first therapeutic infusion of intravenous fluid was provided on May 15, 1832 by Scottish physician Dr. Thomas Latta.[22] The impetus for the new therapy was epidemic cholera. At the time, therapies for cholera included administration of emetics, forced exsanguinations (bleeding), and assorted physical assaults.[23] The novel concept of infusing salt-containing fluids to moribund cholera patients was developed by 22-year-old Irish physician Dr. William Brooke O'Shaughnessy,[24] who initially conceived of treating cholera "by the injection of highly-oxygenated salts into the venous system." This theory was later revised, and in a subsequent report to the Central Board of Health of London (later reviewed by the *Lancet*), O'Shaughnessy[25] concluded that the aims of treatment were to restore the blood to its natural specific gravity and to replace deficient saline matters. He further suggested that this could only be accomplished by "absorption, imbibition or intravenous injection." Thomas Latta infused saline solutions into patients less than 7 weeks after O'Shaughnessy's recommendations were published.[23] Latta's report described a fluid composition (calculated by Awad and colleagues)[26] of Na^+ 48 mmol/L to 68 mmol/L, Cl^- 38 mmol/L to 59 mmol/L, and HCO_3^- 9 mmol/L.[27] Practical experience taught Latta that repeated infusions were often necessary and that large volumes (up to 3.5 L) were needed.[28]

Despite the physiologic correctness of intravenous fluid administration in dehydrated cholera patients, the therapy did not gain popularity until the end of the nineteenth century. Enthusiasm for this new therapy waned when Latta died of tuberculosis in 1833 and when O'Shaughnessy emigrated from England that same year.[26] Practical factors also hampered the uptake of intravenous-fluid therapy. In the early 1830s equipment for intravenous infusion was not well developed, the concepts of bacteria and sterility were unknown, and the fluids used were chemically impure and usually hypotonic.[29] Intravenous fluid infusion was only used in moribund patients, so success was not assured. Large volumes were needed but "...the more fluid was given, even with good intentions, the greater was the chance of bacteremia, pyrogen reactions, and hemolysis."[29] However sound the rationale, the idea was much ahead of contemporary knowledge of physiologic chemistry and microbiology.

Multiple scientific advances over the next 80 years helped intravenous fluid infusion gain acceptance. The pathophysiology of dehydration was described by Carl Schmidt in 1850; Claude Bernard conceptualized the "milieu interieur" in 1859; Jacobus H. Vant Hoff defined osmosis in 1887; E. H. Starling described fluid flux across membranes in 1896 and Starling's "Law of the Heart" had been published by 1915; ionization of electrolytes was discovered in 1903 by S. A. Arrhenius; and hydrogen ion equilibrium was reported by L. J. Henderson between 1906 and 1920.[28] Between 1882 and 1898, research documenting the beneficial effects of saline solutions for the treatment hemorrhage and trauma helped to establish intravenous fluid as a useful therapy.[30,31]

The composition of intravenous fluids developed from careful study and serendipity. After observing that isolated frog hearts performed better when his lab assistant used water supplied by the New River Water Company instead of distilled water, Sydney Ringer (England) (**Fig. 2**) developed a physiologic solution for perfusion in 1876. Ringer determined that New River Company water had significant calcium content, and demonstrated that sodium, potassium, calcium, and chloride in precise proportions are necessary for cardiac contraction.[32,33] Ringer's solution saw widespread use as a perfusion medium, and was modified by the addition of lactate in 1934 by Alexis Hartman (United States) to create Ringer's lactate solution for intravenous infusion.[32,34] Readers interested in more detail on saline infusions are referred to the review by Awad and colleagues on the history of 0.9% saline.[26] A review on the history of vascular access by Dudrick is also suggested.[35]

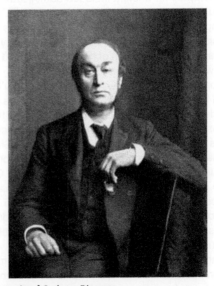

Fig. 2. Photographic portrait of Sydney Ringer.

Fluid Infusion for Shock and Surgery

Albert Landerer (Germany) and Rudolph Matas (United States) pioneered saline infusions in the management of surgical patients.[36,37] Patients had to be extremely ill to receive intravenous fluids and proctoclysis (rectal administration of fluid); hypodermoclysis (subcutaneous isotonic fluid adminstration) and intraperitoneal fluid administration were more established techniques at this time.[34] By the early twentieth century, intravenous saline infusions had become iso- or hypertonic and many contained sodium bicarbonate to combat the acidosis commonly found in shock patients. At the beginning of the century, hypertonic bicarbonate solutions were used in India and the Philippines to reduce mortality in cholera victims.[38,39] In 1918, Walter Cannon (United States) advocated wartime resuscitation with intravenous injection of a 4% (hypertonic) solution of sodium bicarbonate. Cannon[40] was also mindful to the note potential harms associated with aggressive fluid resuscitation, such that, "If the pressure is raised before the surgeon is ready to check any bleeding that may take place, blood that is sorely needed may be lost." Stored whole blood was infused for the first time during World War I, but blood was infrequently transfused because of the popularity of colloid solutions, which were believed to restore intravascular volume and tissue perfusion more rapidly, and with more prolonged effect when compared with crystalloids.[41,42]

An early attempt to use colloid occurred in 1837 when John Macintosh (Scotland)[43] added albumin from eggs to saline infusion solutions in an attempt to "make the fluid resemble the serum of blood." The first synthetic colloid used in human beings was a gelatin solution (1915); however, vegetable colloid solutions (gum arabic, acacia, pectin) were more widely used, given their relative purity and ease of administration.[44] Serious side effects curtailed acacia-based colloid solutions in the early 1920s. Colloid use subsided after World War I, as blood transfusion became more common and saline infusions appeared safer than the available colloids.

World War II was a significant catalyst for intravenous infusion development. During that war a synthetic compound called polyvinylpyrrolidine was produced as a colloid plasma substitute (*Periston*) and was used extensively by the German Army Medical Services until concerns about carcinogenicity and storage within the reticulo-endothelial system curtailed its use.[42,44] Other developments during World War II included: the development of starch-based solutions (amylase degradation however prevented their clinical use); industrial fractionation of blood allowing production of 25% human albumin solutions;[45] and production of dextran solutions.[42,44] Gelatin solutions became viable in the early 1950s as chemical modifications allowed liquidity to 10°C. Hydroxyethyl starch solutions resistant to amylase degradation entered clinical use between 1964 and 1966.[42,44] Colloid solutions grew more popular when it was appreciated that restoration of intravascular volume and tissue perfusion was more rapid and more durable with colloids compared with crystalloids. Despite these characteristics, colloids have never been shown to be superior to crystalloids when important clinical outcomes are considered.[46]

No review of fluid therapy would be complete without acknowledging the contributions of James Gamble (United States), who advanced our understanding of body-fluid physiology by defining the extracellular fluid (ECF) and its response to loss by fasting. Gamble introduced new terms (eg, mEq/l) to describe concentrations in solutions, and graphically related cations and anions via bar graphs, which became known as Gamblegrams.[47] ECF became a focus for investigators from the University of Michigan, and influential studies by Moyer, Coller, and Moore resulted in the practice of fluid restriction during and after surgery on the basis of "postoperative salt intolerance," whereby retained sodium caused water to shift from the intracellular to extracellular spaces.[48,49] Experiments in the early 1960s by Tom Shires in Texas resulted in marked changes in practice after he reported the existence of a "functional extracellular fluid volume deficit" in dogs with hemorrhagic shock. In addition to replacement of the lost blood, Shires advocated for the infusion-balanced salt solutions to correct extracellular fluid deficits.[50] Although Shires' original studies did not use the term, the ECF deficit he postulated came to be known as the "third space."[51]

Shires' work on extracellular fluid deficits profoundly influenced the opinions and practice of fluid therapy. In response to Shires' experimental reports, physicians began to infuse Ringer's lactate in larger and larger quantities to surgical patients and to patients with hemodynamic compromise.[52] Moore and Shires issued a plea for "moderation" in 1967, as they became concerned that perioperative fluid administration was excessive.[53] Recently, investigators have questioned the existence of an ECF deficit or "third space," and some have speculated that Shires' original results may have been artifacts of radioactive sulfate tracers.[54] Shires[55] has disputed this speculation; however, the debate has encouraged new studies of restrictive and hypertonic fluid administration in shock and surgical patients.[56,57]

The field of intravenous fluid therapy continues to evolve in response to new ideas and innovative research. In 1983, Peter Stewart (Canada) described a mathematical approach to acid base balance defining the strong ion difference ($[Na+K]-[Cl]$) as a major determinant of the hydrogen ion concentration. Stewart classified the metabolic acidosis following saline infusion as a decreased strong anion difference acidosis.[58] This approach has encouraged physicians to reconsider the widespread use of 0.9% saline infusions in patients without large chloride losses.[56] Other contemporary influences on fluid administration in ICU patients include William Shoemaker's suggestions to provide resuscitation to "supranormal" goals,[59] and Emanuel Rivers' advocacy of "early goal-directed resuscitation" in patients with septic shock.[60]

The quest for the ideal replacement fluid continues to be a matter of intense research and passionate debate. In 1998, concerns regarding potentially harmful consequences from albumin administration were raised.[61] These concerns were assuaged with the results of the SAFE (saline versus albumin fluid evaluation) trial, which demonstrated the relative safety of 4% albumin compared with 0.9% saline in critically ill patients.[62] Post-hoc analysis of this trial, however, has called into question the safety of albumin in specific patient subgroups, especially those with severe head injury.[63] The safety of hydroxyethyl starch solutions garnered recent attention given the results of the VISEP (volume substitution and insulin therapy in severe sepsis) trial, which demonstrated adverse renal outcomes with hydroxyethyl starch administration in septic shock patients.[64] Though newer, lower molecular-weight starches are now available for use and have been marketed as safer alternatives to previous starch compounds, clinical trials examining relevant clinical endpoints have not yet been conducted.

HISTORY OF THE DEVELOPMENT OF VASOPRESSORS AND INOTROPES

In 1893, Dr. George Oliver, a physician from Harrowgate, England investigated the effects of various glandular extracts on the diameter of the radial artery using a self-made instrument he called an "arteriometer." Using his son as a research subject, Oliver found that the ingestion of sheep adrenal extracts caused vasoconstriction.[65] The following year, further collaboration with acclaimed physiologist Edward Schafer at University College in London led to the discovery of the extract's blood pressure-raising properties in a variety of animal models.[66] Oliver and Schafer isolated the active effects to the adrenal medulla; however, the active constituent was unknown.

Research on vasoactive adrenal extracts continued and, in 1897, both John Jacob Abel (the first Professor of Pharmacology at Johns Hopkins University) and Otto von Furth (from the University of Strasbourg) isolated stable, but mostly inactive, derivatives of the active compound. Von Furth was able to bring his iron-based compound to market as a weak hemostatic agent under the trade name "Suprarenin."[67] Abel claimed his benzoate derivative was the active substance of the adrenal gland and called it "epinephrin,"[68] based on a suggestion that *epinephris* would be the best name for the suprarenal capsule.[69] Unfortunately, Abel's extract never behaved as robustly as the crude adrenal extract.

A pure crystalline form of the active adrenal extract that was 2,000 times more potent than either von Furth's or Abel's compounds was successfully isolated in 1900 by the Japanese chemist Jokichi Takamine[70] (**Fig. 3**). After obtaining a patent for the substance, Takamine[71] published his research in 1901. The product was marketed in the United States by Parke Davis & Co., using the proprietary name "Adrenalin." Epinephrin became the generic name, based on Abel's description of the compound, which he was never able to fully isolate.[69] Interestingly, Takamine visited Abel at his laboratory in late 1900 and discussed the possibility of a simpler isolation process. Takamine, however, had already made significant progress in that regard before that visit.[70,72] Abel would later publish assertions that the chemical structure of Takamine's compound formula was incorrect and not a pure form of epinephrine. Years later it was shown that Takimine's natural epinephrine product was found to contain nearly 40% norepinephrine.[72]

In the United Kingdom, "adrenaline" was used as the generic name. This was due to the influence of Nobel laureate physiologist Henry Dale, who insisted upon the term "adrenaline" because Abel's extract "epinephrine" showed minimal physiologic activity. In 1906, adrenaline became the first hormone to be synthesized de novo due to the

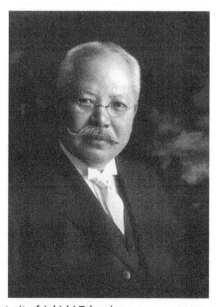

Fig. 3. Photographic portrait of Jokichi Takamine.

work of Friederich Stolz and Fritz Flacher. The first synthetic adrenaline, however, had half the potency of naturally derived adrenaline because of the presence of a weak dextrorotatory isomer. Flacher discovered that the unwanted isomer could be dissolved, leaving the highly active levorotatory isomer. This discovery facilitated the large-scale production of an adrenaline compound with identical activity to that of naturally derived adrenaline.[67]

The first detailed report of the actions of adrenaline on the heart was published in 1905 by Thomas Elliot.[73] Elliot was also the first to describe adrenaline as an excitatory neurotransmitter. In his original communication, Elliot[74] reported that adrenalin was the "chemical stimulant liberated on each occasion when the [axonal] impulse arrives at the periphery." In 1910, the chemist George Barger and pharmacologist Sir Henry Dale studied more than 50 adrenaline-related synthetic amines and proposed the term "sympathomimetic" to describe their actions.[75] There is some evidence to suggest that George Crile, a leading cardiovascular physiologist and surgeon at the turn of the century, may have been the first to use infusions of epinephrine products for the management of shock between 1900–1910.

Japan's first doctorate of pharmacy, Nagojosi Nagai, isolated ephedrine from the extracts of the Ma Huang (Ephedra sinica) plant in 1885. Ephedrine was first chemically synthesized in 1920 and was found to be structurally similar to adrenaline. In 1923, it was shown that ephedrine caused renal vasoconstriction and sustained elevations in blood pressure and heart rate when injected into dogs. Unlike adrenaline, ephedrine was long-acting and orally bioavailable. These properties prompted further research, which lead to its initial widespread use as a bronchodilator for the treatment of asthma.[67]

In 1927, chemist Helmut Legerlotz synthesized the adrenaline analogs synephrine and its isomer phenylephrine. In the United States, phenylephrine was initially marketed as an oral decongestant, although its intravenous form is used widely use as a vasopressor. Synephrine was marketed as a vasoconstrictor by the German company C.H. Boehringer of Ingelheim. In 1941 the company also marketed Aludrin, an isopropyl analog of adrenaline. Aludrin was found to have significant bronchodilatory effects without the hypertensive complications of adrenaline. The clinical utility of this drug was only appreciated after World War II, when it was approved in the United States and renamed Isuprel (isoproterenol).[67] Morris Nathanson and Harold Miller[76] described its selective chronotropic effects in comparison to adrenaline and noradrenaline. Isoproternol use in the treatment of cardiogenic shock was reviewed by Ludwig Eichna in 1968. Its use as an inotropic agent is limited by predominant chronotropic effects.[77] In 1975, Ronald Tuttle and Jack Mills[78] showed that removing isoproterenol's side-chain hydroxyl group resulted in a molecule with potent inotropic properties and less arrythmogenic and vascular side effects. This compound would become known as "dobutamine."

Although noradrenaline was synthesized independently by Friedrich Stolz and Henry Dakin in 1904, its role as the primary sympathetic neurotransmitter in mammals was not elucidated until 1946, by Ulf von Euler.[79] Its clinical use as a vasopressor was not documented until 1949.[80] Evidence supporting noradrenaline as a potent agent for the treatment of hypotension soon followed.[81]

In 1910, George Barger and Arthur Ewins, as well as Carl Mannich, independently reported dopamine synthesis. Various investigators observed that dopamine possessed cardiovascular activity but was less potent than epinephrine or norepinephrine.[82] Its clinical use in shock states was not published until the late 1960s and early 1970s.[83,84] Though the naturietic properties of dopamine are well described, its utility as a renal protective agent (also referred to as "low dose dopamine treatment") has been disproven.[85]

Of utmost importance in the history of adrenergic substances is the landmark article by pharmacologist Raymond Ahlquist,[86] describing his theory of different receptors (alpha and beta) accounting for heterogeneous effects in various tissues in response to the same "adrenotropic" mediators. His explanation and chart summaries are now considered essential introductory pharmacology. Like other revolutionary new discoveries in medicine, Ahlquist had difficulty getting his initial manuscript published and widespread acceptance of his new paradigm took more than a decade.[87]

During the 1950s and 60s, a variety of different drugs were used for the treatment of hypotension, many of which have since fallen out of favor.[88] Metaraminol, an amine with similar direct effects as noradrenaline, and indirect effects secondary to the release of endogenous noradrenaline, was touted as the most beneficial vasopressor.[89] Its prolonged action facilitated administration by intermittent subcutaneous or intramuscular injections without causing tissue necrosis. Metaraminol was also purported to preserve renal perfusion more than other agents.[90] The development of tachyphylaxis, lack of titratability, and poor intravenous cross-compatibility prevented its widespread use. Methoxamine, a potent long-acting pure alpha-adnergic agonist, was found to inhibit cardiac output and cause peripheral edema; its use therefore diminished in favor of phenylephrine.[91] Angiotensin resulted in splanchnic and coronary vasoconstriction and suffered from poor titratibility.[91] Mephentermine was minimally potent as an inotrope or vasopressor and its use was complicated by adverse reaction, such as seizures and neuropsychiatric effects.[92]

Nonadrenal glandular extracts have also resulted in the development of alternate vasopressor agents. In 1895, Oliver and Schafer were able to show that pituitary extracts raised blood pressure.[93] In 1953, Vincent Du Vigneaud determined the chemical structures of the peptide hormones oxytocin and vasopressin, and synthesized these compounds. He was awarded the Nobel Prize in Chemistry for this work in 1955.[67] Although the use of vasopressin for the treatment of hypotension in human beings was reported as early as 1965,[94] clinical trials defining its role have only been recently conducted. A large and definitive randomized, controlled trial comparing vasopressin and norepinephrine in septic shock showed no difference in mortality or in other relevant clinical outcome measures.[95]

In the late 1970s, novel nonadrenergic inotropic agents were being developed by the Sterling-Winthrop Research Institute. Amrinone was originally tested as a bronchodilator and, subsequently, the more potent and less toxic derivative milrinone was developed.[96,97] These bypyridine-derivatives increase intracellular calcium via phosphodiesterase III inhibition and are considered to be inodilators, due to their concomitant vasodilatory properties.

Despite decades of development and a long history of use, debate persists regarding the best choice of vasopressor or inotrope. Current international guidelines suggest the use of dopamine or noradrenaline as first-line agents for the management of septic shock; however, this remains a grade 1C recommendation (strong recommendation, weak evidence).[98] Much progress has been made and many lifesaving compounds now exist, but after more than 100 years we have yet to determine the optimal pharmacologic approach to the failing circulation.

HISTORY OF ANTIMICROBIALS IN CRITICAL CARE

The care of infections in the critically ill has made dramatic strides since the release of the first sulfonamide antibiotic, Prontosil in 1935. World War II provided the initial motivation behind further antibiotic developments, when staphylococcal infections and gas gangrene unresponsive to sulfonamides were killing more men than organ damage from gun fire.[99] After the development of the first penicillins, the story takes on a character analogous to the tale of *Sisyphus* from Greek mythology. As one antibiotic is discovered and used to treat an infectious disease, resistance soon appears, and we roll backward into the preantibiotic era. This story is applicable today, as in the 1940s, with only brief periods of hubris following the advent of broad-spectrum antibiotics in the late 1960s when the United States Surgeon General William H. Stewart declared we can "close the book on infectious disease."[100] Today, critical care medicine has moved beyond simply awaiting the arrival of the next antibiotic to one of improved use of existing agents to better cure disease and simultaneously minimize the expression of drug resistance. Early aggressive intervention, rapidly abbreviated courses of therapy, antibiotic combinations, and pharmacodynamically optimized dosing regimens are all activities directed toward retaining these agents in critical care for many years to come.

In this section, historical perspectives, contemporary uses, and clinical challenges of selected antibiotics are presented. Although the discovery of penicillin by Alexander Fleming in 1928 is the recognized starting point in the history of antimicrobial development, the focus of this review will be limited to the development of recent and novel antimicrobials.

Cephalosporins

The first cephalosporin identified was *Cephalosporium acremonium*, which was isolated near a sewer outlet off the coast of Sardinia in 1948 by Giuseppe Brotzu.[101] Structurally similar to the other beta-lactam antibiotics, cephalosporins appeared to inhibit bacterial cell-wall synthesis in a manner similar to penicillins. The cephalosporins were classified in generations based somewhat on their spectrum of activity.[102]

One of the greatest challenges in the early 1990s in critical care had been the identification of cases of resistance, which developed on therapy with third-generation cephalosporins.[103,104] Especially noted with Enterobacter, it was soon discovered that Amp-C beta-lactamase production resulting from simple exposure to these agents subsequently lead to these failures. Increased stability against the Amp-C beta-lactamases came about with the release of the fourth-generation cephalosporin, cefepime, in 1994. In the spring of 2008, the Food and Drug Administration released an approval letter for ceftobiprole, the latest broad spectrum cephalosporin with excellent activity against methicillin-resistant *Staphylococcus aureus* (MRSA).

Glycopeptides

With the rise in penicillin-resistant staphylococcal infections in the early 1950s, Eli Lilly aggressively pursued a campaign of searching for compounds with greater activity against these pathogens. In 1952, a missionary in Borneo had sent a sample of dirt to his friend, Dr. E. C. Kornfield, who worked for Eli Lilly.[105] From this sample, the organism *Streptomyces orientalis* was identified, which produced a substance referred to as "compound 05,865." This substance had activity confined to gram-positive organisms, including penicillin-resistant staphylococci. To suggest that science was winning the war over penicillin-resistant staphylococcus, or "vanquishing" the enemy, they named the compound "vancomycin."[105] A common misconception was that the drug was made from Mississippi mud, but this term actually came from the very brown color of the original product. As a consequence, it required extensive purification before it was ready for clinical trials.

Vancomycin was introduced into clinical practice in 1958, with its greatest impact being in the management of infections caused by methicillin-resistant Staphylococci *Enterococcus* and *Clostridia*. The significant challenge with vancomycin has been the sudden appearance of vancomycin-resistant enterococci (VRE) in United States hospitals in the late 1980s, vancomycin-intermediately susceptible S. aureus (VISA) in Japan in 1996, and vancomycin-resistant S. aureus (VRSA) in the United States in 2002. The latest glycopeptide discoveries, oritavancin, telavancin, and dalbavancin, have shown favourable activity against some of these resistant gram-positive pathogens, and improved pharmacokinetic and pharmacodynamic properties.[106]

Carbapenems

The carbapenems were a new class of beta-lactam antibiotics first identified as thienamycin in 1977 by workers from England and Ciba-Geigy out of Switzerland.[107] N-formimidolyl thienamycin, renamed imipenem, was the first stable derivative of thienamycin, which was isolated from the natural occurring soil organism, Streptomyces cattleya.[108,109] Workers at the time were focused on agents with increased affinity for penicillin-binding proteins and beta-lactamase stability, and thus more broadly active compounds.[107] Researched by Merck pharmaceuticals in the early 1980s, imipenem was noted to have enhanced activity against aerobic and anaerobic gram-positive and gram-negative bacteria, including Pseudomonas.[110]

The challenge with imipenem in critical care had been that seizures occurred with drug accumulation, especially evident in those with renal failure. Meropenem was released in 1996 as a carbapenem with enhanced gram-negative activity and a better safety profile, particularly as related to a lower potential for seizures.[108] Overall, imipenem retained greater activity against gram-positive pathogens, while meropenem had better activity against gram-negative organisms. Newer carbapenems include ertapenem (with activity comparable to ceftriaxone) and doripenem (with activity comparable to meropenem). The notable exception to the broad activity of this class of drugs is the susceptibility of all the carbapenems to the zinc-metalloenzymes or carbapenemases. First identified within Stenotrophonomas maltophilia, this group of resistance enzymes has begun to migrate to other gram-negative species, particularly Acinetobacter.[99] In critical care, the carbapenems have found the unique role of being the broadest, empiric therapy for serious pneumonia, septicemia, and intra-abdominal sepsis.

Fluoroquinolones

The fluoroquinolones were relatively novel agents developed in the mid-1980s as a result of modifications to their predecessor and first-generation quinolone, nalidixic acid (released in 1962).[111] The basic nalidixic acid structure originated from the liquor remaining after fermentation of quinine from cinchona bark.[112] The hopes at the time in critical care were for a workhorse antimicrobial with a broad spectrum of activity against common infecting gram-negative and gram-positive pathogens. Bayer pharmaceuticals led the effort, pursuing an agent within this class with broad activity, optimal pharmacokinetics, and improved safety over earlier antibiotics. The first broadly used agent of this class was norfloxacin, which was ideal for enteric therapy in that it had very poor gastrointestinal absorption. Subsequently, agents including ciprofloxacin, ofloxacin, and moxifloxacin with better systemic absorption and broader range of activity were successfully introduced to market in the last two decades.

The challenge with the fluoroquinolones has been the very rapid rise in resistance development. Since its introduction to market, ciprofloxacin-resistant Pseudomonas aeruginosa in ICUs in the United States has gone from 11.2% in 1993 up to 28.9% in 2004.[113] Another major challenge with the fluoroquinolone class has been a number of severe postmarketing adverse reactions, leading to rapid market withdrawal of some of the most promising agents within the class. Trovafloxacin had been associated with at least 14 acute toxic liver reactions, while grepafloxacin was associated with cardiotoxicity from QT prolongation, and gatifloxacin with dysglycemic reactions.

Oxazolidinones

The oxazolidinones were developed by DuPont de Nemours & Company in 1978 for the treatment of fungal and bacterial diseases of tomatoes and other plants.[99] With a rise in predominance of gram-positive infections in ICUs in the early 1980s, DuPont had discovered a new class of compounds with strong activity against this spectrum. Their purely synthetic nature raised hopes that bacteria would not be able to easily develop resistance to this class. Failures, however, in finding a compound free of marrow toxicity lead to their early abandonment by the company. With the rise of VRE and MRSA in the late 1990s, Pharmacia & Upjohn saw the potential activity of this class and started to develop safer alternatives with enhanced activity. In 2000, the first marketed compound of the class was linezolid, and it was effective against a wide spectrum of gram-positive pathogens, such as *Enterococcus faecium*, *Staphylococcus aureus*, *Streptococcus pneumoniae*, and *Streptococcus pyogenes*, and some anaerobic pathogens.[114] It had almost no activity on gram-negative bacteria and was unfortunately only bacteriostatic against Enterococcus species.[114] Linezolid also had the advantage over vancomycin of having a systemically available oral formulation. As recognized in the early development of the oxazolidinones, the challenges with linezolid had been bone marrow suppression and severe thrombocytopenia. Although linezolid was identified to have nonselective, monoamine oxidase-inhibiting activity, no reports of serotonin syndrome occurred during early clinical premarket assessment. Since market release however, linezolid has been associated with a number of case reports of serotonin syndrome through drug interaction.[115]

Lipopeptides

Daptomycin was the first cyclic lipopeptide developed by Eli Lilly Company, but it had been on the researcher's bench since the 1980s. Daptomycin structurally resembled the polymyxins, but it was derived from the fermentation of *Streptomyces roseosporus*.[116] In the early years, Eli Lilly was not impressed with a number of clinical failures involving patients with endocarditis and bacteremia and the drug's notorious effects on causing skeletal muscle damage.[117] Eli Lilly ceased further research activities, but the rapid emergence of MRSA in the 1990s forced a re-examination of this compound.[117] Cubist Pharmaceuticals obtained the compound in 1997 and was able to ready it for market by 2003. Interestingly, they had also optimized the dosing regimen to once daily dosing, which diminished its inherent potential toward skeletal muscle damage and rhabdomyolysis.

An advantage in critical care has been daptomycin's potent concentration-dependent, bactericidal activity against most clinically important gram-positive pathogens, including those resistant to beta-lactams and vancomycin, such as MRSA and VRE.[99,116] The greatest challenge with this compound however, has been the potential for drug-induced rhabdomyolysis, mandating weekly monitoring of creatine kinase and myoglobin.

CLOSING REMARKS

As observed from the collective histories of blood transfusion, intravenous fluids, vasopressors/inotropes, and antibiotics, war and armed conflict remain significant catalysts for advances in the field of Critical Care Medicine. In recent years, rapidly escalating health care costs have also begun to drive innovation in health care. While therapeutic advancement must continue, with each newly available therapy comes a responsibility to ensure the timely completion of clinical trials designed to establish the benefits and harms. The recent experience of aprotinin used for cardiac surgery serves as a lasting reminder to clinicians and researchers that multiple small trials of efficacy should be discouraged in favor of clinical trials that are sufficient to uncover anticipated or important harms.[118] Therapeutic advancement is both necessary and welcome, but clinical effectiveness, safety, and cost utility must be the priority as we move forward.

REFERENCES

1. Giangrande PL. The history of blood transfusion. Br J Haematol 2000;110: 758–67.
2. Corwin HL, Gettinger A, Pearl RG, et al. The CRIT study: anemia and blood transfusion in the critically ill—current clinical practice in the United States. Crit Care Med 2004;32:39–52.
3. Rodriguez RM, Corwin HL, Gettinger A, et al. Nutritional deficiencies and blunted erythropoietin response as causes of the anemia of critical illness. J Crit Care 2001;16:36–41.
4. Wise MW, Oleary JP. The origins of blood transfusion: early history. Am Surg 2002;68:98–100.
5. Rivera AM, Strauss KW, van ZA, et al. The history of peripheral intravenous catheters: how little plastic tubes revolutionized medicine. Acta Anaesthesiol Belg 2005;56:271–82.
6. Pelis K. Taking credit: the Canadian Army Medical Corps and the British conversion to blood transfusion in WWI. J Hist Med Allied Sci 2001;56:238–77.
7. Rous P, Turner JR. Preservation of living red blood corpuscles in vitro. II. The transfusion of kept cells. J Exp Med 1916;23:239–48.
8. Robertson LB. The transfusion of whole blood. A suggestion for its more frequent employment in war surgery. Br Med J 1916;2:38–40.
9. Pinkerton PH. Canadian surgeons and the introduction of blood transfusion in war surgery. Transfus Med Rev 2008;22:77–86.
10. Hess JR, Thomas MJ. Blood use in war and disaster: lessons from the past century. Transfusion 2003;43:1622–33.
11. Cohn EJ, Oncley JL, Strong LE, et al. Chemical, clinical, and immunological studies on the products of human plasma fractionation I: the characterization of the protein fractions of human plasma. J Clin Invest 1944;23:417–32.
12. Starr D. Medicine, money, and myth: an epic history of blood. Transfus Med 2001;11:119–21.
13. Yazer MH, Podlosky L, Clarke G, et al. The effect of prestorage WBC reduction on the rates of febrile nonhemolytic transfusion reactions to platelet concentrates and RBC. Transfusion 2004;44:10–5.
14. Blumberg N, Zhao H, Wang H, et al. The intention-to-treat principle in clinical trials and meta-analyses of leukoreduced blood transfusions in surgical patients. Transfusion 2007;47:573–81.
15. Tinmouth AT, McIntyre LA, Fowler RA. Blood conservation strategies to reduce the need for red blood cell transfusion in critically ill patients. CMAJ 2008;178: 49–57.
16. Hebert PC, Wells G, Blajchman MA, et al. A multicenter, randomized, controlled clinical trial of transfusion requirements in critical care. Transfusion requirements

in critical care investigators, Canadian Critical Care Trials Group. N Engl J Med 1999;340:409–17.

17. Natanson C, Kern SJ, Lurie P, et al. Cell-free hemoglobin-based blood substitutes and risk of myocardial infarction and death: a meta-analysis. JAMA 2008;299:2304–12.

18. Zarychanski R, Turgeon AF, McIntyre L, et al. Erythropoietin-receptor agonists in critically ill patients: a meta-analysis of randomized controlled trials. CMAJ 2007; 177:725–34.

19. Borgman MA, Spinella PC, Perkins JG, et al. The ratio of blood products transfused affects mortality in patients receiving massive transfusions at a combat support hospital. J Trauma 2007;63:805–13.

20. Ketchum L, Hess JR, Hiippala S. Indications for early fresh frozen plasma, cryoprecipitate, and platelet transfusion in trauma. J Trauma 2006;60:S51–8.

21. Malone DL, Hess JR, Fingerhut A. Massive transfusion practices around the globe and a suggestion for a common massive transfusion protocol. J Trauma 2006;60:S91–6.

22. Lewins R. Injection of saline solutions in extraordinary quantities into the veins in cases of malignant cholera. Lancet 1832;2:243–4.

23. Howard-Jones N. Cholera therapy in the nineteenth century. J Hist Med Allied Sci 1972;27:373–95.

24. O'Shaughnessy W. Proposal of a new method of treating the blue epidemic cholera by the injection of highly-oxygenated salts into the venous system. Lancet 1831;17:366–71.

25. O'Shaughnessy W. Report on the chemical pathology of the blood in cholera, published by authority of the Central Board of Health. Lancet 1832;17:929–36.

26. Awad S, Allison S, Lobo D. The history of 0.9% saline. Clin Nutr 2008;27:179–88.

27. Latta T. Documents communicated by the Central Board of Health, London, relative to the treatment of cholera by the copious injection of aqueous and saline fluids into the veins. Lancet 1832;18:274–7.

28. Finberg L. The early history of the treatment for dehydration. Arch Pediatr Adolesc Med 1998;152:71–3.

29. Cosnett JE. The origins of intravenous fluid therapy. Lancet 1989;1:768–71.

30. Jennings C. The intravenous injection of fluid for severe haemorrhage: part I. Lancet 1882;120:436–7.

31. Thelwall T. Injection of saline solution in shock. Lancet 1898;152:1390–1.

32. Lee JA. Sydney Ringer (1834–1910) and Alexis Hartmann (1898–1964). Anaesthesia 1981;36:1115–21.

33. Ringer S. A further contribution regarding the influence of the different constituents of the blood on the contraction of the ventricle. J Physiol 1883;4:29–42.

34. Barsoum N, Kleeman C. Now and then, the history of parenteral fluid administration. Am J Nephrol 2002;22:284–9.

35. Dudrick SJ. History of vascular access. JPEN J Parenter Enteral Nutr 2006;30:S47–56.

36. Landerer A. Ueber transfusion und infusion. Verhandl Dtsch Ges Chir 1886;15:280–2 [in German].

37. Matas R. A clinical report on intravenous saline infusion in the wards of the New Orleans Charity Hospital from June 1888, to June 1891. New Orleans Med Surg J 1891;19:1–93.

38. Rogers L. The mortality from post-choleraic uraemia: a 70 per cent reduction though intravenous injections of sodium bicarbonate. Lancet 1917;2:745–6.

39. Sellards A. Tolerance for alkalies in asiatic cholera. Philippine J Sci 1910;5: 363–89.
40. Cannon W, John F, Cowell E. The preventive treatment of wound shock. JAMA 1918;70:618–21.
41. Bayliss W. Methods of raising a low arterial pressure. Proc R Soc Med 1916;89: 380–93.
42. Saddler JM, Horsey PJ. The new generation gelatins. A review of their history, manufacture and properties. Anaesthesia 1987;42:998–1004.
43. Macintosh J. Principles of pathology and practice of physic, vol. 1. Philadelphia: Edward C Biddle; 1837.
44. Hassig A, Stampfli K. Plasma substitutes past and present. Bibl Haematol 1969; 33:1–8.
45. Cohn EJ. Blood proteins and their therapeutic value. Science 1945;101:51–6.
46. Evidence-based colloid use in the critically ill: American Thoracic Society consensus statement. Am J Respir Crit Care Med 2004;170:1247–59.
47. Gamble J, Ross G, Tisdall FF. The metabolism of fixed base during fasting. J Biol Chem 1923;57:633–95.
48. Coller F, Campbell K, Vaughan H, et al. Postoperative salt intolerance. Ann Surg 1944;119:533–41.
49. Moore F. Metabolic care of the surgical patient. Philadelphia: WB Saunders; 1959.
50. Shires T, Coln D, Carrico J, et al. Fluid therapy in hemorrhagic shock. Arch Surg 1964;88:688–93.
51. Jenkins MT. History of sequestered edema associated with surgical operations and trauma. Contemp Anesth Pract 1983;6:1–31.
52. Roth E, Lax L, Maloney JV. Ringer's lactate solution and extracellular fluid volume in the surgical patient: a critical analysis. Ann Surg 1969;169:149–64.
53. Moore F, Shires G. Moderation. Ann Surg 1967;166:300–1.
54. Brandstrup B, Svensen C, Engquist A. Hemorrhage and operation cause a contraction of the extracellular space needing replacement—evidence and implications? A systematic review. Surgery 2006;139:419–32.
55. Shires G. Re: hemorrhage and operation cause a contraction of the extracellular space needing replacement—evidence and implications? A systematic review. Surgery 2007;141:544.
56. Alam HB, Rhee P. New developments in fluid resuscitation. Surg Clin North Am 2007;87:55–72.
57. Kreimeier U, Prueckner S. Small-volume resuscitation from hemorrhagic shock by hypertonic saline dextran—conceptional basis and historical background. Eur Surg Res 2002;34:138–44.
58. Stewart PA. Modern quantitative acid-base chemistry. Can J Physiol Pharmacol 1983;61:1444–61.
59. Shoemaker WC. Prospective trial of supranormal values of survivors as therapeutic goals in high-risk surgical patients. Chest 1988;94:1176–86.
60. Rivers E, Nguyen B, Havstad S, et al. Early goal-directed therapy in the treatment of severe sepsis and septic shock. N Engl J Med 2001;345:1368–77.
61. Human albumin administration in critically ill patients: systematic review of randomised controlled trials. Cochrane Injuries Group Albumin Reviewers. BMJ 1998;317:235–40.
62. Finfer S, Bellomo R, Boyce N, et al. A comparison of albumin and saline for fluid resuscitation in the intensive care unit. N Engl J Med 2004;350:2247–56.

63. Myburgh J, Cooper DJ, Finfer S, et al. Saline or albumin for fluid resuscitation in patients with traumatic brain injury. N Engl J Med 2007;357:874–84.

64. Brunkhorst FM, Engel C, Bloos F, et al. Intensive insulin therapy and pentastarch resuscitation in severe sepsis. N Engl J Med 2008;358:125–39.

65. Bancroft H, Talbot JF. Oliver and Schafer's discovery of the cardiovascular action of suprarenal extract. Postgrad Med J 1968;44:6–8.

66. Oliver G, Schafer EA. The physiologic effects of extracts of the suprarenal capsules. J Physiol 1895;18:230–76.

67. Sneader W. Drug discovery—a history. Chichester, West Sussex (UK): John Wiley & Sons Ltd; 2005.

68. Abel JJ. On epinephrine, the active constituent of the suprarenal capsule and its compounds. Proc Am Physiol Soc 1898;16:3–5.

69. Aronson JK. Where name and image meet—the argument for adrenaline. BMJ 2000;320:506–9.

70. Yasmashima T. Jokichi Takamine (1854–1922), the samurai chemist, and his work on adrenalin. J Med Biogr 2003;11:95–102.

71. Takamine J. Adrenalin: the active principle of the suprarenal gland. Am J Pharm 1901;73:523–31.

72. Davenport HW. Epinephrin(e). Physiologist 1982;25:76–82.

73. Elliot TR. The action of adrenalin. J Physiol 1905;32:401–67.

74. Elliot TR. The action of adrenalin. J Physiol 1904;31:20–1.

75. Barger G, Dale HH. Chemical structure and sympathathomimetic action of amines. J Physiol 1910;41:19–59.

76. Nathanson MH, Miller H. The action of norepinephrine, epinephrine and isopropyl norepinephrine on the rhythmic function of the heart. Circulation 1952;6:238–44.

77. Eichna LW. The treatment of cardiogenic shock III. The use of isoproterenol in cardiogenic shock. Am Heart J 1967;74:48–52.

78. Tuttle RR, Mills J. Dobutamine: development of a new catecholamine to selectively increase cardiac contractility. Circ Res 1975;36:185–96.

79. Bennett MR. One hundred years of adrenaline: the discovery of autoreceptors. Clin Auton Res 1999;9:145–59.

80. Goldenberg M, Apgar V, Deterling R, et al. Nor-epinephrine (arterenol, sympathin N) as a pressor drug. JAMA 1949;140:776–8.

81. Livesay WR, Chapman DW. The treatment of acute hypotensive states with l-norepinephrine. Am J Med Sci 1953;225:159–71.

82. Goldberg LI. Cardiovascular and renal actions of dopamine: potential clinical applications. Pharmacol Rev 1972;24:1–29.

83. MacCannell KL, McNay JL, Meyer MB, et al. Dopamine in the treatment of hypotension and shock. N Engl J Med 1966;275:1389–98.

84. Loeb HS, Winslow EB, Rahimtoola SH, et al. Acute hemodynamic effects of dopamine in patients with shock. Circulation 1971;44:163–73.

85. Marik PE. Low-dose dopamine: a systematic review. Intensive Care Med 2002; 28:877–83.

86. Ahlquist RP. A study of the adrenotropic receptors. Am J Phys 1948;153: 586–600.

87. Bylund DB. Alpha- and beta-adrenergic receptors: Ahlquist's landmark hypothesis of a single mediator with two receptors. Am J Physiol Endocrinol Metab 2007;293:E1479–81.

88. Aviado DM Jr. Cardiovascular effects of some commonly used pressor amines. Anesthesiology 1959;20:71–97.

89. Fankhauser A, Fishman SI, Madonia PF, et al. The use of aramine in clinical shock. Circulation 1956;13:834–6.
90. Weil MH. Current concepts on the management of shock. Circulation 1957;16: 1097–105.
91. Smith NT, Corbascio AN. The use and misuse of pressor agents. Anesthesiology 1970;33:58–101.
92. Zaimis E. Vasopressor drugs and catecholamines. Anesthesiology 1968;29: 732–62.
93. Oliver H, Schafer E. On the physiological action of extracts of the pituitary body and certain other glandular organs. J Physiol 1895;18:277–9.
94. Light GA, Rattenborg C, Holaday DA. A new vasoconstrictor: preliminary studies of phelypressin. Anesth Analg 1965;44:280–7.
95. Russell JA, Walley KR, Singer J, et al. Vasopressin versus norepinephrine infusion in patients with septic shock. N Engl J Med 2008;358:877–87.
96. Farah AE. Historical perspectives on inotropic agents. Circulation 1986;73:III4–9.
97. Alousi AA, Johnson DC. Pharmacology of the bipyridines: amrinone and milrinone. Circulation 1986;73:III10–24.
98. Dellinger RP, Levy MM, Carlet JM, et al. Surviving sepsis campaign: international guidelines for management of severe sepsis and septic shock: 2008. Crit Care Med 2008;36:296–327.
99. Khardori N. Antibiotics—past, present, and future. Med Clin North Am 2006;90: 1049–76.
100. Stewart WH. A Mandate for State Action; presented at the Association of State and Territorial Health Officers, Washington, D.C., Dec 4, 1967. Taken from: Garrett L. The Coming Plague: Newly Emerging Diseases in a World Out of Balance. New York: Penguin Books; 1994. p. 33.
101. Mandell GL, Sande MA. Antimicrobial agents—the cephalosporins. In: Goodman A, Gillman AG, editors. Goodman and Gilman's the pharmacological basis of therapeutics. 7 edition. New York: Macmillan; 1985.
102. Marshall WF, Blair JE. The cephalosporins. Mayo Clin Proc 1999;74:187–95.
103. Chow JW, Fine MJ, Shlaes DM, et al. Enterobacter bacteremia: clinical features and emergence of antibiotic resistance during therapy. Ann Intern Med 1991; 115:585–90.
104. Drusano GL. Infection in the intensive care unit: beta-lactamase-mediated resistance among *Enterobacteriaceae* and optimal antimicrobial dosing. Clin Infect Dis 1998;27(Suppl 1):S111–6.
105. Levine DP. Vancomycin: a history. Clin Infect Dis 2006;42(Suppl 1):S5–12.
106. Aksoy DY, Unal S. New antimicrobial agents for the treatment of Gram-positive bacterial infections. Clin Microbiol Infect 2008;14:411–20.
107. Spratt BG, Jobanputra V, Zimmermann W. Binding of thienamycin and clavulanic acid to the penicillin-binding proteins of *Escherichia coli* K-12. Antimicrobial Agents Chemother 1977;12:406–9.
108. Hellinger WC, Brewer NS. Carbapenems and monobactams: imipenem, meropenem, and aztreonam. Mayo Clin Proc 1999;74:420–34.
109. Norrby SR, Alestig K, Ferber F, et al. Pharmacokinetics and tolerance of N-formimidoyl thienamycin (MK0787) in humans. Antimicrobial Agents Chemother 1983;23:293–9.
110. Shadomy S, May RS. N-formimidoyl thienamycin (MK0787): in vitro study. Antimicrobial Agents Chemother 1981;19:201–4.
111. Walker RC. The fluoroquinolones. Mayo Clin Proc 1999;74:1030–7.

112. Fernandes P. Antibacterial discovery and development—the failure of success? Nat Biotechnol 2006;24:1497–503.
113. Lockhart SR, Abramson MA, Beekmann SE, et al. Antimicrobial resistance among gram-negative bacilli causing infections in intensive care unit patients in the United States between 1993 and 2004. J Clin Microbiol 2007;45:3352–9.
114. Zhanel GG, Shroeder C, Vercaigne L, et al. A critical review of oxazolidinones: an alternative or replacement for glycopeptides and streptogramins? Can J Infect Dis 2001;12:379–90.
115. Huang V, Gortney JS. Risk of serotonin syndrome with concomitant administration of linezolid and serotonin agonists. Pharmacotherapy 2006;26:1784–93.
116. Schriever CA, Fernandez C, Rodvold KA, et al. Daptomycin: a novel cyclic lipopeptide antimicrobial. Am J Health Syst Pharm 2005;62:1145–58.
117. Sauermann R, Rothenburger M, Graninger W, et al. Daptomycin: a review 4 years after first approval. Pharmacology 2008;81:79–91.
118. Fergusson DA, Hébert PC, Mazer CD, et al. A comparison of aprotinin and lysine analogues in high-risk cardiac surgery. N Engl J Med 2008;358(22):2319–31.

A History of Ethics and Law in the Intensive Care Unit

John M. Luce, MD[a,b,*], Douglas B. White, MD, MAS[a,c]

KEYWORDS

- Biomedical ethics • End-of-life care
- Withholding and withdrawing life-sustaining therapy
- Cardiopulmonary resuscitation • Do-not-resuscitate orders
- Critical care medicine

Intensive care units (ICUs) have existed in the United States and other developed countries for approximately 50 years. During that time, many patients have benefited from mechanical ventilation and other medical interventions available in the units. However, these treatments have not been in the past and are not today uniformly effective. According to Angus and colleagues,[1] one-fifth of all Americans now die after using intensive care some time during a terminal hospital admission. Whether they live or die, many ICU patients experience prolonged pain and suffering. At the same time, their care comes at a high price: Multz and colleagues[2] have estimated that in 1998, ICU expenditures in the United States amounted to 34% of hospital budgets, $62 billion in health care costs, and more than 1% of the gross domestic product.

Because they provide potential benefit at great personal and public cost, the ICU and the interventions rendered therein have become symbols of both the promise and the limitations of medical technology. At the same time, the ICU has served as an arena in which many of the ethical and legal dilemmas created by that technology have been defined and debated. This article outlines major events in the history of

Dr. White was supported by a Greenwall Foundation Bioethics Faculty Scholars Award and by NIH Grant K12 RR024130 from the National Center for Research Resources, a component of the NIH Roadmap for Medical Research.
Neither Dr. Luce nor Dr. White has a relationship with a commercial company that has a direct interest in the subject matter or materials discussed in their article or with a company making a competing product.
ᵃ Department of Medicine, University of California, 505 Parnassus Avenue, San Francisco, CA 94143, USA
ᵇ Division of Pulmonary and Critical Care Medicine, San Francisco General Hospital, 1001 Potrero Avenue, Room 5 K1, San Francisco, CA 94110, USA
ᶜ Program in Medical Ethics, University of California, 521 Parnassus Avenue, Suite C126, Box 0903, San Francisco, CA 94143-0903, USA
* Corresponding author. Division of Pulmonary and Critical Care Medicine, San Francisco General Hospital, 1001 Potrero Avenue, Room 5 K1, San Francisco, CA 94110.
E-mail address: john.luce@sfdph.org (J.M. Luce).

Crit Care Clin 25 (2009) 221–237
doi:10.1016/j.ccc.2008.10.002
0749-0704/08/$ – see front matter © 2009 Elsevier Inc. All rights reserved.
criticalcare.theclinics.com

ethics and law in the ICU, covering the following 10 areas: (1) the evolution of ICUs, (2) ethical principles, (3) informed consent and the law, (4) medical decision-making, (5) cardiopulmonary resuscitation, (6) withholding and withdrawing life-sustaining therapy, (7) legal cases involving life support, (8) advance directives, (9) prognostication, and (10) futility and the allocation of medical resources.

Although other countries have contributed to the history covered in this article, the authors highlight the United States because they are most familiar with how ethical principles are applied in the United States and with its laws. In addition, although nurses and other clinicians are invaluable members of the ICU team, the article focuses primarily on the role of physicians in causing and confronting ethical and legal issues. Finally, although some men and women who have addressed these issues and contributed to the authors' knowledge of them are mentioned, many others have not been mentioned because of space limitations.

THE EVOLUTION OF ICUs

The ICU, now commonplace in hospitals in the United States and other developed countries, evolved from three main sources, according to Hilberman.[3] First was the postoperative recovery unit, the first of which was established for neurosurgical patients at the Johns Hopkins Hospital in Baltimore in 1923. The demand for recovery units increased during World War II, with the development of field hospitals and new surgical techniques that kept patients alive but required prolonged recovery. The Ochsner Clinic in New Orleans opened a recovery unit in 1947 so that patients undergoing complicated procedures, such as pneumonectomy and esophagogastrectomy, could be maintained after surgery. This and other recovery units were the forerunners of today's surgical ICUs (SICUs).

The first medical ICUs (MICUs) were created primarily to care for patients with respiratory failure caused by poliomyelitis and other neuromuscular diseases. Negative-pressure ventilation was used for such patients until Ibsen[4] demonstrated the superiority and wider applicability of positive-pressure ventilation during the polio epidemic in Copenhagen, Denmark in 1952. Respiratory care units were opened in Toronto, Canada, Uppsala, Sweden, and at the Baltimore City Hospital in 1958. The Baltimore unit, which was developed by Safar,[5] is regarded by Ayres and Combs[6] as America's first stand-alone ICU.

The first coronary care units (CCUs) were established in 1962 at Toronto General Hospital, Bethany Hospital in Kansas City, and Presbyterian Hospital in Philadelphia.[3] These and the other units that followed were based in large part on advances in electrocardiographic monitoring, which revealed that potentially treatable arrhythmias often caused death in patients with myocardial infarctions, and on resuscitative techniques that could best be used in such patients if they were closely monitored. These advances included AC defibrillation, which was shown to reverse ventricular fibrillation by Zoll and colleagues[7] in 1956; closed-chest cardiac massage, reported by Kouwenhoven and colleagues[8] in 1960, to support patients who arrested while receiving anesthesia; and DC defibrillation, which was demonstrated to be superior to AC defibrillation by Lown and colleagues[9] in 1962.

Specialized units for neonatal and pediatric patients, patients with burns and neurosurgical problems, and patients recovering from heart surgery were developed after SICUs, MICUs, and CCUs were established. Like the earlier units, these new units were justified primarily by studies demonstrating the physiologic effects of mechanical ventilation[10] and other therapies. Few outcome studies were actually available in the 1950s, 60s, and 70s, other than those showing improved survival because of the detection and correction of arrhythmias after myocardial infarction.[11] Nevertheless, because they housed impressive innovations that could reverse physiologic dysfunction and sustain life, ICUs became a standard of care. In the process, physicians and others who practiced in the units witnessed increasing conflicts among the ethical principles applied there.

ETHICAL PRINCIPLES

In 1978, Beauchamp and Childress[12] delineated four principles that they believed could organize physicians' thinking about the ethical practice of medicine: (1) beneficence, the physicians' duty to help patients whenever possible; (2) nonmaleficence, the obligation to avoid harm; (3) respect for autonomy, the patients' right to self-determination; and (4) justice, the fair allocation of medical resources. The principles of beneficence and nonmaleficence underlie the fiduciary relationship through which physicians serve the best interests of their patients and hold those interests in trust. Respect for autonomy allows patients to define and prioritize their interests. Justice situates patients within the larger society and acknowledges the importance of treating similar patients in similar ways. Ethical principles are insufficient by themselves to guide practice, but instead allow physicians to identify circumstances in which ethical goals are in conflict. For example, respect for autonomy and justice may conflict if a patient requests scarce medical resources needed by others who are more likely to benefit from them.

Jonson[13] has observed that beneficence and nonmaleficence are the oldest ethical principles. They were contained in the Hippocratic corpus, wherein there is no consideration of the issues of proper disclosure to patients, some of whom were slaves, or of obtaining their consent before medical interventions. Similarly, Percival's[14] historic *Medical Ethics*, which when published in 1803 was the first work to incorporate "medical ethics" in its title, makes no mention of respect for patients' self-determination or their right to make medical decisions. The first Code of Ethics of the American Medical Association (AMA),[15] published in 1847, was designed largely after Percival's British publication and was based solely on the principles of beneficence and nonmaleficence, along with the virtues of physicians who applied these principles.

According to Faden and Beauchamp,[16] the initial consideration of autonomy as a compelling ethical principle occurred when informed consent found its way into American medicine in the mid-twentieth century. One reason for this appearance was increasing legal appreciation of the right of consent, as will be discussed. Another was growing concern about civil liberties involving ethnic minorities, women, and other groups. A third reason was post-World War II realization of atrocities committed by the Nazis in the name of medical research, and of the lack of informed consent in the Tuskegee Syphilis Study in the United States. The Nuremberg Code of 1947[17] and the World Medical Association's Declaration of Helsinki in 1964[18] grounded the principle of autonomy in biomedical research. The AMA Code of Ethics was revised to incorporate informed consent for both clinical and research purposes around the same time.

INFORMED CONSENT AND THE LAW

The right of patients to consent to or refuse medical treatment has been contained for centuries within English and American common law. Common law also has held that physicians have a number of professional duties to patients, including the duty to endeavor to be beneficent and to avoid harm. Before the twentieth century, courts in both England and the United States did not include informed consent as a duty unless "medical experts testified that such consent comprised an ordinary and beneficial part of medical therapy."[16] On the few occasions when medical experts so testified, they supported informed consent solely on the grounds of beneficence and not because they supported patient autonomy.[19]

The legal obligation of clinicians to obtain consent before treating patients was established by several landmark decisions in the United States in the twentieth century. In the first case, *Schloendorff v. Society of New York Hospitals*,[20] the Court of Appeals of New York in 1914 determined that "Every being of adult years and sound mind has the right to determine what shall be done with his own body…" In the second case, *Salgo v. Leland Stanford University Board of Trustees*,[21] which was heard in 1957, the Court of Appeals of California stated that clinicians must disclose to a patient "all the facts which mutually affect his rights and interests …" in obtaining consent. In the third case, *Cobbs v. Grant*,[22] the Supreme Court of California in 1972 established that "The scope of the physician's communication to the patient, then, must be measured by the patient's need, and that need is whatever information is material to the decision."

MEDICAL DECISION-MAKING

The court cases that clarified informed consent in the United States were a reaction to medical decision-making influenced, if not dominated, by the traditional paternalistic model. Also called "priestly" by Veach[23] in 1975 and "parental" by Burke[24] in 1980, this model is based on the ethical principles of beneficence and nonmaleficence. It allows clinicians to define what is within the best interests of their patients without necessarily knowing what the patients want or consulting them. The paternalistic model is particularly well suited to decision-making in emergency situations, where time is of the essence, patients may be unable to communicate, and consent for treatment (but not research) can be waived because most people would prefer to be treated (but not necessarily enrolled in research) in these situations.

Emanuel and Emanuel[25] have described another model of medical decision-making that supplanted the paternalistic model in the latter half of the twentieth century: the deliberative model. Under this model, clinicians help patients define their best interests, provide treatment alternatives through which the interests can be served, and assist the patients in deciding which alternative is best. The deliberative model is best suited for situations in which clinicians and patients have ample time to discuss alternatives, extensive communication is possible, and consent can be informed. Clinicians need not be neutral under this model, as Ingelfinger[26] noted in 1980. Rather, decision-making by patients and clinicians is shared, a practice that was endorsed as recently as 2003 by the 5th International Consensus Conference in Critical Care.[27]

The deliberative model of medical decision-making initially was predicated on the assumption that clinicians and patients could communicate with one another. Similarly, the Nuremberg Code and the Declaration of Helsinki addressed consent for research only by subjects who could make their own decisions, just as the court cases regarding informed consent for medical purposes considered only patients who were legally competent. The question of whether incompetent patients could refuse treatment fell to courts in the second half of the twentieth century, when ICUs were developed and clinicians began treating large numbers of patients whose cognitive function was impaired by critical illnesses and its treatment, and could not make decisions themselves.

CARDIOPULMONARY RESUSCITATION AND DO-NOT-RESUSCITATE ORDERS

One of the first treatments used in critically ill patients without obtaining their consent was cardiopulmonary resuscitation (CPR). Indeed, after closed-chest cardiac massage and DC defibrillation were introduced in the 1960s, most American hospitals required that they be administered to all patients who suffered cardiopulmonary arrest in- and outside ICUs, as recalled by Burns and colleagues.[28] This universal requirement for CPR was based on the assumptions that the nascent technology would benefit and not harm patients, that not providing CPR constituted "passive euthanasia" and was therefore unethical, and that failure to perform resuscitation might invite civil suits or criminal prosecution.

In 1983, Bedell and colleagues[29] demonstrated that although 44% of hospitalized patients responded initially to CPR, only 14% survived to hospital discharge. Decades before that publication, however, many physicians had already realized that CPR could transiently restore physiologic function in some patients but often prolonged their suffering until they finally died. This led Symmers[30] in 1968 to question whether the new technology was truly sustaining life or merely interfering with the dying process. The realization also led some physicians to decide which patients should or should not be resuscitated and thus to apply this medical resource selectively.

In the early 1980s, alarmed by the death under mysterious circumstances of a patient in a Queens hospital ICU, a New York grand jury discovered that hospital physicians had been ordering that small purple dots be affixed to the charts of patients they did not want to resuscitate. The dots were removed after patients died so that their de facto do-not-resuscitate (DNR) status could not be identified.[31] During the same period, physicians commonly conducted "slow codes" in which they delayed CPR or provided resuscitation in such a fashion that it was destined to fail. According to Gazelle,[32] slow codes were used primarily in patients with terminal illness or dementia and those in a persistent vegetative or other comatose state. The wishes of these patients regarding resuscitation generally were unknown to their physicians, although in some cases the physicians were putting on a show for surrogates who desired that all therapies be used in their loved ones.

Purple dots and slow codes initially were surreptitious responses to universal resuscitation policies that physicians considered maleficent and perhaps wasteful of medical resources. In time, however, physicians and hospital administrators realized that some patients and their surrogates did not want CPR. Although the legal propriety of not resuscitating some patients with their or their surrogate's consent remained uncertain, in 1974 the AMA[33] proposed that DNR decisions be documented in the medical record and argued that "CPR is not indicated in certain situations, such as in cases of terminal irreversible illness where death is not unexpected." Two years later, Massachusetts General Hospital and the Beth Israel Hospital in Boston publicly reported their policies regarding end-of-life care for critically ill patients.[34,35]

Although the Beth Israel Hospital policy only concerned CPR and writing explicit DNR orders, that of Massachusetts General Hospital covered the broader topic of "Optimum care for hopelessly ill patients." It described the on-going application on ICU admission of a system in which patients were divided into four categories: (1) those patients expected to live, who were to receive maximal therapeutic effort; (2) those who might die and should receive maximum effort but be evaluated daily; (3) those who were likely to die and who should receive selective limitation of therapeutic measures; and (4) those with severe neurologic impairment who should have life support discontinued after consultation with and concurrence of the patient's surrogates, who were not considered likely to initiate the process themselves.

WITHHOLDING AND WITHDRAWING OF LIFE-SUSTAINING THERAPY

In an editorial entitled "Terminating life support: out of the closet!" that accompanied these reports, Fried[36] praised Massachusetts General Hospital and the Beth Israel

Hospital for going public with their policies. Few other commentators would argue in print that CPR and other kinds of life support should be withheld or withdrawn from patients in 1976. However, during that year, the Supreme Court of New Jersey, in its decision regarding Karen Ann Quinlan, established that incompetent patients, through their surrogates, could refuse mechanical ventilation. Along with the reports of policies from the Boston hospitals, this landmark legal case prompted a series of publications denoting how life support could be foregone in the ICU.

The first of these publications came from the President's Commission for the Study of Ethical Problems in Medicine and Biomedical and Behavioral Research, which explored the medical, legal, and ethical issues in the determination of death,[37] in the patient-provider relationship,[38] and in deciding to forego life-sustaining treatment.[39] Coming from a body empowered by the President, these publications provided the first consensus-based ethical rationale for limiting unwanted therapy in critically ill patients with terminal illnesses. The Commission's publication on foregoing treatment in 1983 coincided with an editorial by Grenvik,[40] describing how he and his colleagues used a process called "terminal weaning" to discontinue mechanical ventilation and other interventions in the terminally ill. The next year, Wanzer and colleagues[41] described limiting treatment and other aspects of "the physician's responsibility toward hopelessly ill patients" in a follow-up to the 1976 publication from Massachusetts General Hospital.

Withholding and withdrawing mechanical ventilation was the focus of a workshop convened by the National Institutes of Health[42] in 1986; Ruark, Raffin, and the Stanford University Medical Center Committee on Ethics[43] that year; and Schneiderman and Spragg[44] in 1988. In 1989, a second publication on "The physician's responsibility toward hopelessly ill patients" by Wanzer and colleagues[45] acknowledged that DNR orders, advance directives, and professional and public approval of allowing patients with terminal illnesses to forego treatment was now commonplace. These investigators also noted that the courts increasingly were attributing the deaths of such patients to their underlying medical conditions rather than to the withholding or withdrawal of life-sustaining therapy.

In 1990, Smedira and colleagues[46] published the first description of how and why life support was foregone in critically ill patients in the United States. From their observations in two ICUs at hospitals associated with the University of California, San Francisco, these investigators determined that the withholding or withdrawal of mechanical ventilation and other therapies precipitated death in over half of the patients who died in the units during the study year. The primary reason for limiting care was poor prognosis. A small number of the patients were able to make the decision to limit care; the others were incompetent. Family members made decisions for those incompetent patients with families and physicians decided for patients who lacked surrogates.

Subsequent observational studies from other ICUs following this 1990 publication, established that limiting of life support had become a standard practice in the United States,[47] Canada,[48] and Europe.[49] In 1997, Prendergast and Luce[50] reported that the withholding and withdrawal of life support now preceded death in 90% of patients who died in the two ICUs studied by Smedira and colleagues 5 years earlier. Prendergast and colleagues[51] reported in 1998 that of patients who died in 131 ICUs at 110 United States hospitals over a 6-month period, only 23% received full support, including failed CPR. On the other hand, 77% of the dying patients either received full care without CPR or had other kinds of life-sustaining therapy withheld or withdrawn.

In addition to describing how commonly life support was foregone in ICUs, publications, such as that of Wilson and colleagues[52] in 1992, detailed how and to what extent sedatives and analgesics were given to dying patients. Increasingly, commentators focused on providing palliative care while removing unwanted treatment, as highlighted by Brody and colleagues[53] in 1997. At the same time, professional societies, such as the AMA,[33] the Society of Critical Care Medicine (SCCM),[54] the American Thoracic Society (ATS),[55] and the American College of Chest Physicians[56] supported both the ethical and legal propriety of limiting potentially restorative treatment in patients not wanting such treatment, and the necessity of providing palliation to them. These twin principles were captured in the first book on managing death in the ICU, edited by Curtis and Rubenfeld[57] in 2001, which was subtitled "The Transition from Cure to Comfort."

More recently, professional societies and investigators have strived to improve the ICU experience at the end of life not just for patients but also for their families. For example, both the American Academy of Critical Care Medicine[58] and the ATS[59] in their most recent publications include the family as a treatment focus. Curtis and colleagues[60] have demonstrated impairments in communication during physician-family conferences about end-of-life care in the ICU, whereas White and colleagues[61] have explored how communication can be enhanced. In 2006, an entire supplement of Critical Care Medicine, edited by Levy and Curtis,[62] was devoted to "Improving the quality of end-of-life care in the ICU."

LEGAL CASES INVOLVING LIFE SUPPORT

Improving end-of-life care would not have been possible without a series of legal cases involving life support. Of these, the first and most important was *In re Quinlan*,[63] which was decided by the Supreme Court of New Jersey in 1976. It involved Karen Ann Quinlan, a then-22-year-old woman in a vegetative state following a drug overdose, who was receiving mechanical ventilation in a New Jersey hospital ICU. Ms. Quinlan's father petitioned a trial court to be named her guardian, with the avowed intent of ordering that her ventilator be removed. The trial court refused, and the hospital and Ms. Quinlan's physicians sought a restraining order against Mr. Quinlan on the grounds that removing her ventilator would constitute euthanasia. When his appeal was turned down at the Superior Court level, Mr. Quinlan appealed to the New Jersey Supreme Court.

The Court opined that, if Ms. Quinlan were to become miraculously lucid and perceptive of her irreversible condition, she would decide against further mechanical ventilation, which it considered her constitutionally-guaranteed right of privacy. Because Ms. Quinlan could not exercise this right on her own, it could be asserted by her father acting as her guardian. To assuage Ms. Quinlan's physicians and the hospital and to provide legal protection for them, the Court decreed that if the clinicians believed that she was truly vegetative, and if the hospital's Ethics Committee or a like body concurred, her ventilator could be withdrawn without incurring civil or criminal liability. Ms. Quinlan's ventilator subsequently was removed and she died of meningitis and pneumonia in 1985.[64]

Over the 15 years following *In re Quinlan*, according to Annas,[65] courts in almost 20 states recognized the general right of competent patients to refuse treatment, and all but two states acknowledged that the United States Constitution, state constitutions, or common law permitted surrogate decision-making for incompetent patients. One example of this trend was the case of *Bartling v. Superior Court*,[66] in which two California physicians were absolved of murder charges for ordering that fluids and nutrition be removed from a patient with his family's consent. However, New York, in the cases of *In re Storar*[67] and *In re Westchester County Medical Center on behalf of O'Connor*,[68] and Missouri in *Cruzan v. Harmon*,[69] bucked the trend. The Cruzan case went to the United States Supreme Court in 1990 in *Cruzan v. Director, Missouri Department of Health*.[70]

Nancy Cruzan was vegetative as a result of an automobile accident and her subsequent resuscitation, and she required only tube feedings to stay alive in a Missouri state hospital. Having been told earlier by their daughter that she would not want to live unless she could be "at least halfway normal," Ms. Cruzan's parents sought to have her feeding tube removed, with which a trial judge agreed over the objections of the state hospital. Nevertheless, in *Cruzan v. Harmon*, the Missouri Supreme Court reversed the decision on the grounds that, because the state had a legitimate interest in preserving life regardless of its quality, life-sustaining treatment could be removed from Ms. Cruzan only if "clear and convincing evidence" confirmed that she rejected such treatment. Ms. Cruzan's parents in turn appealed this decision to the United States Supreme Court.

Chief Justice Rehnquist, who wrote the Supreme Court's 5 to 4 majority decision in *Cruzan v. Missouri Department of Public Health*, acknowledged that "...for the purposes of this case, we assume that the United States Constitution would grant a competent person a constitutionally protected right to refuse lifesaving hydration and nutrition." Unlike the judges in *In re Quinlan*, however, he based this right not on any right of privacy but rather on the liberty interest delineated in the fourteenth amendment. At the same time, he opined that the Constitution does not prohibit a state from requiring "clear and convincing evidence" of prior wishes, in part because this standard promotes the state's interest in preserving life. Only New York and Missouri still maintain the standard disputed in *In re Cruzan,* and the Court's decision does not diminish a surrogate's authority in foregoing life support in other states. Nancy Cruzan herself died shortly following the decision, after her parents presented additional evidence of her prior wishes regarding resuscitation to the Missouri courts and her feeding tube was removed.

After *In re Cruzan*, the Supreme Court confirmed its approval of the foregoing of life-sustaining treatment in *Washington v. Glucksberg*[71] and *Vacco v. Quill*,[72] and also provided guidelines for administering palliative care. These two cases concerned the constitutionality of laws prohibiting physician-assisted suicide in the states of Washington and New York. In *Washington v. Glucksberg*, the Court decided that patients did not have a liberty interest in receiving a physician's assistance in committing suicide. In *Vacco v. Quill*, the Court drew distinctions between assisted suicide and withholding and withdrawal of life support. Thus, the Court wrote that "When a patient refuses life-sustaining medical treatment, he dies from an underlying disease or pathology; but if a patient ingests lethal medication prescribed by a physician, he is killed by that medication."

In their opinions in these two cases, Justice Breyer indicated that state laws prohibiting physician-assisted suicide might be problematic if they inhibited the provision of palliative care, including the administration of drugs as needed to avoid pain at the end of life, while Justice O'Conner wrote favorably about "relieving pain to the point of unconsciousness." In *Vacco v. Quill*, the Court as a whole sanctioned terminal sedation "based on informed consent and the double effect. Just as a state may prohibit assisted suicide while permitting patients to refuse unwanted lifesaving treatment, it may permit palliative care related to that refusal, which may have the foreseen but unintended double 'effect' of hastening the patient's death."

ADVANCE DIRECTIVES

In the wake of *In re Cruzan*, Congress in 1990 passed the Patient Self-Determination Act[73] to help patients avoid unwanted medical interventions. Sponsored by Senator Danforth, of Ms. Cruzan's home state of Missouri, the Patient Self Determination Act requires that federally funded health care institutions inquire about the presence of advance directives on admission, record patient preferences in the medical record, and assist patients and surrogates in obtaining advance directives if they do not already have them. The Act was the first to promote advance directives on a national level. Nevertheless, both instructional directives (eg, living wills) and proxy directives (eg, the durable power of attorney for health care) had been available at the local level and in many states for many years.

The first living will was developed in 1969 and distributed by the Euthanasia Education Council. In 1976, Bok[74] published a groundbreaking article on "Personal directions for care at the end of life" that cited the plight of Karen Ann Quinlan, described how to prepare a living will, and provided an example of one. Living wills were advocated by clinicians and ethicists, such as Eisendrath and Jonsen[75] in 1983, as devices to promote patient autonomy while removing onerous decision-making about receiving CPR and other interventions from physicians and the patient's surrogates. Nevertheless, these commentators pointed out that living wills could cause confusion if they were vague in terminology and used for patients with uncertain prognoses.

California, which enacted the nation's first "Natural Death Act," allowing for living wills in 1976, created the first comprehensive statute establishing a durable power of attorney (DPOA) for health care in 1983. As described by Steinbrook and Lo[76] 1 year later, the California statute allowed competent patients to delegate medical decision-making, including that involving decisions at the end of life, to surrogates if the patients should become incompetent. Physicians who relied on proxy decisions were granted legal immunity from criminal and civil charges and from professional disciplinary action. If they doubted the surrogate's fidelity to the patient's health-related values, judicial review could be obtained.

Other states followed California in passing statutes authorizing the use of the DPOA for health care, especially after the Supreme Court's *In re Cruzan* decision and passage of the Patient Self-Determination Act in 1990. Among others, Silverman and colleagues[77] remarked that proxy directives might be particularly helpful in states that did not automatically give legal recognition to families as decision-makers for patients who could not make decisions for themselves. Yet a DPOA could not be created if patients lacked suitable surrogates. Furthermore, even if surrogates were available, a DPOA might not be helpful if they and the patients they were speaking for had not discussed end-of-life issues previously.

Despite the wide publicity given to cases like *In re Quinlan* and *Cruzan*, the passage of the Patient Self-Determination Act, and the call for greater use of advance directives by Emanuel and colleagues[78] and others, observational studies conducted in the1990s by investigators such as Danis and colleagues[79] demonstrated that few patients had advance directives and that directives did not affect their care. Schneiderman and colleagues,[80] who hoped that the California DPOA "…might provide a more ethical approach to reducing health care costs," offered it to hospitalized patients with life-threatening illnesses; a control group was not offered advance directives. In 1992, these investigators reported that execution of a DPOA had no effect on the patient's well being, health status, medical treatments, or treatment charges.

In 1984, Levinsky[81] argued that, in the face of public pressure to reduce health care expenditures, "…physicians are required to do everything that they believe may benefit each patient without regard to costs or other societal considerations." After publication of the article by Schneiderman and colleagues, demonstrating a limited impact of the California DPOA, Levinsky[82] questioned whether advance directives were mechanisms for reinforcing informed consent or methods "…whereby physicians shift their role from that of care givers to that of propagandists for limited medical treatment." Although not universally shared, Levinsky's sentiments underscored the conflict between the ethical principles of autonomy and justice that runs through the history of ethics and law in the ICU.

PROGNOSTICATION

One reason for the limited use of advance directives is that patients' preferences are not static but change as their medical conditions evolve, as demonstrated by Somogyi-Zakud and colleagues.[83] In other words, what patients want in terms of attempts at life prolongation varies according to their prognoses.[84] Some prognostic information has been derived from ICU studies of patients with specific disorders, such as chronic obstructive pulmonary disease (COPD),[85] *Pneumocystis* pneumonia, acquired immunodeficiency syndrome,[86] and acute respiratory distress syndrome (ARDS).[87] Other information has come from studies of certain age groups, such as the elderly,[88] or certain interventions, such as mechanical ventilation.[89]

Additional information has been obtained from the use of prognostic scoring systems based largely on physiologic variables and diagnoses on admission to the ICU. Perhaps the best known of these systems, the Acute Physiology and Chronic Health Evaluation (APACHE), was first reported by Knaus and colleagues[90] in 1981 and has since gone through three additional iterations. APACHE and other prognostic scoring systems have been shown to be as accurate (or inaccurate) as clinical assessment by physicians and nurses.[91] They also have demonstrated good calibration in that the overall hospital mortality they predict is comparable to that observed in research studies. Nevertheless, the systems have not discriminated well between individuals who survive and those who die.[92]

Another limitation of prognostic scoring systems is that physicians do not necessarily use the information they provide any more than they rely on advance directives. These behaviors were demonstrated in the Study to Understand Prognoses and Preferences for Outcomes and Risks of Treatment (SUPPORT),[93] published in 1995. SUPPORT was based on a large cohort of hospitalized adult patients with advanced COPD, ARDS, and other serious illnesses. The SUPPORT investigators estimated 6-month survival using a prognostic scoring system similar to APACHE, elicited patient and family preferences, and facilitated advance care planning and patient-physician communication in an intervention group. Despite these measures, however, the incidence of timing DNR orders, physicians' knowledge of their patients' preferences not to be resuscitated, and number of days spent in an ICU receiving mechanical ventilation or in a comatose state was the same in the intervention group as in controls.

FUTILITY AND THE ALLOCATION OF MEDICAL RESOURCES

Among other things, SUPPORT showed that providing prognostic information and advance-care planning did not reduce the use of medical resources or their cost. Reducing resource use or allocating medical resources to patients most likely to benefit from them has been a concern—if not an agenda item—in ICUs almost since their inception. As an example, when the Massachusetts General Hospital and Beth Israel Hospital policies regarding resuscitation were reported in 1976, Fried[36] questioned at which social good the policies were aimed: "...freeing the patient from the tyranny of a technologic (or bureaucratic-professional) imperative to keep alive at all costs" or "...freeing society from the burden and expense of caring for a growing multitude of extravagantly demanding moribund persons?"

Debates about the proper allocation of medical resources in the ICU are as old as the ICU itself. Sparking the debates are the realizations that ICU resources are limited, as captured in Teres's[94] paradigm of "the last bed"; that patients and families generally want ICU care despite its negative aspects, as demonstrated by Danis and colleagues;[95] and that ICU rationing is therefore inevitable and ethical, as discussed by Engelhardt and Rie.[96] Indeed, limiting ICU admission of patients with chest pain who were unlikely to have myocardial infarctions and of patients with medical problems but few physiologic derangements was demonstrated in the 1980s by both Singer and colleagues[97] and Strauss and colleagues[98] during times of decreased bed availability in the their ICUs.

Observational studies documenting the preclusion of ICU admission of patients with advanced illnesses and severe physiologic disturbances have not been performed. Nevertheless, prognostic scoring systems could be used for this purpose, and Asch and colleagues[99] have demonstrated that some surveyed critical care physicians acknowledge withholding or withdrawing life-sustaining therapies without the knowledge or consent of patients and their surrogates or over their objections. The rationale for this behavior, as cited in the title of an article[100] on the subject, is that "Physicians do not have a responsibility to provide futile or unreasonable care if a patient or family insists."

According to Helft and colleagues,[101] the concept of medical futility and its use to rationalize unilateral decision-making by physicians was introduced in the late 1980s. In 1987, Blackhall[102] noted that CPR was unsuccessful in restoring life in many situations and advocated that physicians administer it selectively. In 1990, Schneiderman and colleagues[103] defined futility quantitatively as a medical intervention that had not been useful in the last 100 cases, and qualitatively as interventions that merely preserve permanent unconsciousness or dependence on intensive medical care. In 1996, Rubenfeld and Crawford[104] argued that evidence-based guidelines could be developed for limiting the use of life support for patients, such as bone marrow transplant recipients with hepatic or renal failure and a requirement for vasopressors, none of whom survived ICU admission.

The major problems with futility as a concept are summarized by Truog and colleagues.[105] Outside the rare circumstances of strict physiologic futility, it is a value-laden concept about which a consensus has not been achieved. Moreover, physicians sometimes invoke futility to hide what are really implicit resource allocation decisions that should be discussed explicitly. These problems were acknowledged in 1997 by the SCCM,[106] which argued that "Treatments should be defined as futile only when they will not accomplish their intended (physiologic) goal. Treatments that are extremely unlikely to be beneficial, are extremely costly, or are of uncertain benefit may be considered inappropriate and hence inadvisable, but should not be labeled futile."

The AMA[107] took a stance similar to that of the SCCM two years later. In addition, it urged that decisions regarding interventions physicians considered futile or inappropriate be made through an extra-judicial conflict-resolution process involving both physicians and patients and their families. This process, which was first implemented in hospitals in Houston,[108] was incorporated into the Texas Advance Directives Act[109] in 1999. It allows a physician to ask an ethics or ad-hoc medical committee to review a patient or surrogate request for treatment the physician considers inappropriate. If the committee agrees that the request is inappropriate and no other facility will accept the patient in transfer, the treatment may be withheld or withdrawn. Despite its apparent popularity among physicians, this policy has been criticized as being disproportionately applied to disenfranchised minorities. It also implies that in debates over value-laden decisions about life and death, physicians' values can trump those of their patients.[110]

Within the last year, in widely publicized cases in Australia[111] and Canada,[109,112–114] surrogates have asked courts to prevent ICU physicians from limiting life-sustaining therapy in relatives under circumstances that did not meet the criteria of physiologic futility. In all but one[112] of these cases, the courts allowed the physicians to exercise clinical judgment, and life support was withheld or withdrawn. Australia and Canada differ from the United States in that both countries provide universal health coverage, and physicians in them may consider themselves empowered to decide life-and-death issues regardless of surrogates' requests. It is not clear that American physicians currently are so empowered, or that they would be empowered even if the United States were to provide universal coverage. Nevertheless, the apparently increasing frequency of contentious legal cases in other countries suggests that the debate over who decides if treatment should be provided is likely to intensify in the United States.

SUMMARY

Over 30 years ago, the New Jersey Supreme Court established through its *In re Quinlan* decision that patients and their surrogates can refuse unwanted therapies, thereby giving the principle of respect for autonomy a privileged position in American bioethics. Today, a different movement is afoot: physicians concerned about their own prerogatives and about the just distribution of health care resources are challenging whether their patient's right to self-determination must compel the physicians to provide treatment they consider inappropriate. Given our limited ICU resources, the introduction of new potentially life-saving technologies, patient demand for them, and the aging of our population, such challenges will become more commonplace in the future, as will conflicts among ethical principles in the ICU.

REFERENCES

1. Angus DC, Barnato AE, Linde-Zwirble WT, et al. on behalf of the Robert Wood Johnson Foundation ICU End-of-Life Peer Group. Use of intensive care at the end of life in the United States: an epidemiologic study. Crit Care Med 2004; 32:638–43.
2. Multz AS, Chalfin DB, Samson IM, et al. A "closed" medical intensive care unit (MICU) improves resource utilization when compared with an "open" MICU. Am J Respir Crit Care Med 1998;157:1468–73.
3. Hilberman M. The evolution of intensive care units. Crit Care Med 1975;3: 159–65.
4. Ibsen H. The anaesthetist's viewpoint on treatment of respiratory complications in poliomyelitis during the epidemic in Copenhagen. Proc R Soc Med 1954;47: 72–81.
5. Safar P, Kornfield T, Pierson JM. Intensive care unit. Anaesthesia 1961;16: 275–84.
6. Ayres SM, Combs AH. A tale of two intensive care units? All intensive care units are not the same. Crit Care Med 1992;20:727–8.
7. Zoll PM, Linenthal AJ, Norman LR. Treatment of unexpected cardiac arrest by external electrical stimulation of the heart. N Engl J Med 1956;541:996–1002.
8. Kouwenhoven WB, Jude JR, Knickerbocker GG. Closed-chest cardiac massage. JAMA 1960;173:1064–7.
9. Lown B, Newman J, Amarasingham R. A new method of termination of cardiac arrhythmias. JAMA 1962;182:548–55.
10. O'Donohue WJ, Baker JP, Gell GM. The management of acute respiratory failure in a respiratory intensive care unit. Chest 1970;58:608–20.
11. Marshall RM, Blount SG, Centon R. Acute myocardial infarction: influence of a coronary care unit. Arch Intern Med 1968;122:427–35.
12. Beauchamp TL, Childress JF. Principles of biomedical ethics. Oxford (UK): Oxford University Press; 1978.

13. Jonsen AR. The birth of bioethics. Oxford (UK): Oxford University Press; 1998.
14. Percival T. Medical ethics: or, a code of institutes and precepts, adapted to the professional conduct of physicians and surgeons. Manchester (UK): S. Russell; 1803.
15. American Medical Association. Code of medical ethics. Chicago: American Medical Association; 1847.
16. Faden RR, Beauchamp TL. A history and theory of informed consent. Oxford (UK): Oxford University Press; 1986.
17. Trials of war criminals before the Nurenberg military tribunals under control council law N. 10. Washington, DC: U.S. Government Printing Office; 1948–1949.
18. Declaration of Helsinki: recommendations guiding medical doctors in biomedical research involving human subjects. N Engl J Med 1964;271:473–80.
19. Luce J. Is the concept of informed consent applicable to clinical research involving critically ill patients? Crit Care Med 2003;31:S153–60.
20. Schloendorff v. Society of New York hospitals, 211 NY 125, 105 NE:1915.
21. Salgo v. Leland Stanford Jr. Board of Trustees, 317 PZA 170, 1957.
22. Cobbs v. Grant, 8 Cal 3d 229; 502P: 2d 1, 1972.
23. Veach RM. Models for ethical medicine in a revolutionary age. Hastings Cent Rep 1975;2:3–5.
24. Burke G. Ethics and medical decision-making. Prim Care 1980;7:615–24.
25. Emanuel EJ, Emanuel LL. Four models of the physician-patient relationship. JAMA 1992;267:2221–6.
26. Ingelfinger FJ. Arrogance. N Engl J Med 1980;303:1507–11.
27. Thompson BT, Cox PN, Antonelli M, et al. Challenges in end-of-life care in the ICU: statement of the 5th International Consensus Conference in Critical Care: Brussels, Belgium, April 2003: executive summary. Crit Care Med 2004;32:1781–4.
28. Burns JP, Edwards J, Johnson J, et al. Do-not-resuscitate order after 25 years. Crit Care Med 2003;31:1543–50.
29. Bedell SE, Delbanco TL, Cook EF, et al. Survival after cardiopulmonary resuscitation in the hospital. N Engl J Med 1983;309:569–76.
30. Symmers WS. Not allowed to die. BMJ 1968;1:442.
31. Baker R. The legitimization and regulation of DNR orders. In: Baker R, Strosberg MA, editors. Legislating medical ethics: a Study of the New York state do-not-resuscitate law. Boston: Kluwer Acadfemic; 1995. p. 33–101.
32. Gazelle G. The slow code—should anyone rush to its defense? N Engl J Med 1998;338:467–9.
33. American Heart Association: Standards and guidelines for cardiopulmonary resuscitation (CPR) and emergency cardiac care (ECC): medicolegal considerations and recommendations. JAMA 1974;227(Suppl):864–6.
34. Clinical Care Committee of the Massachusetts General Hospital. Optimum care for hopelessly ill patients: a report of the clinical care committee of the Massachusetts General Hospital. N Engl J Med 1976;295:362–4.
35. Rabkin MT, Gillerman G, Rice NR. Orders not to resuscitate. N Engl J Med 1976; 295:364–6.
36. Fried C. Terminating life support: out of the closet. N Engl J Med 1976;295:390–1.
37. President's Commission for the Study of Ethical Problems in Medicine and Biomedical and Behavioral Research. Defining death. A report on the medical, legal, and ethical issues in the determination of death. Washington, DC: US Government Printing Office; 1981.
38. President's Commission for the Study of Ethical Problems in Medicine and Biomedical and Behavioral Research. Making health care decisions. A report on the

ethical and legal implications of informed consent in the patient-practitioner relationship. Washington, DC: US Government Printing Office; 1982.

39. President's Commission for the Study of Ethical Problems in Medicine and Bio-medical and Behavioral Research. Deciding to forego life-sustaining treatment. A report on the ethical, medical, and legal issues in treatrment decisions. Washington, DC: US Government Printing Office; 1983.

40. Grenvik A. "Terminal weaning": discontinuance of life-support therapy in the terminally ill patient. Crit Care Med 1983;11:394–6.

41. Wanzer SM, Adelstein SJ, Cranford RE. The physician's responsibility toward hopelessly ill patients. N Engl J Med 1984;310:955–9.

42. Hyers TM, Briggs DD, Hudson LD, et al. NIH workshop summary: withholding and withdrawing mechanical ventilation. Am Rev Respir Dis 1986;134:1327–30.

43. Ruark JE, Raffin TA, the Stanford University Medical Center Committee on Ethics. Initiating and withdrawing life support: principles and practices in adult medicine. N Engl J Med 1988;318:25–30.

44. Schneiderman LJ, Spragg RG. Ethical decisions in discontinuing mechanical ventilation. N Engl J Med 1988;318:984–8.

45. Wanzer SH, Federman DD, Adelstein SJ, et al. The physician's responsibility toward hopelessly ill patients: a second look. N Engl J Med 1989;320:844–9.

46. Smedira NG, Evans BH, Grais LS, et al. Withholding and withdrawal of life support from the critically ill. N Engl J Med 1990;322:309–15.

47. Lee DKP, Swinburne AJ, Fedullo AJ, et al. Withdrawing care: experience in a medical intensive care unit. JAMA 1994;271:1358–61.

48. Hall RI, Rocker GM. End-of-life care in the ICU: treatments provided when life support was or was not withdrawn. Chest 2000;118:1424–30.

49. Vincent J-L, Parquier J-N, Presier J-C, et al. Terminal events in the intensive care unit: review of 258 fatal cases in one year. Crit Care Med 1989;17:530–3.

50. Prendergast TJ, Luce JM. Increasing incidence of withholding and withdrawal of life support from the critically ill. Am J Respir Crit Care Med 1997;155:15–20.

51. Prendergast TJ, Claessens MT, Luce JM. A national survey of end-of-life care for critically ill patients. Am J Respir Crit Care Med 1998;158:1163–7.

52. Wilson WD, Smedira NG, Fink C, et al. Ordering and administering of sedatives and analgesics during the withholding and withdrawal of life support from critically ill patients. JAMA 1992;267:949–53.

53. Brody H, Campbell ML, Faber-Langendoen K, et al. Withdrawing intensive life-sustaining treatment—recommendations for compassionate clinical management. N Engl J Med 1997;652–7.

54. Task Force on Ethics of the Society of Critical Care Medicine. Consensus report on the ethics of foregoing life-sustaining treatments in the critically ill. Crit Care Med 1990;18:1435–9.

55. American Thoracic Society. Withholding and withdrawing life-sustaining therapy. Am Rev Respir Dis 1991;144:726–31.

56. ACCP/SCCM Consensus Panel. Ethical and moral guidelines for the initiation, continuation, and withdrawal of intensive care. Chest 1990;97:949–58.

57. Curtis JR, Rubenfeld GD, editors. Managing death in the intensive care unit: the transition from cure to conmfort. Oxford (UK): Oxford University Press; 2001.

58. Truog RD, Campbell ML, Curtis JR, et al. Recommendations for end-of-life care in the intensive care unit: a consensus statement by the American Academy of Critical Care Medicine. Crit Care Med 2008;36:953–63.

59. Lanken PN, Terry PB, DeLisser HM, et al. on behalf of the ATS End-of-Life Care Task Force. An official American Thoracic Society clinical policy statement:

palliative care for patients with respiratory diseases and critical illnesses. Am J Respir Crit Care Med 2008;177:912–27.

60. Curtis JR, Engelbeerg RA, Wenrich MD, et al. Missed opportunities during family conferences about end-of-life care in the intensive care unit. Am J Respir Crit Care Med 2005;171:844–9.

61. White DB, Braddock CH, Bereknyei S, et al. Toward shared decision making at the end of life in intensive care units: opportunities for improvement. Arch Intern Med 2007;167:461–7.

62. Levy MM, Curtis JR. Improving end-of-life care in the intensive care unit. Crit Care Med 2006;34:S301.

63. In re Quinlan, 755 A2A 647 (NJ), cert denied, 429 70 NJ 10, 355 A2d 647 (1976).

64. Kinney HC, Korein J, Panigrahy A, et al. Neuropathological findings in the brain of Karen Ann Quinlan—the role of the thalamus in the persistent vegetative state. N Engl J Med 1994;330:1469–75.

65. Annas GJ. Nancy Cruzan and the right to die. N Engl J Med 1990;323:670–3.

66. Bartling v. Superior Court.

67. In re Storar, 52 NY 2d 363, 420 NE, cert denied, 454 US 858 (1981).

68. In re Westchester County Medical Center on Behalf of O'Connor, 581 NE 2d 607 (NY, 1988).

69. Cruzan v. Harmon, 760 SW 2d 408 (Mo, 1988) (en banc).

70. Cruzan v. Director, Missouri Dept. of Health. 110 S Ct 2841 (1990).

71. Washington v. Glucksberg, 521 US 702 (1997).

72. Vacco v. Quill, 521 US 793 (1997).

73. Omnibus Budget Reconciliation Act of 1990. Public Law No. 101–508.

74. Bok S. Personal directions for care at the end of life. N Engl J Med 1976;295: 367–9.

75. Eisendrath SJ, Jonsen AR. The living will: help or hindrance. JAMA 1983;249: 2054–8.

76. Steinbrook R, Lo B. Decision making for incompetent patients by designated proxy: California's new law. N Engl J Med 1984;310:1598–601.

77. Silverman HJ, Vinicky JK, Gasner MR. Advance directives: implications for critical care. Crit Care Med 1992;20:1027–31.

78. Emanuel LL, Barry MJ, Stoeckle JD, et al. Advance directives for medical care— a case for greater use. N Engl J Med 1991;324:889–95.

79. Danis M, Multran E, Garrett JM, et al. A prospective study of the impact of patient preferences on life-sustaining treatment and hospital cost. Crit Care Med 1996;24:1811–8.

80. Schneiderman LJ, Kronick R, Kaplan RM, et al. Effects of offering advance directives on medical treatment and costs. Ann Intern Med 1992;117:599–606.

81. Levinsky NG. The doctor's master. N Engl J Med 1984;311:1573–5.

82. Levinsky NG. The purpose of advance medical planning—autonomy for patients or limitation of care? N Engl J Med 1996;335:741–6.

83. Somogyi-Zalud E, Zhong Z, Lynn J. Dying with acute respiratory failure or multiple organ system failure with sepsis. J Am Geriatr Soc 2000;48:S140–5.

84. Fried TR, Bradley EH, Towle VR, et al. Understanding the treatment preferences of seriously ill patients. N Engl J Med 2002;346:1061–6.

85. Conners AF, Dawson NV, Thomas C. Outcomes following acute exacerbations of chronic obstructive lung disease. Am J Respir Crit Care Med 1996;154:959–67.

86. Wachter RM, Luce JM, Safrin S. Cost and outcomes of intensive care for patients with AIDS, *Pneumocystis carinii* pneumonia, and severe respiratory failure. JAMA 1995;273:230–5.

87. Fowler AA, Hamman RF, Zerbe GO. Adult respiratory distress syndrome: prognosis after onset. Am Rev Respir Dis 1985;132:472–8.

88. Ely EW, Evans GW, Haponik EF. Mechanical ventilation in a cohort of elderly patients admitted to an intensive care unit. Ann Intern Med 1999;131:96–104.

89. Gillespie DJ, Marsh HMM, Divertie MB. Clinical outcome of respiratory failure in patients requiring prolonged (>24 hours) mechanical ventilation. Chest 1986;90:364–9.

90. Knaus WM, Zimmerman JE, Wagner DO, et al. APACHE—acute physiology and chronic health evaluation: a physiologically based classification system. Crit Care Med 1981;9:591–7.

91. Kruse JA, Thill-Baharozian MC, Carlson RW. Comparison of clinical assessment with APACHE II for predicting mortality risk in patients admitted to a medical intensive care unit. JAMA 1988;260:1739–42.

92. Zimmerman JE, Wagner DP, Draper EA, et al. Evaluation of acute physiology and chronic health evaluation III* predictions of hospital mortality in an independent database. Crit Care Med 1998;26:1317–26.

93. The SUPPORT Principal Investigators. A controlled trial to improve care for seriously ill hospitalized patients: the Study to Understand Prognoses and Preferences for Outcomes and Risks of Treatment (SUPPORT). JAMA 1995;274:1591–8.

94. Teres D. Civilian triage in the intensive care unit: the ritual of the last bed. Crit Care Med 1993;21:598–606.

95. Danis M, Patrick DL, Southerland LI, et al. Patients' and families' preferences for medical intensive care. JAMA 1988;260:797–802.

96. Engelhardt HT, Rie MA. Intensive care units, scarce resources, and conflicting principles of justice. JAMA 1986;255:1159–64.

97. Singer DE, Carr PL, Mulley AG, et al. Rationing intensive care—physician responses to a resource shortage. N Engl J Med 1983;309:1155–60.

98. Strauss MJ, LeGerfo JP, Yeltatzie JA, et al. Rationing of intensive care unit services: an everyday occurrence. JAMA 1986;255:1143–6.

99. Asch DA, Hansen-Flaschen J, Lanken PN. Decisions to limit or continue life-sustaining treatment by critical care physicians in the United States: conflicts between physicians' practices and patients' wishes. Am J Respir Crit Care Med 1995;151:288–92.

100. Luce JM. Physicians do not have a responsibility to provide futile or unreasonable care if a patient or family insists. Crit Care Med 1995;23:760–6.

101. Helft PR, Siegler M, Lantos J. The rise and fall of the futility movement. N Engl J Med 2000;343:293–6.

102. Blackhall LD. Must we always use CPR? N Engl J Med 1987;317:1281–5.

103. Schneiderman LJ, Jecker NS, Jonsen AR. Medical futility: its meaning and ethical implications. Ann Intern Med 1990;112:949–54.

104. Rubenfeld GD, Crawford SW. Withdrawing life support from mechanically ventilated recipients of bone marrow transplants: a case for evidence-based guidelines. Ann Intern Med 1996;125:625–33.

105. Truog RD, Brett AS, Frader J. The problem with futility. N Engl J Med 1992;326:1560–4.

106. The Ethics Committee of the Society of Critical Care Medicine. Consensus statement of the Society of Critical Care Medicine's Ethics Committee regarding futile and other possibly inadvisable treatments. Crit Care Med 1997;25:887–91.

107. Council on Ethical and Judicial Affairs, American Medical Association. Medical futility in end-of-life care: report of the Council on Ethical and Judicial Affairs. JAMA 1999;281:937–41.
108. Halevy A, Brody BA, For the Houston city-wide Task Force on Medical Futility. A multi-institutional collaborative policy on medical futility. JAMA 1996;276:571–4.
109. Smith ML, Gremillion G, Slomka J, et al. Texas hospitals' experience with the Texas Advance Directives Act. Crit Care Med 2007;35:1271–6.
110. Truog RD. Tackling medical futility in Texas. N Engl J Med 2008;357:1–3.
111. Melo v. Superintendent of Royal Darwin Hospital 2007, NTSC 71.
112. Golubchuk v. Salvation Army Grace General Hospital, et al. 2008 MBQB 49.
113. Rotaru v. Vancouver General Hospital intensive care unit 2008, BcSC 318.
114. I.H.V. (Re), 2008, ABQB 250.

Evolution of the Intensive Care Unit as a Clinical Center and Critical Care Medicine as a Discipline

Ake Grenvik, MD, PhD, FCCM*, Michael R. Pinsky, MD CM, Dr hc, FCCP, FCCM

KEYWORDS

- Intensive care unit • Critical care medicine
- Critical care registered nurses
- Societies and Congresses of critical care medicine

Intensive care medicine owes its roots to the support of failing ventilation. Of great importance for the establishment of respiratory intensive care, was the development of positive pressure ventilation. In 1543 Vesalius published his classical work "De Humani Corporis Fabrica"[1] and described an experiment in which an animal was kept alive by rhythmic insufflation of air into the trachea using bellows. This is the first known application of intermittent positive pressure ventilation (IPPV) under controlled conditions. Matas in 1902[2] was the first to describe an automatic respiratory apparatus. In the beginning he used a double pump giving intermittent positive-negative pressure ventilation (IPNPV), but later abandoned suction during expiration as unnecessary.

In 1904, Sauerbruch[3] introduced his low-pressure chamber for use in thoracic surgery. Both the surgeon and the patient were inside the chamber with only the patient's head exposed through an airtight sealing collar around the neck. This method provided continuous positive airway pressure ventilation (CPAP). It was soon realized that CPAP caused ineffective gas exchange and oxygen had to be given to prevent cyanosis. Volhard[4] claimed that it was this oxygen supply rather than the differential pressure method per se that was responsible for the success of Sauerbruch's method. However, the patient's spontaneous breathing efforts could not move sufficient air in and out of the lungs with the chest open. Thus, CPAP was

Department of Critical Care Medicine, University of Pittsburgh, Room 646 Scaife Hall, 3550 Terrace Street, Pittsburgh, PA 15261, USA
* Corresponding author.
E-mail address: grenvik@comcast.net (A. Grenvik).

Crit Care Clin 25 (2009) 239–250
doi:10.1016/j.ccc.2008.11.001
0749-0704/08/$ – see front matter © 2009 Elsevier Inc. All rights reserved.

correctly identified as a form of apneic diffusion oxygenation. This term was introduced by Holmdahl[5] in his extensive study of this technique, which also documented the obligatory accumulation of carbon dioxide in the body.

Giertz in 1916[6] clearly demonstrated that artificial ventilation by rhythmic insufflation was superior to the differential pressure method introduced by Sauerbruch. His successor, Crafoord,[7] a renowned cardiothoracic surgeon in Sweden, ended the dominance of Sauerbruch's method by introducing "the Spiropulsator" in thoracic surgery.

Traditionally, British nurse Florence Nightingale[8] is considered to be the first to have used an intensive care unit (ICU). She served with the British side in the Crimean War, 1854 to 1856 she collected the sickest and worst injured soldiers in an area close to her nursing station where she could maintain a constant eye on their condition and provide quick help when most needed. There are no reports on similar efforts until 1929 when Dr. Walter Dandy[9] of the Johns Hopkins Hospital in Baltimore described the use of a special postoperative unit for his neurosurgical patients. No other similar efforts involving intensive care were reported until the worldwide epidemic of poliomyelitis in the early 1950s. Information is particularly available from Los Angeles, Boston, and Copenhagen during that epidemic,[10] all using the so-called "iron lung" for treatment of those advanced polio patients who lost the ability to breathe adequately as a result of bulbar invasion of the polio virus.

The iron lung was introduced by Harvard medical researchers Philip Drinker and Shaw[11] in 1927. John Emerson[12] improved on Drinker's invention and designed an iron lung that cost half as much to manufacture. These machines supported ventilation by intermittent negative pressure ventilation (INPV) produced around the body in a chamber surrounding the patient except for the head with an airtight collar around the patient's neck similar to what Sauerbruck used. However, the system was not very efficient in totally paralyzed patients. Danish anesthesiologist Ibsen[13] therefore suggested tracheostomy and manual bag ventilation with intermittent positive pressure ventilation (IPPV) of the patient. During the poliomyelitis epidemic in Denmark, such patients were brought to the University Hospital in Copenhagen. The medical school was closed and the students were called on to manually ventilate the patients in shifts. This approach resulted in a drop in mortality as the respiratory ICU was initiated.

Mörch[14] presented his piston ventilator in 1947 primarily for use in the operating room during thoracic surgery, but it was Bjork and Engstrom[15] who in 1955 introduced the use of prolonged mechanical ventilation by a machine in the postoperative period after lung surgery. At that time, Engstrom[16] had already demonstrated the advantage of his ventilator in the treatment of totally paralyzed polio victims during the Copenhagen epidemic.

The success of the above technique spread quickly and respiratory intensive care units were established in many university medical centers especially in Europe and North America. During the late 1950's, the Danish anesthesiologists Bendixen and Pontoppidan[17] who had both participated in manual ventilation of polio victims in Copenhagen, immigrated to Boston and established the reputable respiratory ICU at Massachusetts General Hospital. At about the same time, Reuben Cherniak in Winnipeg's General Hospital in Manitoba, Canada and Arthur Scott at Toronto General Hospital in Ontario, Canada (each veterans of the polio epidemics of the era) developed their own Intensive Care Units with an emphasis on multidisciplinary staffing. Peter Safar, the Austrian anesthesiologist who with Elam[18] introduced mouth-to-mouth ventilation replacing outdated and inefficient traditional techniques used in emergencies, such as drowning victims with apnea, started the first American round the-clock physician-covered ICU at Baltimore City Hospital[19] and later established the first fellowship training program in Critical Care Medicine at Presbyterian University Hospital in Pittsburgh after moving to this city from Baltimore in 1961. Safar is best known as "The Father of Cardiopulmonary Cerebral Resuscitation" (CPCR)[20] having introduced and outlined the relevant steps of CPCR, all of special importance in CCM. Parallel with the development of respiratory ICU services, advanced postoperative care centers also evolved into ICUs. This was initially the case for postoperative open-heart surgery patients where the combined issues of hemodynamic instability, volume shifts, and arrhythmias made recovery safer in a highly monitored environment. Initially most ICUs were either medical (MICU), mostly treating acute respiratory failure, or surgical (SICU) primarily treating postoperative surgical patients. In addition, cardiologists introduced separate coronary care units (CCU). Today many ICUs in smaller centers are combined medical-surgical ICUs, although the separation of care by patient diagnosis persists in large medical centers.

CRITICAL CARE NURSES AND ALLIED HEALTH PROFESSIONALS

As indicated earlier in this article, the first ICU was introduced by a nurse, and critical care nurses remain the most important personnel category in our ICUs. They are essential for continuous intensive care of the critically ill and injured patients throughout the world. Although for decades constrained to acting only under direct physician order, it was soon realized that critically ill patients required nurses with special skills and knowledge to take action. Initially, dependent on physician instruction, nurses developed their own insights and procedures. In the United States in the late 1960s, groups of ICU and coronary care nurses were meeting to exchange experiences and in 1969, the American Association of Cardiovascular Nurses (AACN) was created.[21] However in 1971, the name was changed to the American Association of Critical Care Nurses keeping the acronym to ABCN. This Association began holding annual meetings and the membership has grown enormously in recent years. The AACN also provides for specialty certification upon examination of qualifying nurses, who then become critical care registered nurses (CCRN). Initially, ICU nurses were prevented from performing any medical intervention without a direct order from a physician but protocols were developed and agreed on among physicians and nurses that not only permit but actually require ICU nurses to intervene in various crisis situations, particularly cardiac arrest.

Another important ICU personnel category, especially in the United States and Canada are respiratory therapists.[22] Respiratory therapists supervise and manage the function of mechanical ventilators and monitor the patients' respiratory function during mechanical ventilation and weaning from these devices as well as spontaneously breathing patients until they can be discharged from the ICU. In Europe and in most other countries outside North America, these duties are provided by critical care nurses in addition to all other aspects of patient care in the ICU. It is unclear if the presence of registered respiratory therapists (RRTs) in North America has resulted in better respiratory care than in the rest of the world, since mortality rates for acute respiratory failure are similar across the developed world. However, the development of a strong respiratory therapy arm in critical care medicine in North America has certainly helped advance artificial ventilation development worldwide. In addition to the categories of caregivers to the critically ill and injured patients, social workers, nutritionists, clinical pharmacologists, clergy, and others have become important for the complex management of ICU patients.

FROM GENERAL ICUS TO SPECIALTY CRITICAL CARE MEDICINE UNITS

Initially, although most general ICUs admitted medical and surgical patients of all kinds, they tended to favor certain types of patients based on the nature of the hospital patient mix and specialization of the ICU medical teams. Notably absent from this initial progress was the presence of pediatric ICUs. Pediatric intensive care became relevant in pediatric departments and major hospitals for sick children; and then separately for neonatal support. In the 1950s, newborn babies weighing less than 4 pounds were put in incubators and merely observed. Gradually, the knowledge and technology was developed for intubation and mechanical ventilation of smaller newborns who were frequently premature and the neonatal ICU was established.

In the United States, medical ICUs split off as separate units in large, particularly tertiary care hospitals and became the domain of pulmonary specialists with increasing emphasis on broader aspects of care of critically ill patients. However, this is not typical for the rest of the world outside the United States. Canada, for example, has maintained a significant tradition of multidisciplinary ICUs staffed by intensivists of varying background training in many academic centers. Because of the greater need for intensive care of surgical patients, especially postoperatively after increasingly complex procedures, large hospital facilities in the United States established separate ICUs for general surgery, cardiothoracic surgery, trauma, neurosurgery, burns, and transplantation.[23] Initially, these units were frequently directed by anesthesiologists, but increasingly specialty surgeons and internists became involved in the management of these patients.

In 1959, the American Hospital Association (AHA) began to collect statistical information on ICUs. At that time there were 238 ICUs in short-term acute-care hospitals. However within 6 years, over 90% of large American hospitals with more than 500 beds had ICUs. Today, practically all acute-care hospitals not only in the United States but throughout the world have at least one ICU. Furthermore, with the change in health care economics, patients are being discharged sooner increasing the average disease severity of the remaining ICU patients. Furthermore, since maximal throughput of care usually requires some short-term stays in ICUs, the proportion of hospital beds being allotted to ICUs has continued to increase worldwide.

MOBILE ICUS AND TRANSPORT CRITICAL CARE MEDICINE

During the Napoleon era, special horse-drawn vehicles were used for evacuation of battle casualties. Railroad cars were used for transport of injured soldiers during the American Civil War. Critically ill soldiers were transported by air to hospitals away from the front lines during World War I. In World War II, the US Air Force transported hundreds of victims by fixed wing aircraft. Furthermore, long-distance, overseas transportation of injured soldiers was also used during World War II, such as bringing patients to the Walter Reed Hospital in Washington, DC.

In the early 1960s, European hospital physicians, particularly anesthesiologists, implemented physician-staffed mobile ICUs especially in Germany. A similar system with mobile ICUs was initiated in Pittsburgh by Dr. Peter Safar. This Freedom House Enterprise ambulance project was started in 1967.[24] The ambulances were manned by hospital-trained emergency medical technicians and paramedics. Guidelines for the design of such ambulances and standards for paramedic training were developed during this time in Pittsburgh and implemented both in Europe and the United States. Special mobile ICUs were introduced for patients with acute chest pain and called mobile coronary care units, first used in Belfast, Ireland, and in New York City by Dr. William Grace. The term "critical care transport" was coined in 1970, referring to the use of medical transport teams including ICU personnel in these mobile ICUs. Following the military development with emergent helicopter transportation of soldiers with life-threatening injuries in recent wars, establishment of hospital-based helicopter services at major hospitals has become commonplace throughout developed countries worldwide. The first neonatal transport of a critically ill infant had previously occurred in 1934 in the United States, but there was no significant change in this technique for many years. Critically ill newborns were transferred in small hand-carried incubators when it was noticed in Quebec, Ontario, that infants cared for in community hospitals had double as high mortality as those transferred to regional centers. Regionalization of neonatal critical care was gradually initiated with guidelines developed for transportation of neonates to these regional centers. Pediatric transport medicine became recognized as a special area of expertise. Other categories of patients necessitating emergent transportation to special centers are the trauma and burn victims.

CRITICAL CARE MEDICINE SOCIETIES AND CONGRESSES

As part of the process of maturing as a discipline, specialists from diverse origins with common interests in critical care medicine came together to form societies with the goal of defining core competencies for ICU physicians, providing relevant training and creating advocacy groups to promote the specialty. Their efforts over the years have resulted in many major milestones in the advancement of critical care medicine as a medical specialty associated with a list of core competencies and expected roles in the acute-care setting.

At the 1968 Federation of American Societies of Experimental Biology Congress in Atlantic City, Drs. Max Harry Weil, Peter Safar, and William Shoemaker met and discussed the need and suitability for the creation of a society for those interested in intensive care.[25] Interestingly, Max Harry Weil, MD, PhD, an internist and cardiologist directing a shock research unit in Los Angeles, CA; Peter Safar, MD, founding chairman of the Department of Anesthesiology at the University of Pittsburgh and initial director of the ICU at Presbyterian University Hospital in that city; and William Shoemaker, MD, trauma surgeon and director of traumatology and intensive care at Cook County Hospital of Chicago, represented three completely different medical specialties but all had the same common interest in intensive care of the critically ill and injured patients. The following year, Dr. Weil, in connection with his annual Shock Symposium in Los Angeles, arranged a meeting of specially invited physicians with documented interest in intensive care. Including the three initiators, this was a group of 28 physicians. This group of founding individuals decided to form the Society of Critical Care Medicine (SCCM), which was incorporated in 1971. That same year, the Society started its journal "Critical Care Medicine" with Dr. Shoemaker as the founding editor. He served as the Society's third president, preceded by Drs. Weil and Safar. From the onset, SCCM has held annual meetings, for the first 6 years alternating in a piggyback fashion between Dr. Weil's Shock and Intensive Care Symposium in Los Angeles and Dr. Safar's Emergency and Critical Care Medicine (CCM) meeting in Pittsburgh. In 1976, SCCM held its first free-standing meeting in New York City. In the past 40 years, this Society has grown from the initial 28 members to a current membership of 15,000, representing 80 different countries with not only physicians but also nurses, respiratory therapists, PhD researchers, technologists, veterinarians, industrial leaders, social workers, pharmacists, and other professionals with interest in intensive care. The CCM journal has grown to become the prime publication of critical care medicine–related topics for individuals throughout the world, currently with Joseph Parrillo, MD of the University of Medicine and Dentistry of New Jersey as chief editor. In 2001 Dr. Patrick Kochanek, of the University of Pittsburgh was elected founding editor of a new spinoff journal, Pediatric Critical Care Medicine. Almost every developed nation over the next 10 years created its own national intensive care medicine societies with a strong focus on patient advocacy, continuing medical education, and setting local standards for ICUs, training, and certification.

In 1974, Drs. Alan Gilston, a British anesthesiologist in London, England, and Iain McA Ledingham, of Glasgow, Scotland, organized the First International Congress on Intensive Care Medicine in London. At the time, a Constitution Advisory Committee of seven international members was formed and the decision made to have world congresses of intensive and critical care medicine every 4 years beginning in Paris in 1977. The proposed constitution was approved, thereby starting the World Federation of Societies of Intensive and Critical Care Medicine (WFSICCM). Dr. Alberto Villazon, a renowned critical care surgeon from Mexico City was elected first president of WFSICCM. Different from SCCM and some other societies with individual membership, the World Federation from the onset involved national and regional societies as its members.

Anesthesiologists were frequently the initiators of ICUs throughout the world. This is because resuscitation, emergency intubation, and mechanical ventilation are particular areas of expertise among anesthesiologists.[26] Furthermore, prolonged mechanical ventilation postoperatively after increasingly complex surgical interventions, such as open heart procedures and various forms of major organ transplantations, also was managed by anesthesiologists as a continuation of their care for these patients in the operating room. In some countries, particularly in Europe and especially in the north, intensive care became included in the primary specialty of anesthesiology. Thus, in Scandinavia there is a regional Society for Anesthesiology and Intensive Care Medicine. Australia and New Zealand formed their own Australia–New Zealand Intensive Care Society (ANZICS) in 1975 followed by the formation of the Canadian Critical Care Society in 1977.[27] Another federation was established in the western hemisphere: the Pan American Federation of Societies of Intensive Care Medicine. Similarly, the western pacific area saw the creation of the Western Pacific Association of Critical Care Medicine (WPACCM) with its first meeting in Singapore in 1981 and regional congresses held thereafter every 2 years. In 2003, the Republic of China became a member of WPACCM. However, when India joined in 2005, the Federation changed its name to the Asia Pacific Association of Critical Care Medicine (APA CCM).

The advantage of forming regional societies of like-minded intensivists spread. Just after ANZICS was formed, the European Society for Intensive Care Medicine (ESICM) in 1982 with Peter Suter, MD, as its first president. In their 25th year of existence, they now boast over 4000 active members making them the second largest CCM society behind SCCM. Importantly, fully 18% of their membership are from outside the European Union. The ESICM has approached intensive care medicine education and credentialing as part of the primary mission with certification examinations given annually at their annual fall congress.

Later still, the American Thoracic Society (ATS) under pressure from its regular members established a Critical Care Assembly in the late 1980s. The Critical Care Assembly grew in 2 years to become the second largest primary assembly in the ATS behind the Structure and Function Assembly. Later, in recognition of the major role that critical care medicine was playing in this Society and that a majority of the physicians certified in critical care medicine also have subspecialty boards in respiratory diseases, the ATS changed the name of its flagship journal from the American

Review of Respiratory Disease to the American Journal of Respiratory and Critical Care Medicine. About the same time, the ESICM and the ATS created joint conferences to develop consensus on critical care issues. Perhaps the most successful were the three-part series entitled the ATS-ESICM Consensus Conferences on the Acute Respiratory Distress Syndrome. The SCCM and ESICM have established more general critical care consensus conferences.

EDUCATION AND BOARD CERTIFICATION

In the United States, the need for separate and advanced training in CCM became evident early on. Peter Safar in Pittsburgh was the first to introduce a fellowship training program in CCM for anesthesiologists. In 1968, Dr. Ake Grenvik, certified in general and cardiac surgery in Sweden, joined Safar and initiated inclusion of other specialists in this training program.

Through SCCM, a recommendation was made in the late 1970s to the American Board of Medical Specialties to establish a board certification process in CCM.[28] A national committee was formed with the initial intention to have one common certification examination of qualifying physicians.[29] However, representatives of the American Boards of Anesthesiology, Internal Medicine, Pediatrics, and Surgery did not agree on the details of required training in relation to each specialty background. Therefore, each of these four specialty boards applied for separate certification examinations which started in 1986. Within Internal Medicine the decision was made to require 2 years of training in CCM unless the individual already held certification in another subspecialty, commonly pulmonary medicine, in which case 1 year of CCM training would suffice. The common denominator was for all physicians seeking certification examination in CCM to have a minimum of 5 years of postgraduate training. With anesthesiology having a 4-year residency and general surgery 5 years, these two specialties required only 1 year of CCM fellowship. However, the American Board of Pediatrics (ABP), with 3 years of residency for ABP certification, decided not only to require 2 years of CCM fellowship but in addition 1 year of research in pediatric CCM–related topics. In Canada a similar requirement for total training held but all base specialties were able to agree on a single unified two year Critical Care training program following primary subspecialty training with a single conjoint examination (excluding pediatrics).

In Spain and most Latin American countries, a similar approach was taken, declaring intensive care medicine a separate primary specialty with 5 years of training required; including rotations in anesthesiology, internal medicine, pediatrics, and surgery. ESICM arranged a certification approach similar to, but different from the United States. The ESICM requirements are primary specialty certification with 2 years of training in ICM followed by first a written and then an oral examination for certification. This process is not limited to anesthesiology, internal medicine, pediatrics, and surgery. Therefore, physicians with a different primary specialty background in the United States, such as emergency medicine physicians with 2 years of training in CCM, may apply for and take the ESICM diploma examination.

To address the need for standardization across countries, the ESICM under the leadership of Dr. Julian Bion from Manchester, UK, developed a core competency program for intensive care medicine in 2006. Called CoBaTrICE, the program emphasizes that the practice of critical care medicine carries with it a defined set of core skills and medical competencies. CoBaTrICE has five components including (1) establishing a European forum for national intensive care medicine training organizations that functions as an expert group, and acquires ownership over future developments through the Division of Professional Development to the European Board of Intensive Care Medicine; (2) surveying current education and training provisions and needs in intensive care medicine at national levels so as to identify current challenges for trainers and trainees and develop a database for benchmarking and accreditation; (3) developing minimum training program standards for quality assurance (monitoring and accreditation) using consensus techniques and attempting to harmonize minimum accreditation standards across the European Union; (4) reviewing workplace-based methods of assessment of individual competence, including case-based discussions, simulation techniques, multisource feedback, link assessment methods to competencies, and identifying quality indicators; and finally (5) creating Web-based tools for evaluation and testing support and lifelong learning for trainers and trainees. With the support of CoBaTrICE, the ESICM successfully lobbied the European Commission via the Union Européenne des Médecins Spécialistes (UEMS) to approve the European Board of Intensive Care Medicine in 2008, making it the first international certifying board for critical care medicine.

Many critical care medicine symposia have been developed to support the CME needs of this rapidly growing specialty. The largest of these symposia are the Society of Critical Care Medicine Annual Congress held in a North American city and the International Symposium of Intensive Care and Emergency Medicine (ISICEM) held anually in Brussels. Each boasts approximately 5000 participants annually. Several smaller but also high-quality symposia have been developed, like the Canadian Critical Care Forum held annually in Toronto, Canada, the SMART conference in Milan and the ISICEM for Latin America in Sao Paulo, Brazil. Many other high-quality smaller conferences also exist allowing practicing intensivists ample opportunity to remain abreast of the most recent advances and best practices in this field.

SIMULATION IN CRITICAL CARE MEDICINE TRAINING

Simulators were introduced in education as a tool to make advanced training standardized, less expensive, and without danger to those involved. In the United States, Edward Link presented in 1922 his homemade flight simulator, which later became commonplace in both military and civilian aviation, known as the "Link Trainer." However, several decades passed before this form of training became accepted in medicine.

Asmund Laerdal, a Norwegian entrepreneur, was advised by Dr. Bjorn Lind, an anesthesiologist who had heard Dr. Peter Safar's presentation in 1958 at a Norwegian congress of the mouth-to-mouth ventilation technique, to design a suitable training tool for this technique. At that time, Kouwenhoven and colleagues[30] published their observation demonstrating that intermittent closed chest compressions could produce bloodflow in cardiac arrest victims. Dr. Safar combined these two techniques and established the ABC of cardiopulmonary resuscitation (CPR), ie, an open airway, mouth-to-mouth breathing, and external cardiac compressions. He advised Mr. Laerdal to include these aspects in his production of a full-size (CPR) training manikin, which became known worldwide as "Resusci Anne."[31]

In the late 1960s, an anesthesia simulator was developed and produced by the Sierra Engineering Company together with physicians at the University of Southern California. This device was called "Sim-One." It could sense the insertion of an endotracheal tube and a computer program was used for control of the logic. Several simulators were developed in subsequent years by different groups in the United States and Europe. In 1986, David Gaba and colleagues[32] started work on the comprehensive anesthesia simulation environment (CASE). Later it became commercially available through the University of Washington, which sold the device to MedSim-Eagle Simulator. Another simulator was produced at the University of Florida in Gainesville by Drs. Good and Gravenstein. This was further developed by Medical Education Technologies in Sarasota, Florida, and has become known as "Meti." It was developed into a high-fidelity simulator but the high cost prevented the widespread use that it otherwise deserved. Laerdal Medical in Norway entered the competition in 2000 by developing further its Resusci Anne into a multipurpose computerized simulator (Sim Man) at much lower cost, which popularized its worldwide distribution.

In 2008, not only Meti and Laerdal's Sim-Man but also pediatric derivatives from both companies as well as a multitude of partial task trainers had become available, and most American medical centers had established simulation centers for training not only of physicians and nurses but also of other health care providers such as respiratory therapists and paramedics. Not only is sophisticated training of invasive procedures varying from endotracheal intubation to laporascopic surgery now available, but also the ability to evaluate the skills and knowledge of trainees, and provide team training programs for groups of individuals involved in code situations such as cardiac arrest and multiple trauma patients in the emergency department. In short, simulation training has become a most important component of training in critical care medicine at large.

EVIDENCE-BASED CRITICAL CARE MEDICINE

Evidence-based medicine requires the systematic and rational use of the best available evidence for clinical decision making in the ICU. However, evidence obtained from the literature has to be critically appraised with attention to clinical relevance and validity in CCM. Many guidelines have been published for the practice of critical care and are continuously updated. Such guidelines exist for many conditions such as in the areas of cardiovascular, airway, pulmonary, hemodynamic monitoring, burns, infectious disease, sepsis, acute renal failure, and trauma care. The American College of Critical Medicine has been particularly active in designing such guidelines, which however are not always based on evidence-based material. Presently, joint consensus conferences sponsored by SCCM, ESICM, and ATS have addressed broad issues like hemodynamic monitoring, sepsis, and the like using experts and naïve intelligent jury reviews. These consensus panel reports are also jointly published in the respective sponsoring societies journals.

RESEARCH AND PUBLICATIONS

A fundamental aspect of the maturation of a new specialty is its development of a durable knowledge base and the growth of a robust and well-funded research arm to advance its field. In the early days of critical care medicine, there were no comprehensive textbooks to which trainees and practitioners could refer. Because critical care medicine from its inception was rapidly growing, this need was acute. Although today there are numerous textbooks specializing on specific facets of the field of CCM, like pulmonary, nephrology, surgery, trauma, anesthesiology, and emergency medicine, then there was none. To address this issue Drs. William Shoemaker (surgery), Ake Grenvik (anesthesiology), Peter Holbrock (pediatrics), and Steven Ayers (internal medicine) edited the first Textbook of Critical Care in 1984, and continued to edit this textbook through subsequent editions in 1989, 1995, and 2000.[33] The Textbook of Critical Care is now in its 5th edition with new editors. However, today the student of critical care medicine has an impressive array of superb comprehensive textbooks to choose from and many more focused critical care volumes.

From a research and publication perspective, critical care medicine evolved from a descriptive discipline that tended to categorize symptoms and disease states, describing hemodynamic and metabolic patterns linked closely to the use of cardiopulmonary resuscitation, artificial ventilation, and pulmonary artery catheter. From these humble roots, the specialty has advanced into a field based on disease, process of care, and outcomes, whose publications routinely appear in major medical journals like Journal of the American Medical Association, the New England Journal of Medicine, and Lancet. Many of the studies in these journals relates to clinical research performed through collaborative, intensivist-led research organizations such as the Canadian Critical Care Trials Group, the ANZICS Group and the ARDSnet group. Furthermore, critical care medicine basic science research often appears in Journal of Clinical Investigation, Nature Medicine, Biochem Biophys Res Acta, Journal of Immunology, American Journal of Physiology, Journal of Applied Physiology, Circulation, and many others, stressing the high quality and exactness that the foundations of critical care medicine enjoy. Finally, most critical care–related studies are published in a small group of high-impact factor specialty journals, listed in order of their ratings, as American Journal of Respiratory and Critical Care Medicine, Critical Care Medicine, Intensive Care Medicine, Critical Care and Shock.

As managed care and cost containment force the less sick to be discharged much earlier and optimizing throughput of patients becomes an economic survival practice for hospitals, critical care medicine has become the epicenter of acute-care medicine. Accordingly, process of care research, patient safety, ethics of life support, and health care economics have evolved into major areas of expertise and research for critical care physicians. In fact, critical care medicine research interests and productivity compare as equals to any other specialty, an impressive statement considering that the first ICUs were introduced only some 50 years ago.

FUTURE CHALLENGES

The challenges of critical care medicine are numerous and important for all acute-care medicine. However, three challenges stand out above the rest. First, now that critical care medicine is firmly established as a specialty with defined competencies and training programs and roles in the acute hospital plus national and European certification, it is essential that it maintains its leadership role in all areas. Specifically, leadership in quality care, patient safety, optimizing effective care delivery, and quantifying these effects are major goals and will become the crowning accomplishments of the specialty as a clinical practice. Second, although the major American medical specialties of medicine, surgery, pediatrics, and anesthesiology confirm critical care medicine special competency certification, primary CCM certification in its own specialty needs to be established so that residencies can become part of the training program. Emergency medicine physicians need to be granted full membership into the specialty. This is not just a North American issue but an international one, and hopefully by defining core competencies and skills within a clinical framework both national and international standards can be developed and used to define certification eligibility. And, third, as critical care research moves more toward basic mechanisms of disease, it is important if not essential to stress the absolute need for translational research and patient-centered outcome studies to both define the field and aid in the most tangible way those who critical care medicine is here to serve, the critically ill.

ACKNOWLEDGMENT

Recommendations by James V. Snyder, MD, Professor of Critical Care Medicine and Anesthesiology at the University of Pittsburgh are greatly appreciated.

REFERENCES

1. Vesalius A. De Humani corporis fabrica. Basel 1543 (Bibl. Waller 9899), p. 659, Basel 1555.
2. Matas R. An experimental automatic respiratory apparatus. Am Med 1902, January 18.
3. Sauerbruch F. Zur Pathologie. d. offenen Pneumothorax und die Grundlagen meines Verfahrens zu seiner Ausschaltung. Mitt. Grentzgeb. Med. u. Chir 1904; 13:399.
4. Volhard F. Ueber künstliche Atmung durch Ventilation der Trachea und eine einfache Vorrichtung zur rhytmischen künstlichen Atmung. München Med Wchnschr 1908;55:209.
5. Holmdahl MH. Pulmonary uptake of oxygen, acid-base metabolism, and circulation during prolonged apnoea. Acta Chir Scand 1956;212(Suppl).
6. Giertz KH. Studier över tryckdifferensandning enlight Sauerbruch och over konstgjord andning (rytmisk luftinblasning) vid intrathoracala operationer. Upsala Lakarefor forhandl 1915;(Suppl 22).
7. Crafoord C. On the technique of pneumonectomy in man. Acta Chir Scand 1938;(Suppl 54).
8. Nightingale F. Notes on hospitals. In: Longman, Green, Longman, editors. 3rd Edition. London: Longman; 1863. p. 89.
9. Hanson CW III, Durbin CG Jr, Maccioli GA, et al. The anesthesiologist in critical care medicine: past, present, and future. Anesthesiology 2001;95(3):781–8.
10. Berthelsen PG, Cronqvist M. The first intensive care unit in the world: Copenhagen 1953. Acta Anaesthesiol Scand 2003;47(10):1190–5.
11. Drinker P, Shaw LA. An apparatus for the prolonged administration of artificial respiration. J Clin Invest 1929;7(2):229–47.
12. Emerson JH. The evolution of "Iron Lung." Cambridge (MA): J.H. Emerson Co.; 1978.
13. Ibsen B. Treatment of respiratory complications in poliomyelitis. Dan Med Bull 1954;1:9.
14. Mörch ET. Controlled respiration by means of special automatic machines as used in Sweden and Denmark. Proc R Soc Med 1947;40:39.
15. Björk VO, Engström CG. The treatment of ventilatory insufficiency after pulmonary resection with tracheostomy and prolonged artificial ventilation. J Thorac Surg 1955;30(3):356–67.
16. Engström CG. The clinical application of prolonged controlled ventilation. Acta Anaesthesiol Scand 1963;(Suppl 13).
17. Bendixen HH, Egbert LD, Hedley-Whyte J, et al. Respiratory care. St Louis (MO): The C.V. Mosby Company; 1965.
18. Safar P, Elam J. Manual versus mouth-to-mouth methods of artificial respiration. Anesthesiology 1958;19:111–2.
19. Safar P, DeKornfeld TJ, Pearson JW, et al. The intensive care unit. A three-year experience at Baltimore City Hospitals. Anaesthesia 1961;16:275–84.
20. Safar P. Cerebral resuscitation after cardiac arrest: a review. Circulation 1986; 74(Suppl IV):138–53.
21. Fairman J, Lynaugh JE. Critical care nursing: a history. Philadelphia: University of Pennsylvania Press; 1998.
22. Grenvik A. Role of allied health professionals in critical care medicine. Crit Care Med 1974;2(1):6–10.
23. Safar P, Grenvik A. Critical care medicine: organizing and staffing intensive care units. Chest 1971;59(5):535–47.

24. Benson DM, Esposito G, Dirsch J, et al. Mobile intensive care by "unemployable" blacks trained as emergency medical technicians (EMTs) in 1967–69. J Trauma 1972;12:408–21.

25. Weil MH. The Society of Critical Care Medicine, its history and its destiny. Crit Care Med 1973;1(1):1–4.

26. Holmdahl MH. Respiratory care unit. Anesthesiology 1962;23:559–68.

27. Trubuhovich RV, Judson JA. Intensive care in New Zealand—a history of the New Zealand region of ANZICS. Auckland: Trubuhovich and Judosn; 2001; 1–4.

28. Grenvik A. Certification of specialty competence in critical care medicine as a new subspecialty: a status report. Crit Care Med 1978;6(6):335–59.

29. Grenvik A, Leonard JJ, Arens JF, et al. Certification as a multidisciplinary subspecialty. Crit Care Med 1981;9(2):117–25.

30. Kouwenhoven WB, Jude JR, Knickerbocker GC. Closed chest cardiac massage. JAMA 1960;173:1064.

31. Grenvik A, Schaefer J. From Resusci-Anne to Sim-Man: the evolution of simulators in medicine. Crit Care Med 2004;32(2 Suppl):S56–7.

32. Gaba DM. A brief history of mannequin-based simulation & application. In: Dunn William, editor. Chap in simulators in critical care education and beyond. Chicago: Soc of Crit Care Med; 2004.

33. Shoemaker WC, Thompson WL, Holbrook PR, editors. The Society of Critical Care Medicine Textbook of Critical Care. Philadelphia: WB Saunders; 1984.

Index

Note: Page numbers of article titles are in **boldface** type.

A

Acute myocardial infarction, mechanical complications of, historical perspective on, 109–110

Adult respiratory distress syndrome (ARDS), PEEP for, history of, 193–194

Advance directives, history of, 228–229

Airway(s), in cardiopulmonary resuscitation, history of, 134–135

Airway pressure release ventilation (APRV), history of, 195

Allied health professionals, evolution of, 241

Angiography, pulmonary, in pulmonary embolism diagnosis, history of, 119–120

"Animacules," discovery of, 84–85

Antibiotic(s), early, history of, 88–90

Antimicrobial drugs, history of, 214
    carbapenems, 213
    cephalosporins, 212
    described, 211–212
    fluoroquinolones, 213–214
    glycopeptides, 212–213
    lipopeptides, 214
    oxazolidinones, 214

APRV. See *Airway pressure release ventilation (APRV)*.

ARDS. See *Adult respiratory distress syndrome (ARDS)*.

Arterial blood gases, in pulmonary embolism diagnosis, history of, 118

B

Bhopal disaster, preparedness lessons from, 49–51

Blood transfusion, in critical illness
    future challenges, 205
    history of, 202–205
        recent developments, 204
        war-related, 203–204

Board certification, in ICU and critical care medicine, evolution of, 245–246

C

Calcineurin era: cyclosporine and FK-506: 1983-present, in solid organ transplantation, 170–172

Carbapenems, history of, 213

Cardiac death, organ donation after, 174–177

Crit Care Clin 25 (2009) 251–260

doi:10.1016/S0749-0704(09)00013-X

0749-0704/09/$ – see front matter © 2009 Elsevier Inc. All rights reserved.

criticalcare.theclinics.com

Moving?

Make sure your subscription moves with you!

To notify us of your new address, find your **Clinics Account Number** (located on your mailing label above your name), and contact customer service at:

E-mail: elspcs@elsevier.com

800-654-2452 (subscribers in the U.S. & Canada)
314-453-7041 (subscribers outside of the U.S. & Canada)

Fax number: 314-523-5170

Elsevier Periodicals Customer Service
11830 Westline Industrial Drive
St. Louis, MO 63146

*To ensure uninterrupted delivery of your subscription, please notify us at least 4 weeks in advance of move.

Printed and bound by CPI Group (UK) Ltd, Croydon, CR0 4YY

03/10/2024

01040452-0012